THE FOOT AND ANKLE

Clinical Applications

A.L. LOGAN SERIES IN CHIROPRACTIC TECHNIQUE

The Knee: Clinical Applications
The Foot and Ankle: Clinical Applications
The Low Back and Pelvis: Clinical Applications

THE FOOT AND ANKLE
Clinical Applications

A.L. Logan Series in Chiropractic Technique

Alfred L. Logan

With a contribution by Lindsay J. Rowe

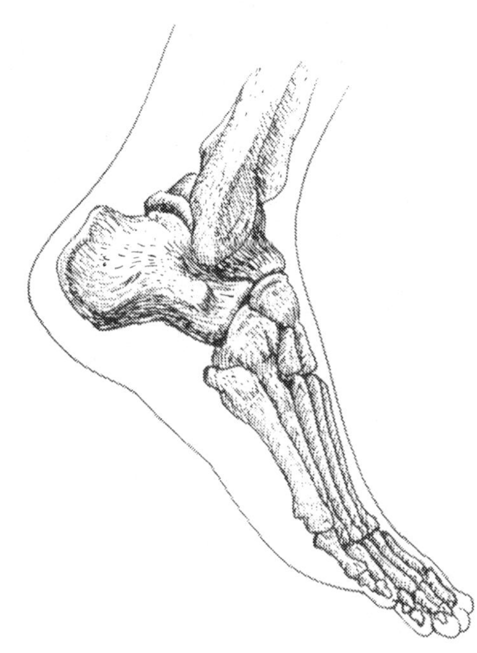

Alfred L. Logan, DC
Formerly associated with
Los Angeles College of Chiropractic
Whittier, California

and

Anglo-European College of Chiropractic
Bournemouth, England

**Lindsay J. Rowe, MAppSc (Chiropractic),
MD, DACBR (USA), FCCR (CAN),
FACCR (AUST), FICC**
Newcastle, Australia

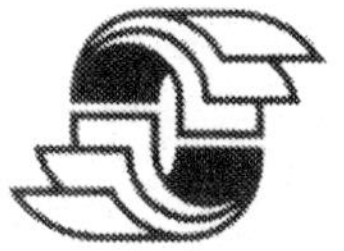

AN ASPEN PUBLICATION®
Aspen Publishers, Inc.
Gaithersburg, Maryland
1995

Library of Congress Cataloging-in-Publication Data
Logan, Alfred L.
The Foot and Ankle: clinical applications/Alfred L. Logan.
p. cm. — (A.L. Logan series in chiropractic technique)
Includes bibliographical references and index.
ISBN: 0-8342-0605-6
1. Foot—Diseases—Chiropractic treatment.
2. Ankle—Diseases—Chiropractic treatment.
3. Foot—Wounds and injuries—Chiropractic treatment.
4. Ankle—Wounds and injuries—Chiropractic treatment.
I. Title. II. Series.
RZ265.F6L64 1995
617.5'85062—dc20
94-3554
CIP

The author has made every effort to ensure the accuracy of the information herein. However, appropriate information sources should be consulted, especially for new or unfamiliar procedures. It is the responsibility of every practitioner to evaluate the appropriateness of a particular opinion in the context of actual clinical situations and with due consideration to new developments. The author, editors, and the publisher cannot be held responsible for any typographical or other errors found in this book.

Editorial Resources: Amy R. Martin

Library of Congress Catalog Card Number: 94-3554
ISBN: 0-8342-0605-6

Printed in the United States of America

1 2 3 4 5

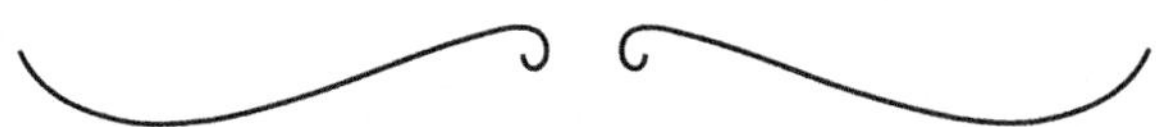

Anyone who has been to school can remember at least one teacher whose influence inspired him to learn more fully, to appreciate the subject being taught, and perhaps to realize a life's work. I have been fortunate enough to have had several such teachers. In high school, my biology teacher moved me into the sciences, and a humanities teacher instilled in me the desire to think and reason. While studying chiropractic, I found Dr. A.L. Logan. I first met him when he voluntarily did clinical rounds at the Los Angeles College of Chiropractic (LACC).

Roy Logan had a capacity to understand how the human body works, and a curiosity about it that kept him constantly searching and researching for ways to help heal it. The profession is full of personalities teaching a variety of techniques, some insisting theirs is the only way, but it has few true professors who can cull the various teachings, and present to the student a clear and concise way to approach a patient, without personality and ego getting in the way. Roy had these abilities, and, fortunately for us, he had a desire to teach others. He never missed an opportunity.

He saw the need in our profession for a way to link the rote clinical sciences and the various ways of executing an adjustment. He gave us an answer to the commonly asked question of when and where to adjust. He was constantly pushing the profession to realize the importance of effective clinical application of chiropractic principles at a time when there seemed to be more emphasis on fitting into the health care industry by wearing a white coat and using big words.

Around the world, students of Dr. Logan use his methods of diagnosis and treatment every day and are reminded of his wonderful contributions to the profession. He lectured repeatedly before several state associations, and taught an eight month post-graduate course at LACC for eight years. He was Chairman of the Technique Department at the Anglo-European College of Chiropractic for five years.

In spite of his many contributions, Roy's work remains unfinished. He passed away in April of 1993, after fighting a terminal illness. He was working hard on his textbooks up to the end, hoping to transfer as much of his knowledge and wisdom to paper as he could.

Dr. Logan has a number of students dedicated to continuing his work and seeing it evolve in the way he envisioned. There is no "A.L. Logan Technique," but rather a compilation of various teachings, combined with a unique understanding of the interdependencies of the human structure. We hope to do his work justice and see more students of chiropractic become as effective as possible in the treatment of human disorders.

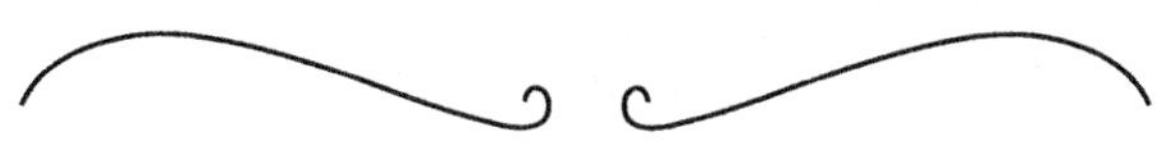

Table of Contents

"... The application of principles ... involves higher mental processes than their memorizing; every student should be given a thorough drill in clinical analysis in which he should be made to see the relationship which exists between the fundamental facts and their clinical application."

Francis M. Pottenger, MD

The education that a modern chiropractor undergoes includes the clinical sciences and the manipulative arts. A graduate doctor of chiropractic has a thorough grasp of the diagnostic and clinical skills and is trained in basic manipulative techniques. With this knowledge, the practicing doctor begins to gain the experience that makes the application of this knowledge successful. A successful doctor is one who continues to learn beyond what is minimally required, for he or she is constantly renewed and stimulated.

Dr. A.L. Logan was a successful chiropractor, a doctor that, like D.D. Palmer, continued to expand his understanding of the human body in health and disease. He studied the works of many of the chiropractic profession's leading educators. He researched and developed his own theories which he applied in his practice, and like most chiropractors, developed a successful, diversified approach to diagnosing and treating his patients. Dr. Logan recognized the need for a practical way to blend basic and advanced manipulative techniques with clinical skills.

From this recognition came over 20 years of teaching. It was his hope that his ideas would generate continued dialogue and interest in expanding the clinical application of chiropractic principles.

Dr. Logan did clinical rounds at the Los Angeles College of Chiropractic, since the early seventies. He lectured often for various state associations, and taught at the Anglo-European College of Chiropractic. During this time Dr. Logan continued to learn and grow as a clinician and teacher. His decision to write a series of texts on the clinical application of chiropractic principles came out of his experience in teaching undergraduate technique at AECC and seeing the difficulty upper division students had in understanding when, where, and why they should adjust.

This series of textbooks will be a comprehensive reference on chiropractic clinical applications. Dr. Logan believed this approach should be the basis for an undergraduate course in adjustive and clinical technique. It is, at the same time, a welcome addition to the knowledge of any practitioner.

Pottenger FM. *Symptoms of Visceral Disease*. St. Louis: Mosby; 1953.

Chris Hutcheson, DC
Auburn, California

The feet would seem the logical place to start in the study of the human body and its function. In building a structure, the foundation is the most important part, supporting and stabilizing all above it. Dysfunction of the foundation affects the rest of the structure. In the human body, however, dysfunction of the body may affect the foundation as well.

This text about the ankle and foot is the second text, not the first, in a series. It has been my opinion for many years that the lower extremities should be taught in chiropractic colleges before the spine and pelvis (some colleges still do not do so). Teaching the spine and pelvis and then the lower extremities makes it difficult for the student to grasp the overall functional anatomy, especially in the presence of an anatomic or functional short leg.

My first text was on the knee, which, in my opinion, is the best place to begin learning the skills of palpation, examination, testing for range of motion, detecting fixations, and beginning manipulation. The knee is the largest joint in the body. It is easy to palpate because it is readily available and there are two of them. After the knee and its relationship to the rest of the body are comprehended, the complex foot and ankle are not as formidable as they would be as a starting place.

As in the first text on the knee, I have attempted to write this book in a manner suitable for the beginner as well as the practitioner.

No book is written without a number of people being involved. The amount of time and effort requires an encroachment on the lives of friends, associates, and family. I would like to thank the following individuals:

My wife, Judy A. Logan, DC, for her many roles over the months; her patience throughout; her encouragement from the beginning to the end; and her hours of reading, commenting on, and editing the text.

Michael Weisenberger, DC, Geelong, Australia, for his encouragement, if not downright insistence, that I write this series of books, and for his invaluable advice and assistance.

Our son, S/Sgt Stephen Hillenbrand, USAF, for his many hours and expertise in producing the photography that made most of the illustrations possible.

A special thanks to Paula Regina Rodriques de Freitas Hillenbrand, our model throughout, for her many hours of posing for us, which made the illustrations possible.

Lindsay J. Rowe, DC, MD, for his invaluable contribution to the text, which allowed coverage of everything except surgery within the one text.

Herbert I. Magee, Jr., DC, for his invaluable assistance in editing the text.

Merrill Cook, DC, for the use of his library, his advice when asked, and his support.

Niels Nilsson, DC, MD, for his suggestions and assistance in editing.

William Remson, DC, for his suggestions and assistance in editing.

Reed B. Phillips, DC, PhD, for reviewing the text and for his suggestions.

Inger F. Villadsen, DC, for her encouragement throughout and for her help in the final edit.

Chris Hutcheson, DC, for his review and editorial support in the later stages of production.

Chapter 1

Anatomy

Shands and Raney[1] state that the functions of the foot are to serve as a support for the weight of the body and to act as a lever to raise and propel the body forward in the act of walking and running. Mennell[2] states that the foot has three basic functions: support (which includes posture), propulsion (which includes gait and dexterity), and dexterity (beyond the dexterity of ambulation). Dexterity is intrinsic and is usually developed only in people without hands. Mennell states further that if the above functions are performed correctly pain will not develop in the normal foot, at least not until the foot is encased in an ill-designed shoe.

Hiss[3] lists the seven fundamentals of foot functions as follows:

1. *Support*—the resistance of bones and ligaments against superimposed body weight.
2. *Balance*—the control of body weight over the center of gravity.
3. *Locomotion*—the coordination of muscles to move joints for the purpose of propelling the body through space.
4. *Adaptability*—the coordination of support, locomotion, and balance to compensate for changed position.
5. *Distribution*—the control of contact pressure made by the sole of the foot on the ground as the load moves through the foot during locomotion.
6. *Vitality*—life itself, which is manifested in the feet as well as in the rest of the body. Vitality embodies intelli-

gence under switchboard control and maintenance by a sustaining metabolism supplied by circulation of the blood.
7. *Power*—the action of muscles.

Schultz[4] states that in childhood the feet are a delicate part of the anatomy. The growth centers unite gradually as development progresses, with the general form being completed at about year 10. The epiphysis for the posterior aspect of the calcaneus appears at year 10 and unites with the rest of the bone soon after puberty. The phalanges are not completely ossified before year 18.

D'Ambrosia[5] states that the calcaneal epiphyses appear at 6 years in girls and at 8 years in boys. The first metatarsal sesamoids appear at 10 years in girls and at 13 years in boys.

As the foot develops, it responds to stresses, in most cases remaining fully functional in spite of injuries and distortions due to incorrect footwear and abnormal posture. Hiss stated,

> There is reasonable, clinical proof that a foot may be greatly changed in physical structure, may be deformed and have hypertrophic changes but still be comfortable. This comfort depends upon sufficient foot function to support the activity necessary each day.
>
> The range of activity that nature has provided in feet is far beyond necessary requirements. Foot deformity and pathological changes may be present to a considerable extent before the range of necessary function is encroached upon.[3(p21)]

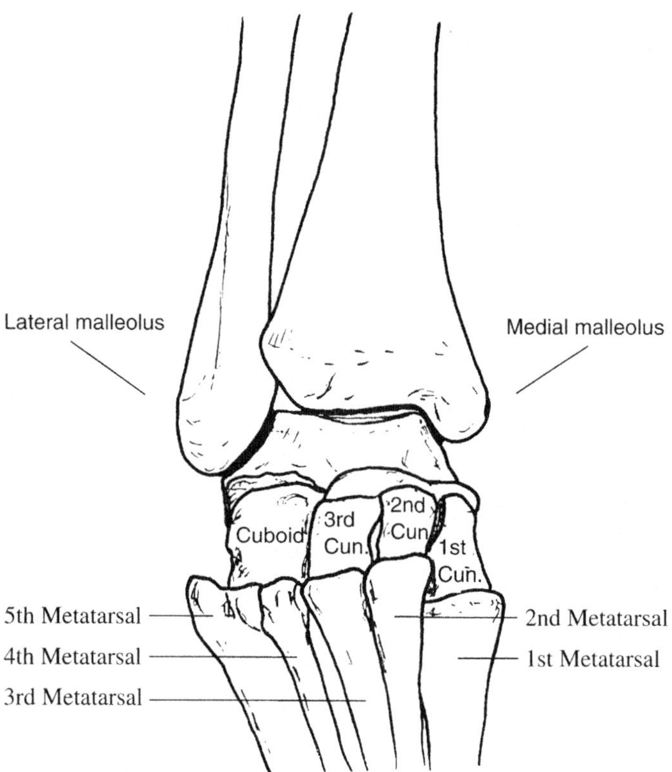

Fig. 1–1 Right ankle, plantar flexed, anterior view.

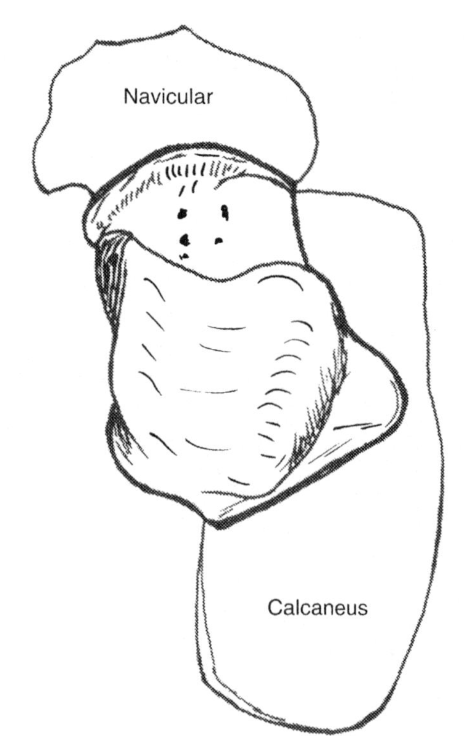

Fig. 1–2 Right talus from above.

Hiss further stated, "The presence of gross distortions and pathology does not necessarily mean the foot is dysfunctional. . . . The absence of pathological conditions also, must not lead the examiner to assume there is no dysfunction. *Comfort varies directly with function* (my emphasis)."[3(p21)]

Over the past 35 years, I have treated feet that looked as though they could not bear their own weight, much less the 200 or more pounds of body that brought them into my office. Often, in spite of gross distortions, minimal therapy on the feet, the back, or both has restored the patient to comfort, allowing a return to normal activities.

Patients may present with foot pain resulting from a problem in the foot or from problems with posture or gait. They may present with back pain resulting from dysfunction of the foot even though the foot is asymptomatic. A patient may complain of back and foot symptoms, with each contributing to the other.

A functional examination of the foot is necessary in any of the above conditions, no matter what its appearance. A beautifully formed foot with one or two fixations may interrupt normal function, making it impossible for the patient to bear weight. The same foot with two fixations may be symptom free yet interfere with normal posture and produce back symptoms. An understanding of anatomy and function therefore is necessary to recognize dysfunction and to relate symptoms to their ultimate cause.

The weight of the body transmits through the tibia to the talus where it is distributed to the rest of the foot. The tibia flares at the distal end, with the medial malleolus projecting along the medial surface of the talus (Fig. 1–1). Articular cartilage is present on the lateral surface of the medial malleolus and the inferior surface of the tibia for articulation with the talus. On the lateral surface of the distal end is the fibular notch. The notch provides the space for passage of the fibula to its articulation with the lateral surface of the talus.

The tibia and fibula form the mortise (socket) into which the talus fits, forming the hinge joint. The talus constitutes the link between the leg and the rest of the foot. The superior articular surface is covered with cartilage for articulation with the medial malleolus portion of the tibia, the inferior surface of the tibia, and the medial surface of the fibula. The trochlea is wider across the anterior than the posterior surface, which provides greater security with the ankle dorsiflexed than plantar flexed (Fig. 1–2).

Anterior to the trochlear surface are the neck and head of the talus. The anterior surface is covered with articular cartilage (Figs. 1–3 and 1–4). Inferiorly, the navicular articular surface continues to become the anterior articulation with the calcaneus. The middle (smallest) articulation is directly posterior. The largest talocalcaneal articulation lies posterior and lateral to the others (Fig. 1–5). Although the talus is the

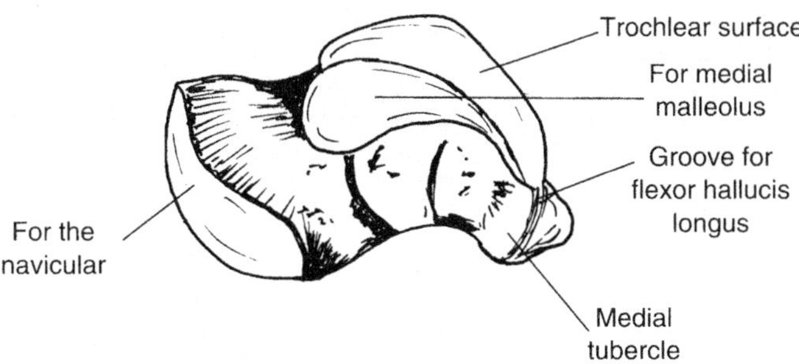

Fig. 1–3 Right talus, medial view.

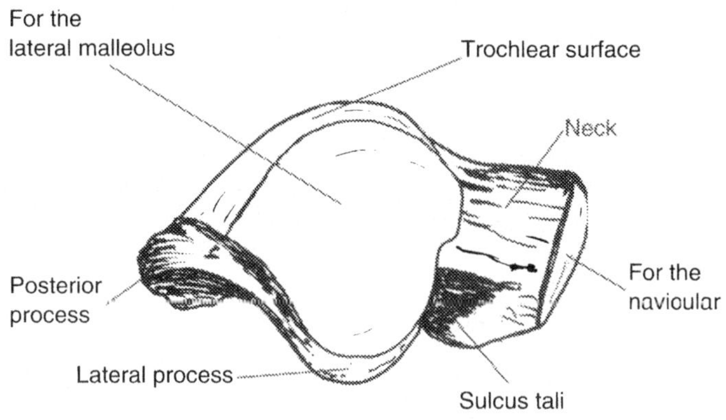

Fig. 1–4 Right talus, lateral view.

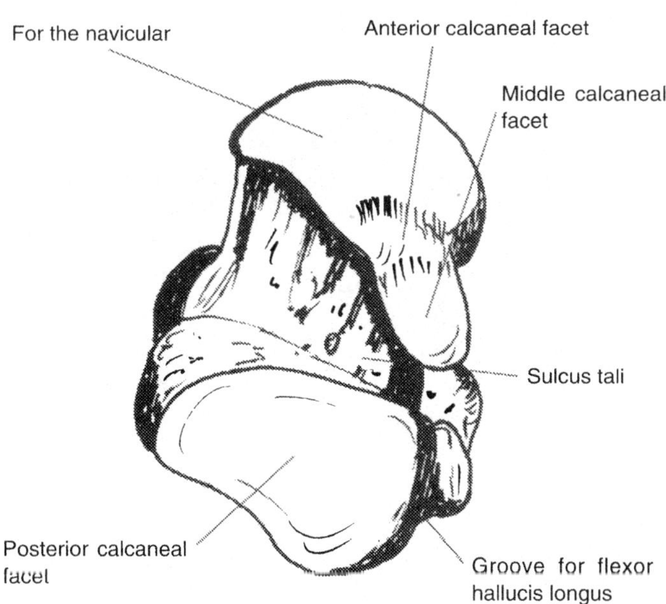

Fig. 1–5 Right talus, inferior view.

keystone to the foot, no muscles attach to it. Therefore, its displacement or malfunction is a result of factors other than direct muscle influence.

There are 26 bones in the foot: the 7 tarsals (talus, calcaneus, navicular, cuboid, and the 3 cuneiforms), the 5 metatarsals, and the 14 phalanges (Figs. 1–6 and 1–7).

Calliet[6] and Scholl[7] divide the foot into three functional segments: the posterior, consisting of the talus at the apex of the foot, making up part of the ankle, and the calcaneus as the hind part of the foot in contact with the ground; the middle, consisting of the navicular, cuboid, and the 3 cuneiforms; and the anterior, consisting of the 5 metatarsals and 14 phalanges.

The calcaneus is the largest bone in the foot, and in the standing position it is the major contact with the ground. The body weight is distributed from the tibia through the talus by way of the three calcaneal articulations. The posterior facet is the largest, situated inferior and lateral to the other talar articular facets (Fig. 1–8). The sustentaculum tali, the medial projection, provides support for the talus (Fig. 1–9). The middle talar facet is on the superior surface of the sustentaculum tali, and just posterior is the groove for the flexor hallucis longus muscle. The calcaneus articulates with the cuboid anteriorly.

The body weight is first distributed through the talus to the calcaneus and then forward from the calcaneus to the cuboid. It is also distributed from the talus to the navicular. Note that the calcaneocuboid articulation is inferior to the talonavicular articulation as well as all the talocalcaneal articulations (Fig. 1–10).

On the medial view, the sustentaculum tali is just below the medial malleolus, where it may be palpated (Fig. 1–11). It provides the support shelf for the middle talar articulation above and the groove for the flexor hallucis longus muscle below. It lies just in front of the groove on the posterior talus for the same muscle.

Figure 1–12 demonstrates the anterior aspect of the ankle with the forefoot flexed. The important anatomic considerations are the mortise joint along with the positioning of the talus relative to the navicular, the navicular and its articulations with the three cuneiforms, and the calcaneus and its articulations with the cuboid and the fourth and fifth metatarsals.

Viewed posteriorly, the sustentaculum tali is a medial projection of the calcaneus (Fig. 1–13). The head of the talus is in line with the most medial aspect of the medial malleolus.

The trochlea of the talus is gripped by the medial malleolus on one side and laterally by the fibula. The structure is secured by ligaments medially, laterally, and posteriorly but not anteriorly. The trochlea of the talus is wider anteriorly and therefore is more secure in dorsiflexion as it becomes wedged between the medial malloleus and the fibula.

The mediolateral axis of the ankle joint is not parallel with the knee joint. The lateral malleolus is larger and slightly posterior to the medial malleolus, producing approximately 10° of toe-out.

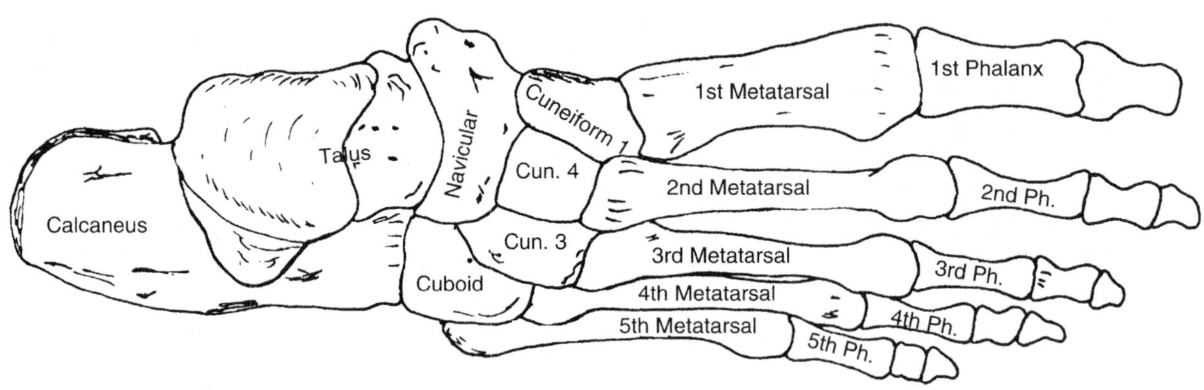

Fig. 1–6 Right foot from above.

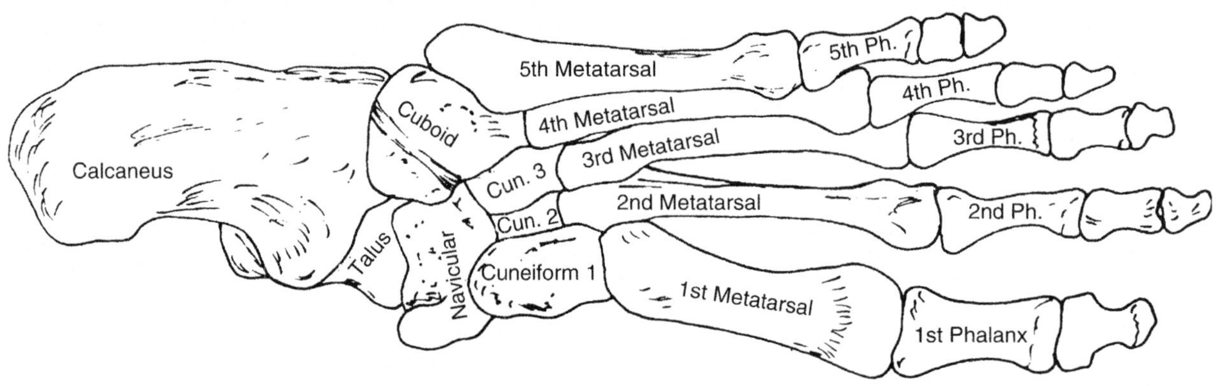

Fig. 1–7 Right foot from below.

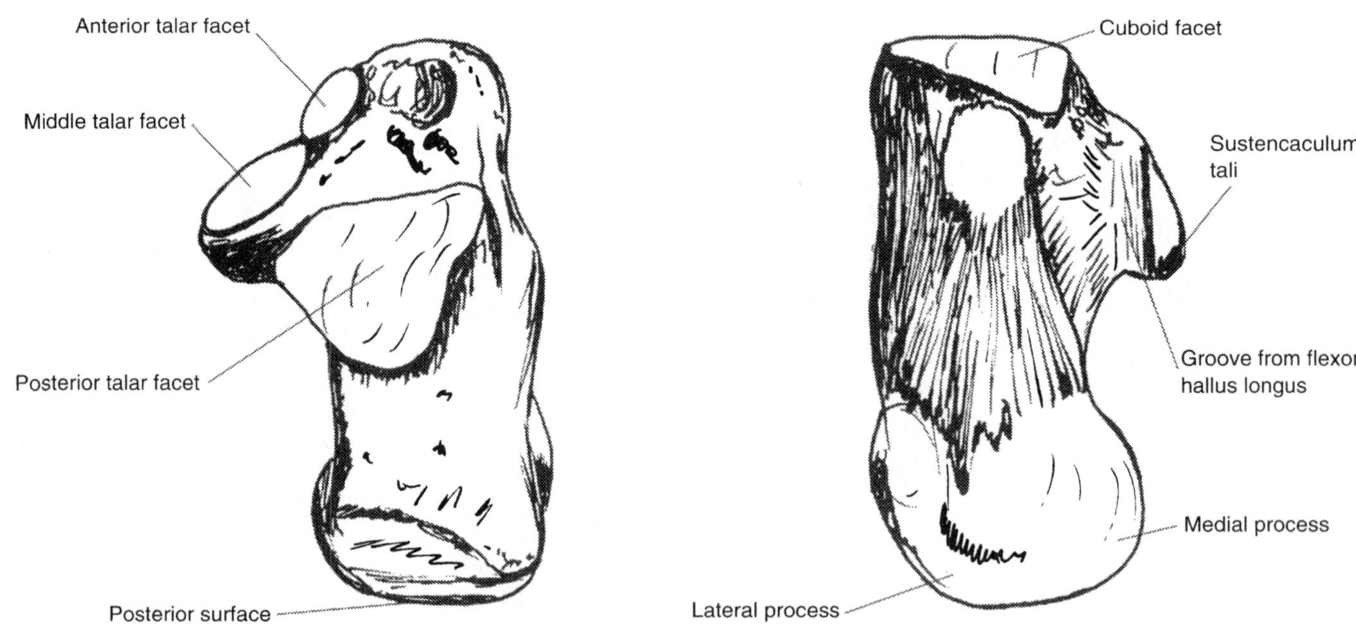

Fig. 1–8 Right calcaneus from above.   **Fig. 1–9** Right calcaneus from below.

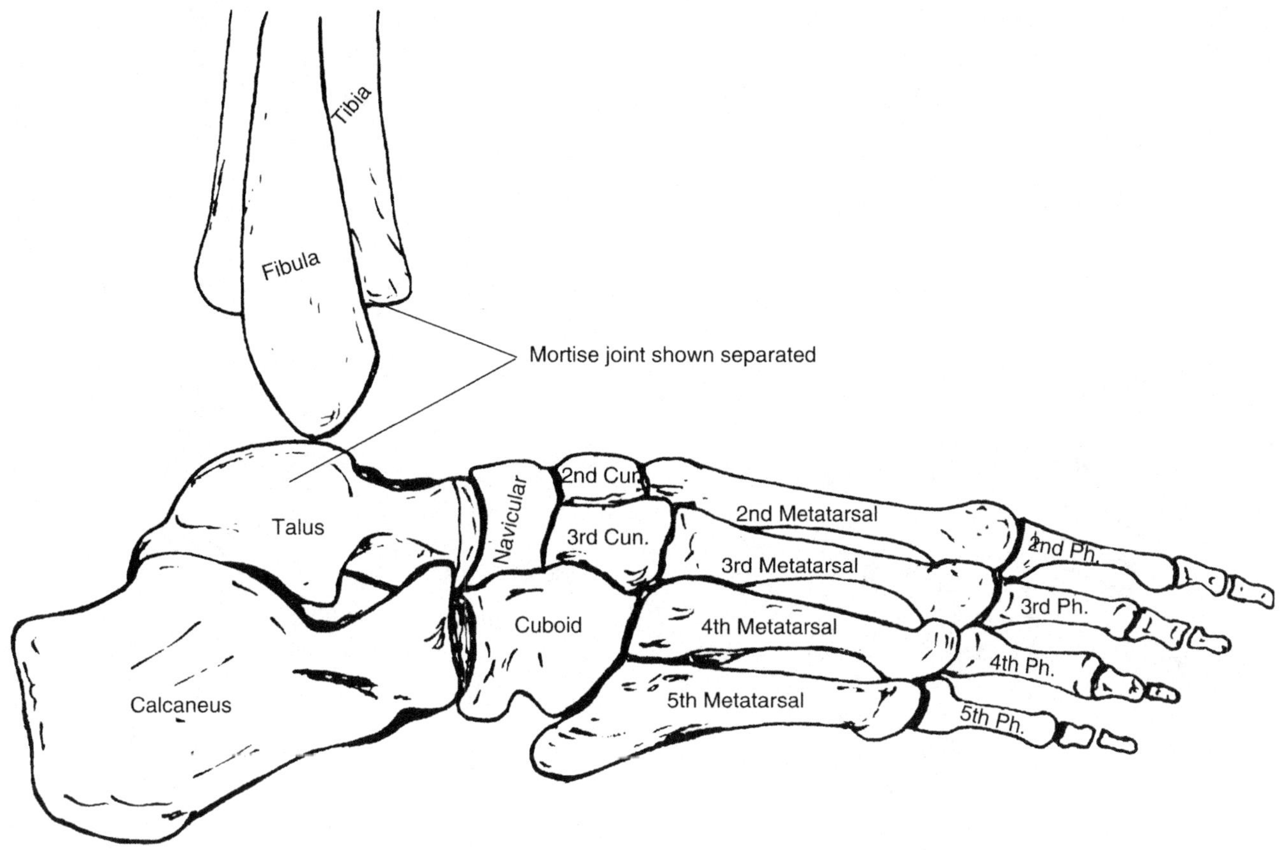

Fig. 1–10 Right foot, lateral view.

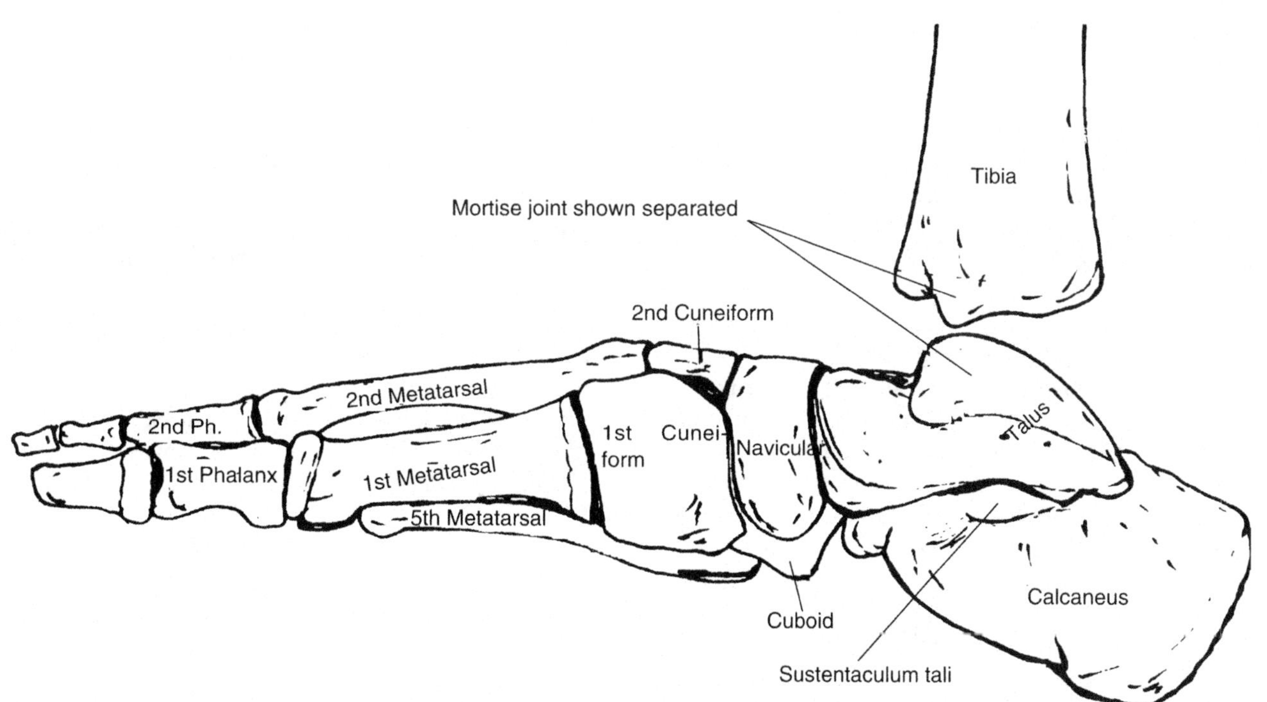

Fig. 1–11 Right foot, medial view.

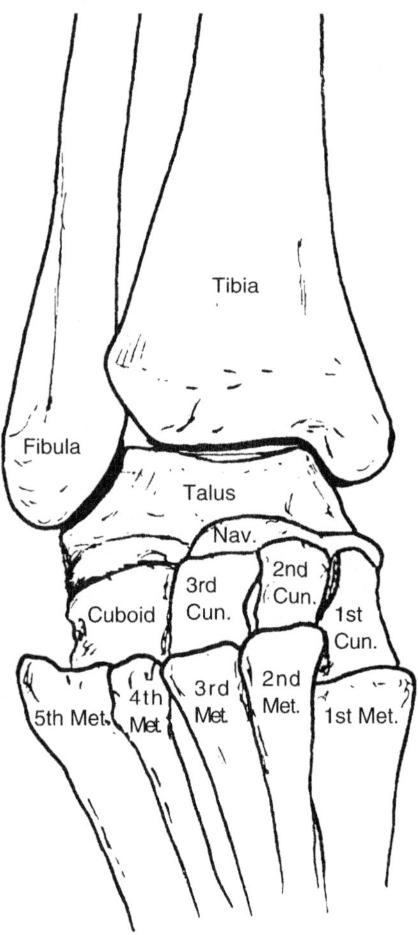

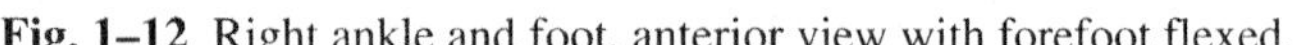

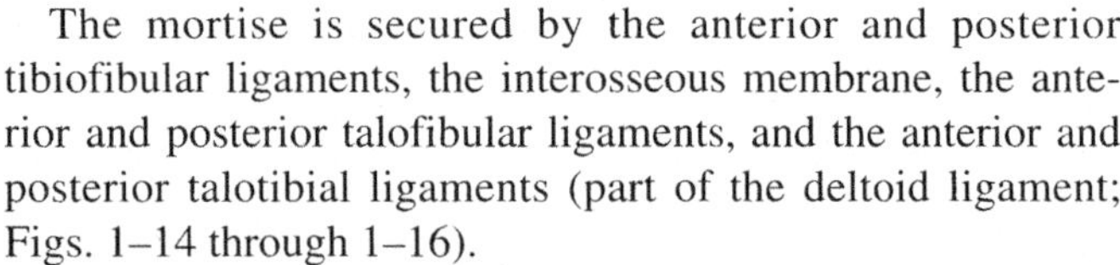

Fig. 1–12 Right ankle and foot, anterior view with forefoot flexed.

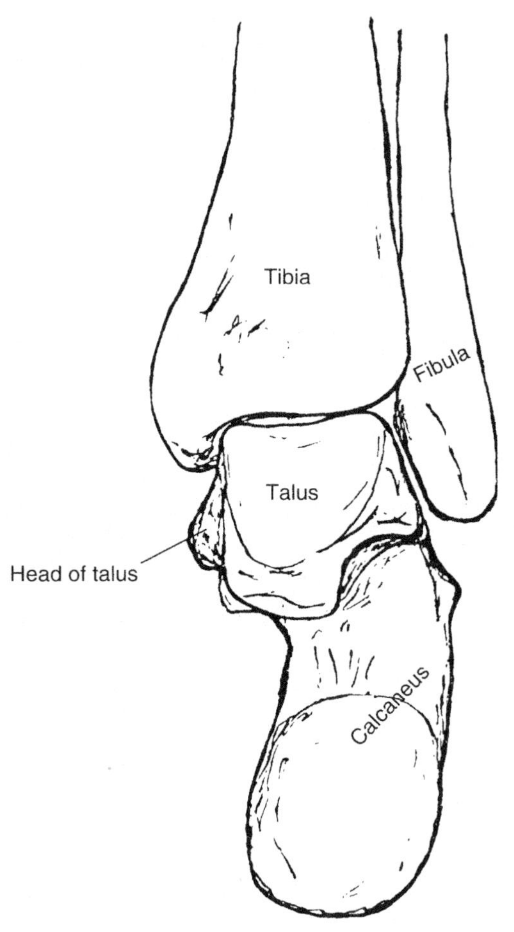

Fig. 1–13 Right ankle and foot, posterior view.

The mortise is secured by the anterior and posterior tibiofibular ligaments, the interosseous membrane, the anterior and posterior talofibular ligaments, and the anterior and posterior talotibial ligaments (part of the deltoid ligament; Figs. 1–14 through 1–16).

Anteriorly the ankle joint is devoid of ligaments, allowing the full range of motion. It is less secure in full plantar flexion because of the smaller width of the talar trochlea, but it is secured from anterior movement by the anterior talofibular and talotibial ligaments (Fig. 1–15). The ankle joint is surrounded by a fibrous capsule lined with a synovial membrane.

The subtalar joint structure, although considered separately, is secured by ligaments from the calcaneus to the talus, tibia, and fibula. The subtalar joint is surrounded by a fibrous capsule lined with a synovial membrane. The capsule does not communicate with any other joint.

The interosseous ligament of the subtalar joint runs from the sulcus tali on the underside of the talus. It separates the anterior from the posterior joint structures, running downward and laterally to the sulcus calcanei on the superior surface of the calcaneus. The most lateral fibers (the cervical ligament) connect the calcaneus with the neck of the talus (Fig. 1–16). The interosseous ligament is the major security of the subtalar joint. With most of its fibers traversing laterally and inferiorly, it prevents excessive inversion. The cervical ligament is palpated easily on the surface of the calcaneus just inferior and anterior to the lateral malleolus (Fig. 1–16).

The posterior talocalcaneal ligament (Fig. 1–14) secures the posterior process of the talus (sometimes referred to as the posterior malleolus) to the calcaneus. Netter[8] describes the posterior talocalcaneal ligament, as do Scholl[7] and Kapandji.[9] Mennell[2] and *Dorland's*[10] list the ligament. *Gray's Anatomy*[11] neither shows nor refers to it, and Calliet,[6] D'ambrosia,[5] and Kessler and Hertling[12] do not list the ligament. It is considered by some part of the joint capsule, however.

The medial talocalcaneal ligament (Fig. 1–17) connects the posterior talus to the sustentaculum tali. The lateral talocalcaneal ligament connects the lateral process of the talus to the calcaneus (Fig. 1–16).

The deltoid ligament (Fig. 1–17) is made up of the posterior tibiotalar, the tibiocalcaneal, the tibionavicular, and the anterior tibiotalar ligaments. It may be referred to as the medial

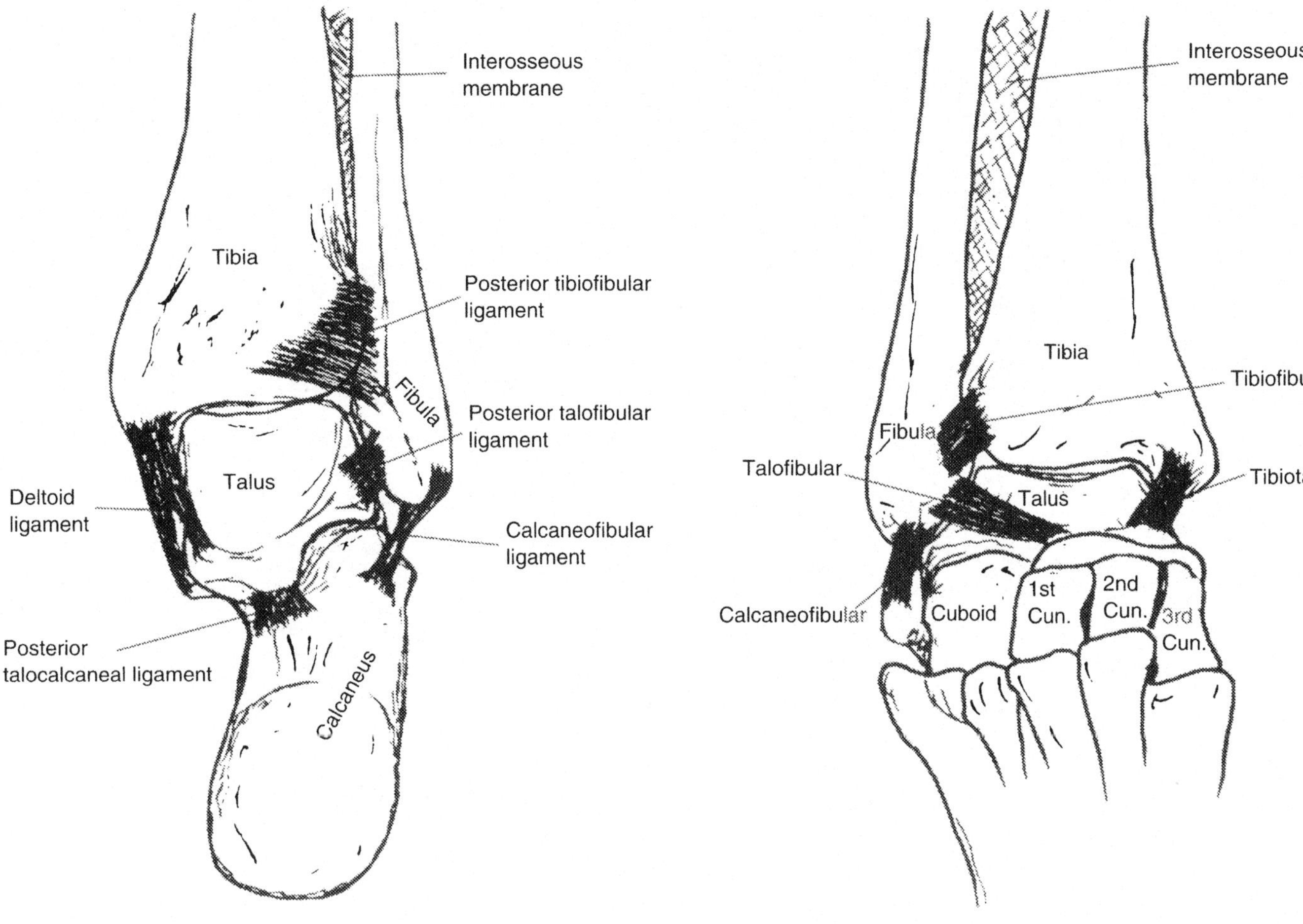

Fig. 1–14 Right ankle and foot, posterior view showing ligaments.

Fig. 1–15 Right ankle and foot, anterior view with the foot plantar flexed and showing ligaments.

collateral ligament of the ankle. The three bands on the lateral malleolus (Fig. 1–16)—the posterior tibiotalar, the calcaneofibular, and the anterior talofibular ligaments—are sometimes referred to as the lateral collateral ligament of the ankle.

The talocalcaneonavicular joint includes the concave navicular bone, the rounded convex head of the talus, the middle and anterior talocalcaneal facets, and the upper portion of the plantar calcaneonavicular or spring ligament (Figs. 1–17 and 1–18). The capsule is sparse, and the posterior portion becomes a part of the interosseous ligament.

The joint is supported directly only by the fibrous capsule and the dorsal talonavicular ligament (Fig. 1–17). It is supported indirectly by the navicular potion of the bifurcate ligament (Fig. 1–16) laterally. Medially the tibionavicular ligament (anterior part of the deltoid ligament) and the spring ligament (from the sustentaculum tali to the navicular tubercle) provide indirect support. On the plantar surface, the plantar calcaneonavicular ligament provides support (Fig. 1–19).

The lack of direct ligamental support allows the great range of motion necessary for the talonavicular joint, yet the joint is provided with stability and restraint by the indirect ligaments. The movements include gliding and rotation (allowing dorsiflexion), plantar flexion, mediolateral gliding, and rotation.

The calcaneocuboid articulation has a fibrous capsule that thickens over the dorsal surface of the joint to become the dorsal calcaneocuboid ligament (Fig. 1–16). It is supported further on the dorsal surface by the cuboid portion of the bifurcated ligament. On the plantar surface these are connected by the short plantar ligament as well as by fibers from the long plantar ligament (Fig. 1–19).

The cuboidonavicular joint is supported by the dorsal ligament (Fig. 1–16), the plantar ligament (Fig. 1–19), and an interosseous ligament connecting the two rough surfaces.

The anterior navicular surface, although convex, is divided into three distinct facets for articulation with the cuneiforms.

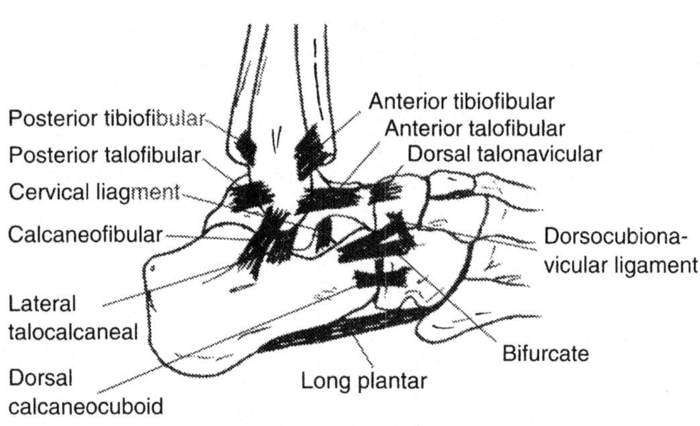

Fig. 1–16 Right ankle and foot, lateral view showing ligaments.

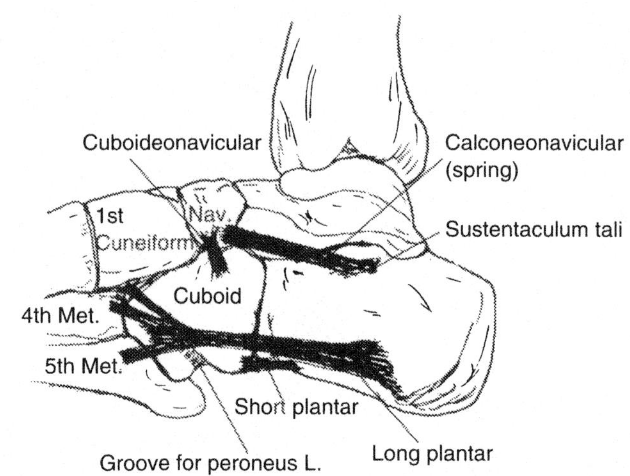

Fig. 1–18 Right ankle and foot, medial and plantar view showing ligaments.

Movement is much more restricted compared with the talonavicular joint and is limited to dorsoplantar movement with minimal rotation during inversion and eversion.

The tarsometatarsal articulations have dorsal, plantar, and interosseous ligaments. The first metatarsal–first cuneiform articulation has an independent joint capsule. The second and third communicate with each other and the intercuneiform capsule. The fourth and fifth are separated from the third by an interosseous ligament. The ligament traverses from the lateral cuneiform to the base of the fourth metatarsal.

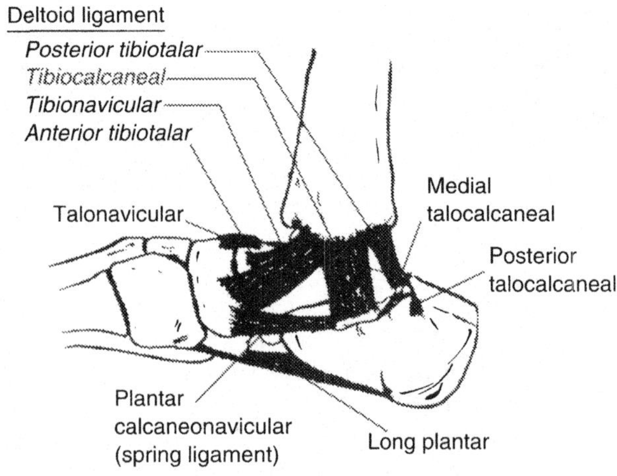

Fig. 1–17 Right ankle and foot, medial view showing ligaments.

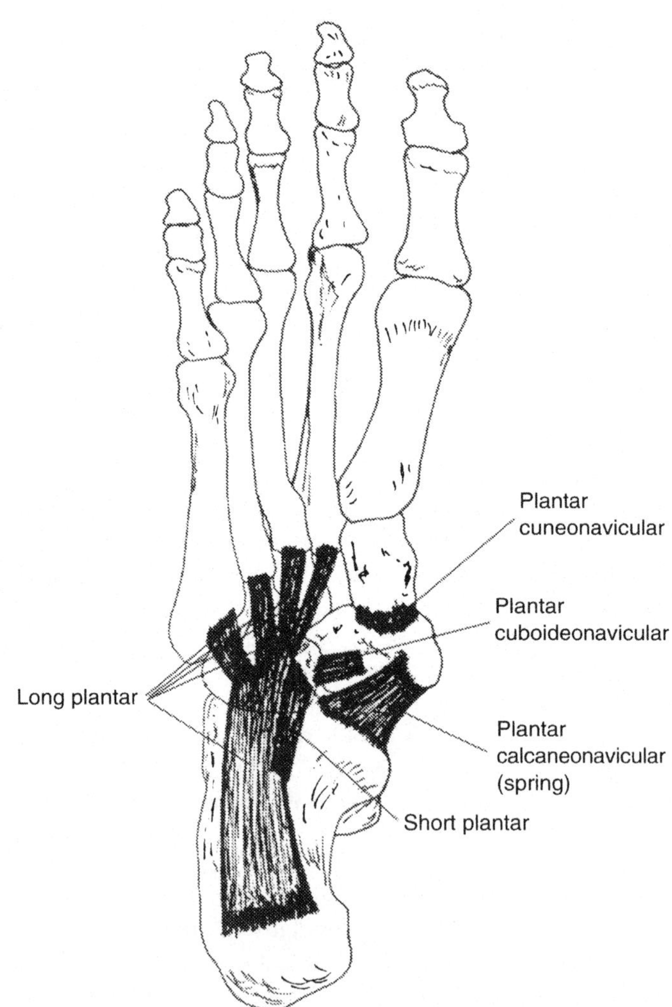

Fig. 1–19 Right foot, ligaments on the plantar surface.

ARCHES OF THE FOOT

Clinicians refer to the arches of the foot, but over these a great deal of controversy exists. The controversy concerns not only which structures they include but their significance as well.

Shands and Raney[1] describe two arches: the longitudinal arch, which is divided into the medial (extending from the calcaneus to the head of the first metatarsal) and the lateral (extending from the calcaneus to the fourth and fifth metatarsals); and the anterior arch, also known as the transverse or metatarsal arch, which includes the metatarsal heads (with primary ground contact by the first and fifth) and is flattened with weight bearing.

Mennell[2] refers to the same divisions with their tripod of weight bearing from the calcaneus to the first and fifth metatarsals yet dismisses them. The existence of the arches is not in doubt, but their significance is questioned. Consider that a great number of pain-free feet exist with no amount of arch present. A great number of patients present with what appear to be normal arches yet are experiencing great pain.

Hiss[3] states that no anterior arch exists. He also states that a dropped arch or flatfoot is not acquired after the first few years of development. He cites a study in which 150 lb was applied to a cadaver foot with no change in contour. When an additional 150 lb was applied, it produced only a mild decrease in the angle. Upon release of the weight, the arch returned to normal with no tissue damage.

Hiss[3] further states that the foot is divided longitudinally (Fig. 1–20) into an outer, weight-bearing arch and an inner, spring arch. The outer arch is the primary weight bearer and stabilizer in walking and standing. The inner arch is a curved structure whose main function is to adjust the body weight, keeping it balanced on the outer weight-bearing part of the foot.

Kessler and Hertling[12] compare the foot to a twisted plate (Fig. 1–21). The calcaneus is at one end, positioned vertically, and the metatarsal heads are positioned horizontally when making contact with the ground. To demonstrate this, they suggest constructing a model with cardboard and twisting it so that one end lies flat on the table. The arching produced by the model is analogous to the arching of the foot. The medial arch is dependent upon the twisted configuration and not on the architectural shape of the bone structure. The lateral arch represents a true architectural arch with the cuboid wedged between the calcaneus and the metatarsals. When the untwisting occurs, the arch flattens.

Kessler and Hertling[12] seem to agree with Hiss[3] in their opinion on the longitudinal arch. They also agree that no transverse arch exists at the metatarsal heads. The use of their model demonstrates the presence of a transverse arch component in the tarsals.

Kapandji[9] states that the medial longitudinal arch is maintained only with the help of the ligaments and muscles. He states that the lateral longitudinal arch consists of the calcaneus, the cuboid, and only the fifth metatarsal; Hiss[3] considers the fourth metatarsal as well. They both agree that the lateral arch has greater stability to provide the transmission of the body weight forward. Hiss[3] and Kapandji[9] point out that a transverse arch component is present at the level of the cuboid.

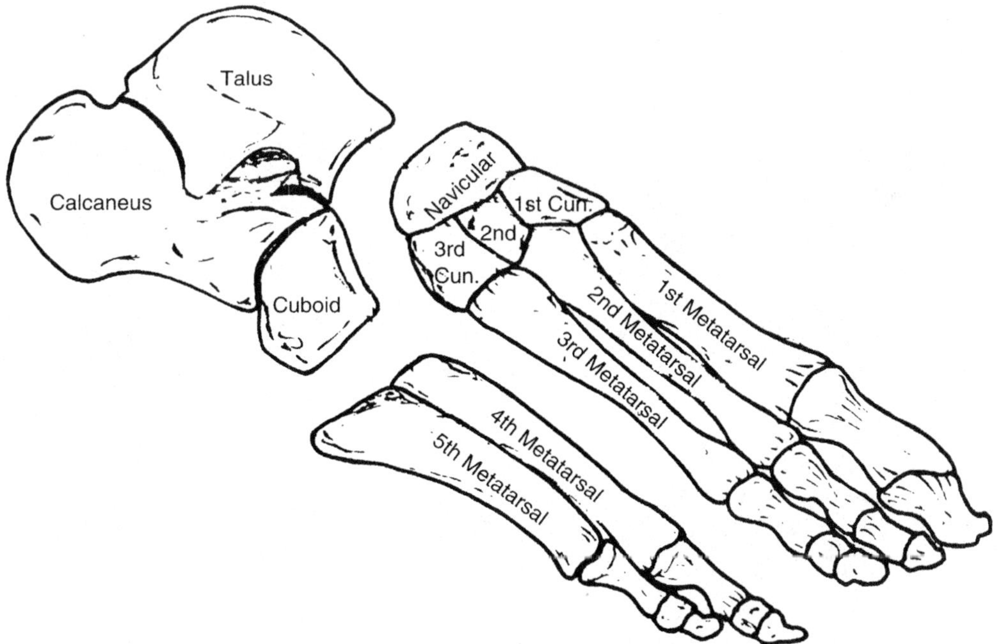

Fig. 1–20 The three units of the right foot.

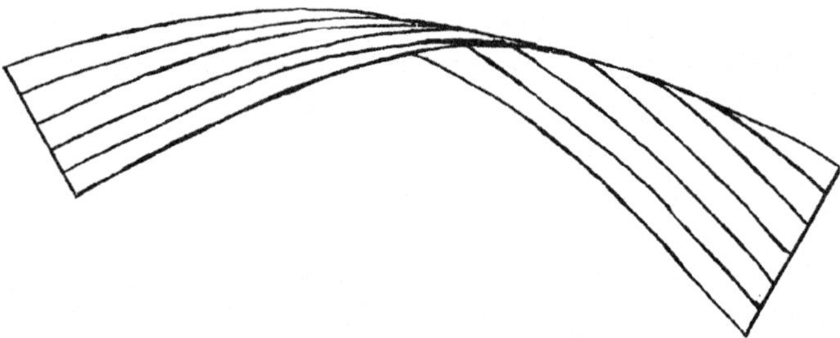

Fig. 1–21 Bending of a long piece of cardboard to simulate the longitudinal arch.

In the normal standing foot the cuboid–third cuneiform articulation angle is 45° (Fig. 1–22). This increases at the beginning of the stride as the medial arch is lifted, causing the navicular to overhang the cuboid, and the weight of the cuneiforms is applied downward onto the cuboid.

Kapandji[9] states that in the normal foot the head of the first metatarsal rests on the ground through the two sesamoid bones. An arch is formed across the metatarsal heads to the fifth, with the second metatarsal head acting as the keystone.

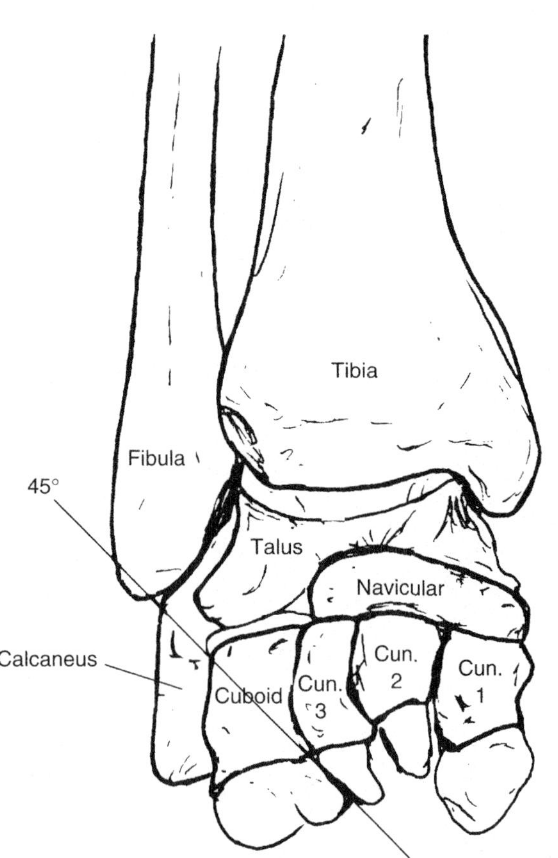

Fig. 1–22 Cross-section of the right foot with the metatarsals removed.

The arch is relatively flat while resting on the ground, being cushioned by the soft tissues.

MOVEMENTS OF THE ANKLE AND FOOT

Normal dorsiflexion (backward bending) is 20° (Fig. 1–23). It is limited by the triceps surae (gastrocnemeus, soleus, and plantaris muscles) and by the encroachment of the talus neck on the tibia. Normal plantar flexion (toward the sole) is 30° at the ankle joint (Fig. 1–23) and 50° if the entire foot is included. It is limited by the dorsiflexors and by encroachment of the posterior process of the talus on the calcaneus.

Terminology varies from text to text. The terms *valgus* and *varus* are no exception. Valgus has been described variously as a deviation away from the midline or a condition in which the apex of the angle points toward the midline.[6] In a valgus deviation, the heel is everted or rotated outward on its longitudinal axis, or the angulation is away from the midline.[10] Varus may be described as the distal member being bent toward the midline.[6] In a varus deviation, the heel is rotated inward on its longitudinal axis or is inverted.

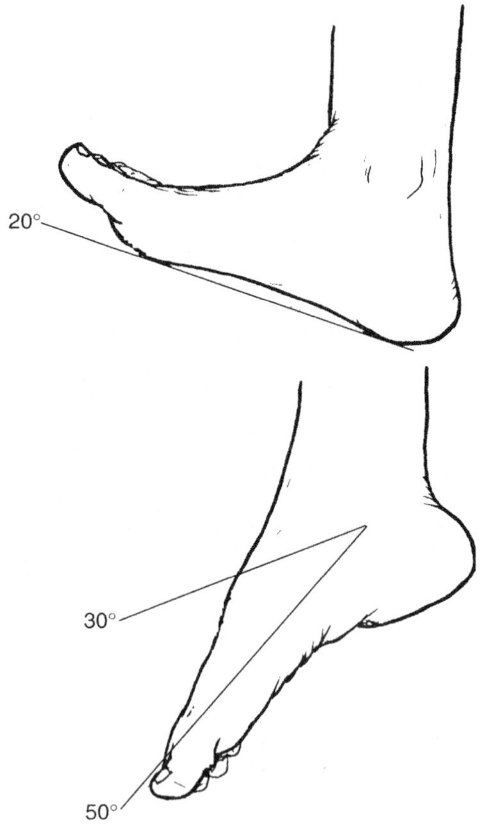

Fig. 1–23 Normal dorsiflexion and plantar flexion of the ankle.

Shands and Raney[1] describe eversion as equaling valgus, the plantar surface of the heel or forefoot being rotated outward. Inversion would be equal to varus, with the plantar surface facing medially (heel or forefoot). Michaud[13] adds dorsiflexion to pronation and plantar flexion to supination.

Rather than add to the confusion, for the purposes of this text the terms *valgus* and *varus* are not used. The other movements are defined as follows:

- *adduction*—movement toward the midline (Fig. 1–24)
- *abduction*—movement away from the midline (Fig. 1–25)
- *supination*— movement produced by raising the medial longitudinal arch, or movement allowing the plantar surface to face medially (Fig. 1–26)
- *pronation*—movement produced by lowering the medial longitudinal arch and elevating of the lateral longitudinal arch, or movement allowing the plantar surface to face laterally (Fig. 1–27)
- *inversion*—a combination of moves including adduction, supination, and some plantar flexion (Fig. 1–28)
- *eversion*—a combination of moves including abduction, pronation, and some dorsiflexion (Fig. 1–29)

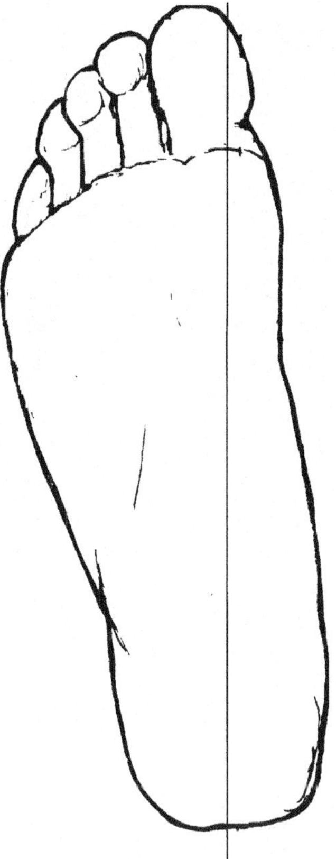

Fig. 1–25 Abduction of the right forefoot.

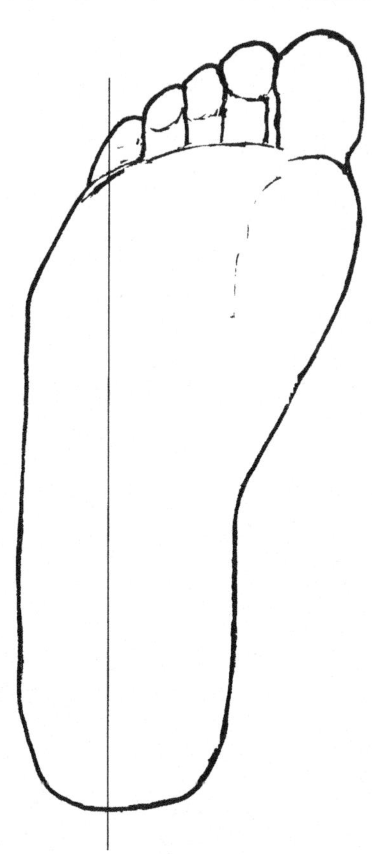

Fig. 1–24 Adduction of the right forefoot.

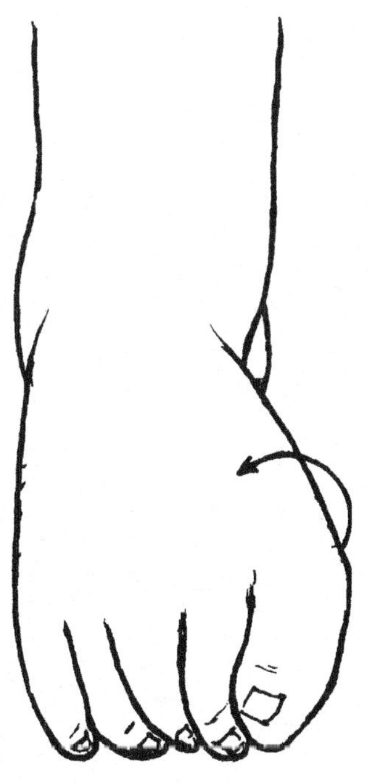

Fig. 1–26 Supination of the right foot.

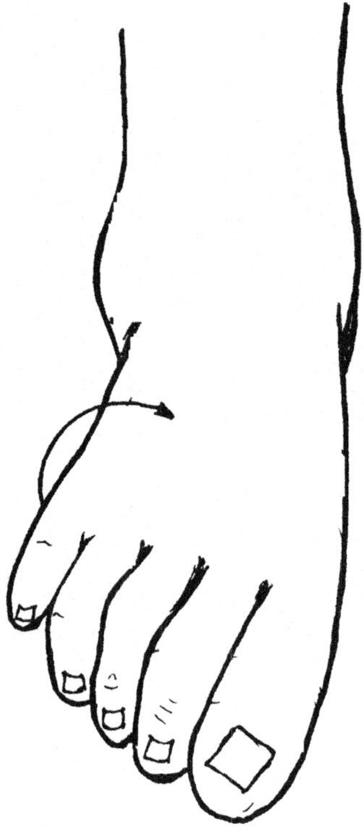

Fig. 1–27 Pronation of the right foot.

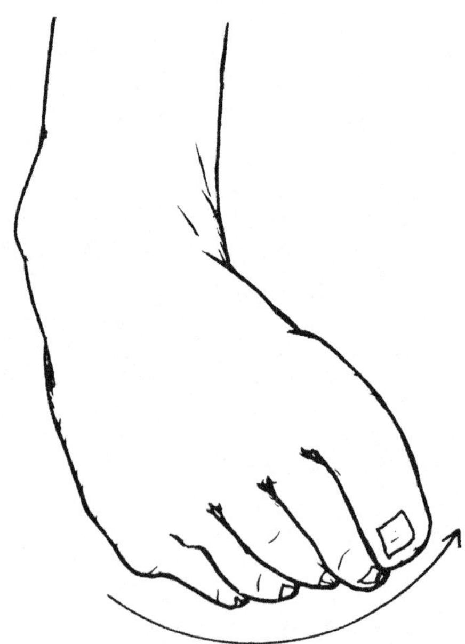

Fig. 1–28 Inversion (adduction, supination, or plantar flexion) of the right foot.

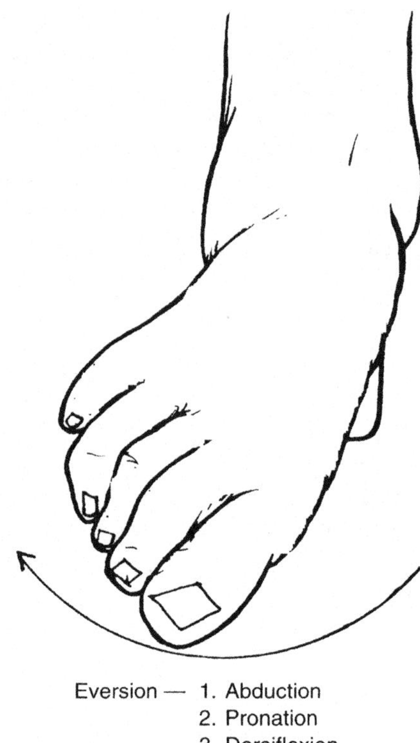

Fig. 1–29 Eversion (abduction, pronation, or dorsiflexion) of the right foot.

MUSCLES AND TENDONS

The foot actually begins at the knee, with the gastrocnemius and plantaris originating on the femur. The muscles are generally divided into the anterior, lateral, and posterior crurals. They may also be divided into the extrinsic muscles (those originating above the ankle) and the intrinsic muscles (those originating in the foot).

Anterior Muscles

The following description of the muscles may include the tendons extending into the foot. It is my intention to discuss the tendons of the foot separately, however, the better to convey their function.

The most superficial muscle on the anterior leg is the anterior tibialis (Fig. 1–30). It originates on the tibia and the interosseous membrane, passing inferomedially under the retinaculum, and inserts into the medial and inferior first metatarsal head and the first cuneiform. *Gray's Anatomy*[11] states that variations include insertions into the talus, the base of the first metatarsal, and the first phalanx.

The belly of the anterior tibialis may be palpated immediately lateral to the sharp anterior ridge of the tibia about one third of the way below the knee. Restraint of the foot with a

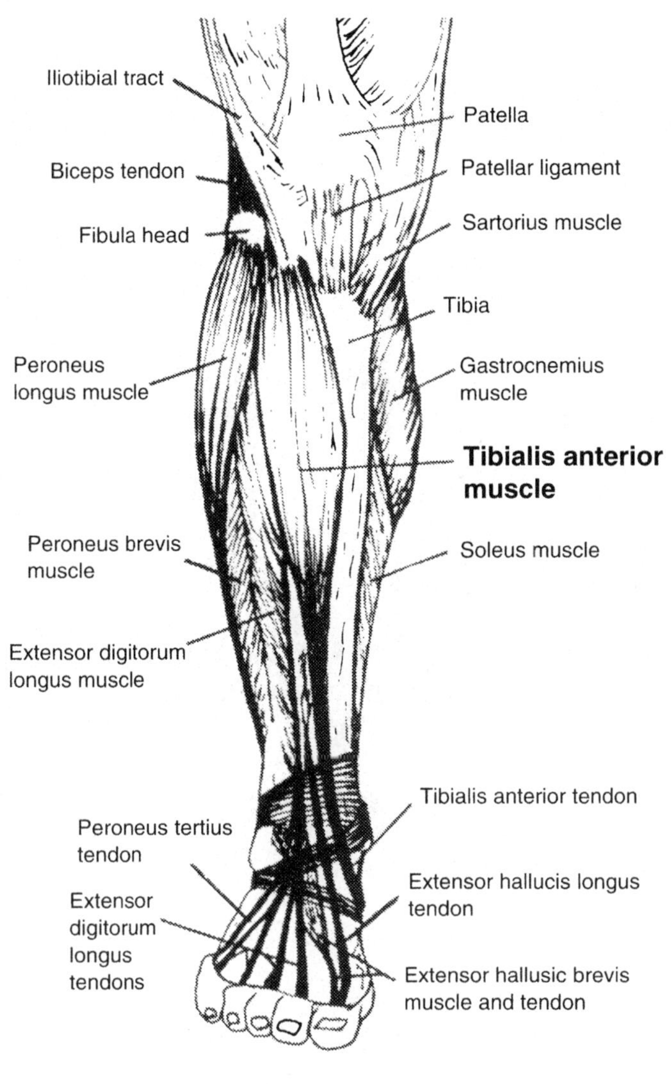

Fig. 1–30 Right leg, ankle, and foot, anterior view.

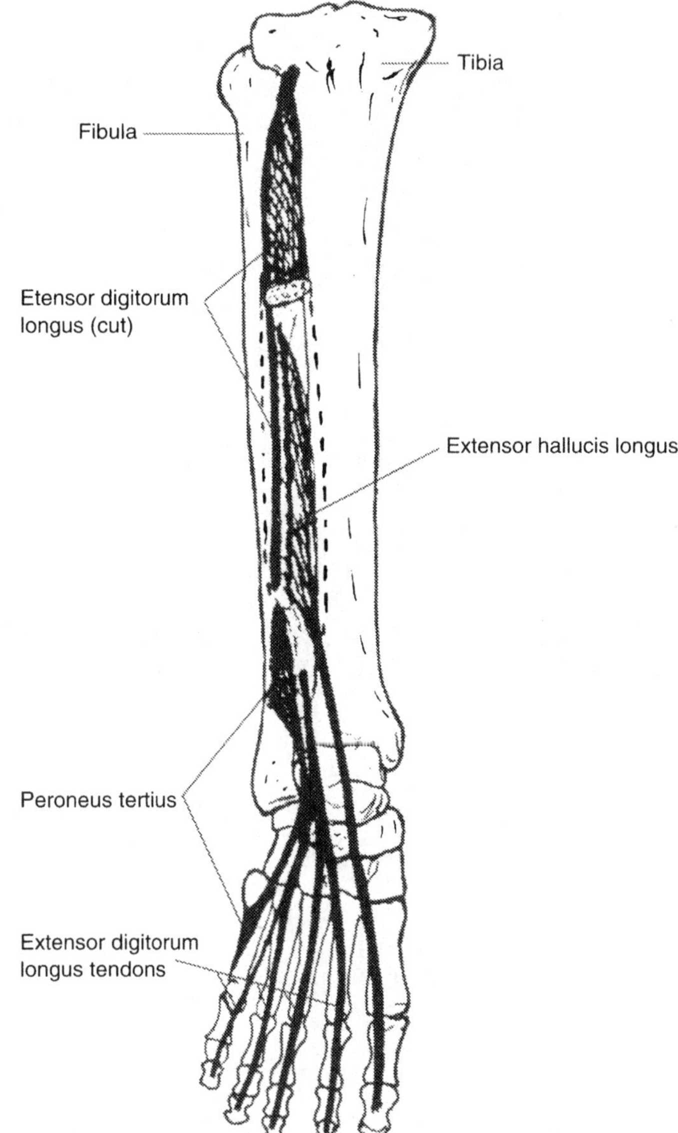

Fig. 1–31 Right leg and foot showing extensor muscles.

mild attempt to invert and dorsiflex the foot several times makes palpation easy.

The extensor digitorum longus muscle (Fig. 1–31) originates from the lateral condyle of the tibia, the upper three quarters of the medial surface of the fibula, and the interosseous membrane. The peroneus tertius muscle originates from the lower third of the medial surface of the fibula, and its tendon becomes a part of the extensor digitorum tendon. The tendons pass under the anterior retinaculum at the ankle. The peroneus tertius portion separates below the ankle and is inserted into the dorsal surface of the base and shaft of the fifth metatarsal. The belly of both muscles may be palpated from half to two thirds of the way from the knee to the ankle. They become apparent with extension of the four lesser digits.

The extensor hallucis longus muscle (Fig. 1–32) originates between and deep to the anterior tibialis and extensor digitorum longus muscles on the middle half of the fibula and the interosseous membrane. Its tendon passes under the anterior ankle retinaculum and inserts into the distal phalanx of the great toe. Palpation of the belly during function is at best difficult.

The tendons of the anterior muscles may be palpated as they pass under the ankle retinaculum (Fig. 1–30) by palpating the anterior surface of the medial malleolus and sliding the finger laterally. The first tendon is the anterior tibialis; it is followed by the extensor hallucis longus and then the extensor digitorum longus and peroneus tertius tendons.

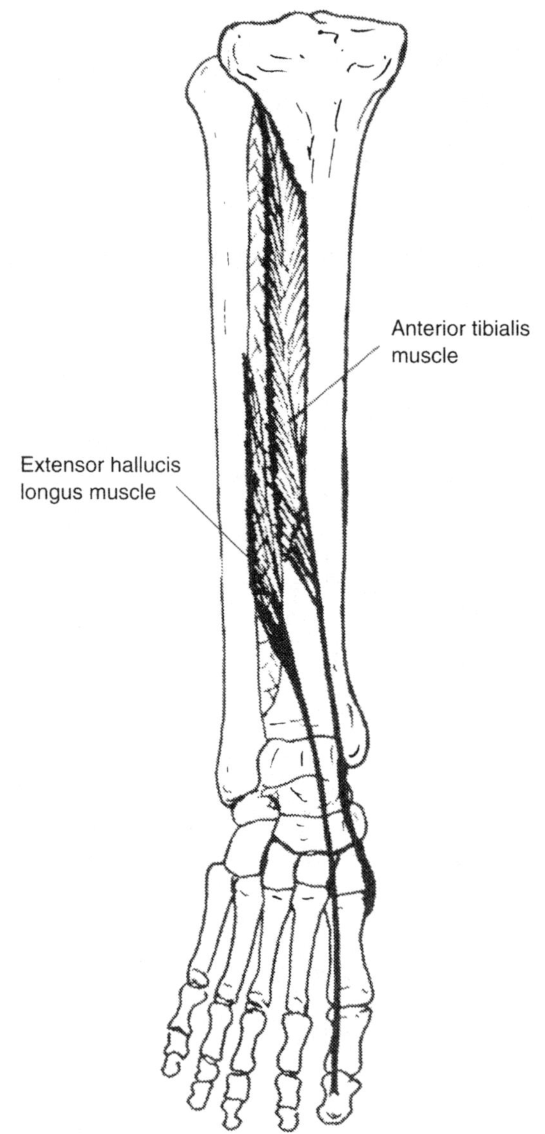

Fig. 1–32 Right leg and foot showing extensor hallucis longus and anterior tibialis muscles.

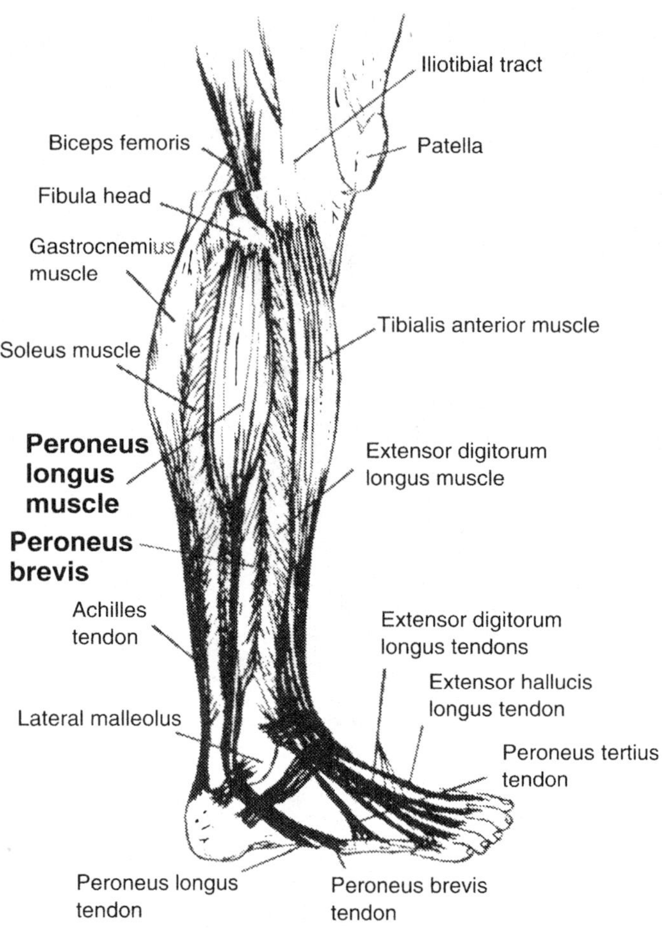

Fig. 1–33 Right leg, ankle, and foot showing muscles and tendons.

Lateral Muscles

Lateral to the anterior tibialis is the peroneus longus muscle, originating from the lateral head and the upper two thirds of the fibula (Fig. 1–33). Its tendon passes posteriorly behind the lateral malleolus in a groove shared with the peroneus brevis and covered by the superior peroneal retinaculum. Both tendons pass under the inferior peroneal retinaculum as well. The peroneus longus continues to the cuboid, where it passes underneath in a groove to insert on the lateral side of the first cuneiform and the base of the first metatarsal. The peroneus longus muscle may be palpated about a quarter of the way inferior to the knee and lateral to the anterior tibialis. On re-

straint of the foot with a mild attempt to plantar flex and evert the foot several times, the muscle contraction becomes apparent.

The peroneus brevis muscle arises from the lower two thirds of the lateral surface of the fibula anterior to the peroneus longus (Fig. 1–33). Its tendon passes posterior to the longus tendon behind the lateral malleolus. Along with the longus tendon, it passes under the peroneal retinaculum, crosses over the longus tendon, and inserts into the tubercle on the base of the fifth metatarsal. Both tendons may be palpated as they traverse posteriorly on the fibula and as they pass behind the lateral malleolus along their course below the peroneal retinaculum. Each tendon may be distinguished by alternately plantarflex-everting and everting alone.

Posterior Muscles

The gastrocnemius arises from two heads (Fig. 1–34). One arises behind the adductor tubercle on the posterior surface of

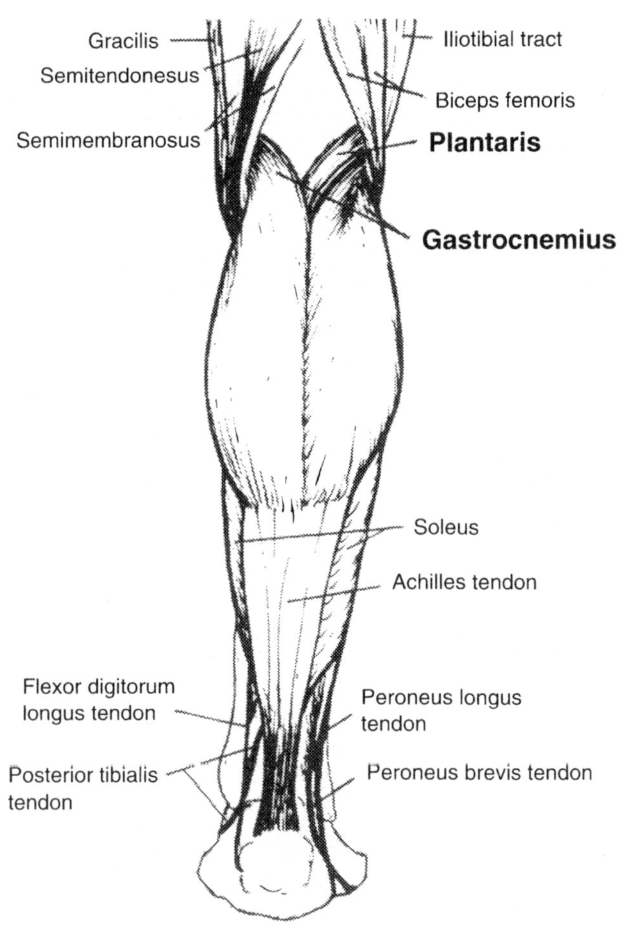

Fig. 1–34 Right leg, posterior view.

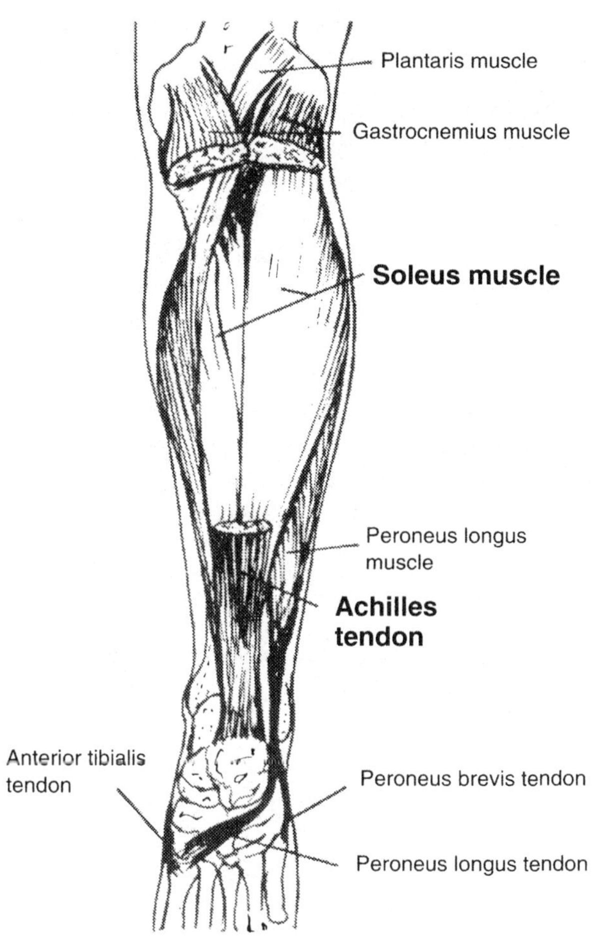

Fig. 1–35 Right leg and ankle, posterior view with the ankle plantar flexed.

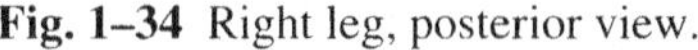

the medial femoral condyle. The other head arises from the lateral and posterior surface of the lateral femoral condyle. Both also arise from the capsule of the knee. The two heads remain separate until they join the soleus and plantaris muscles to form the Achilles tendon.

The plantaris muscle (Fig. 1–35) arises from the lateral supracondylar line of the femur and from the oblique popliteal ligament. Its tendon passes between the gastrocnemius and soleus muscles and inserts into the Achilles tendon.

The soleus muscle (Figs. 1–35 and 1–36) arises deep to the gastrocnemius from the head and upper quarter of the posterior shaft of the fibula. It also arises from the soleal line and the middle third of the medial border of the tibia. Its tendon joins the gastrocnemius to form the Achilles tendon and inserts into the calcaneus.

The Achilles tendon (Fig. 1–35) is formed with the soleus fibers, inserting into the anterior portion almost at the end. During descent the fibers twist on themselves, with the more medial fibers inserting on the lateral portion of the calcaneus.

Palpation of the muscle function may be done while plantar flexing. On mild plantar flexion laterally, greater contraction occurs on the medial head of the gastrocnemius, and an increased tension is applied on the lateral portion of the Achilles tendon. On plantar flexing medially, the opposite occurs.

The peroneus longus and brevis tendons (Figs. 1–34 through 1–36) may be palpated as they pass through the groove posterior to the lateral malleolus and under the peroneal tubercle on the lateral side of the calcaneus. From the tubercle they go their separate ways, with the brevis inserting into the tubercle on the base of the fifth metatarsal. The peroneus longus traverses the calcaneus inferior to the brevis and passes under the cuboid within the peroneal groove, where it is retained by the long plantar ligament. The longus inserts into the lateral side of the bases of the first cuneiform and first metatarsal, directly opposing the anterior tibialis insertion.

Both tendons may be palpated while the foot is fixed and movement toward plantar flexion and eversion is attempted.

Place one finger on the fifth metatarsal base and another on the proximal border of the cuboid. To identify the brevis even further, add abduction to the movement.

The flexor digitorum longus muscle (Fig. 1–36) arises medial to the flexor hallucis longus on the posterior surface of the tibia. It arises medial to the posterior tibialis, with the fibers originating to within 7 to 8 cm of the distal end of the bone. Its tendon crosses the tendon of the posterior tibialis, passing behind the medial malleolus in a groove shared with the posterior tibialis tendon. It then passes inferiorly and anteriorly along the side of the sustentaculum tali on its way to the distal phalanges of the second through fifth digits. The muscle may be palpated just medial to the Achilles tendon on the posterior surface of the tibia 5 to 6 in above the medial malleolus. The tendon may be palpated as it passes behind the medial malleolus between the posterior tibialis and the flexor hallucis longus tendons. To isolate its function, gently flex the four digits while holding the great toe in extension (eliminating the flexor hallucis longus).

The flexor hallucis longus muscle (Figs. 1–36 and 1–37) arises from the inferior two thirds of the posterior surface of the fibula and the lower part of the interosseous membrane. Its tendon passes obliquely to the medial side of the tibia, where it occupies a groove. It then passes under the sustentaculum tali on its way to its insertion into the distal phalanx of the great toe. The muscle belly may be palpated on the posterior fibula approximately a quarter of the way superior from the heel while the great toe is flexed. The tendon may be palpated just in front of the medial border of the Achilles tendon on the posterior surface of the tibia. It may also be palpated during its passage inferoanteriorly below the sustentaculum tali.

The posterior tibialis muscle (Figs. 1–36 and 1–38) arises between the flexor hallucis longus and the flexor digitorum

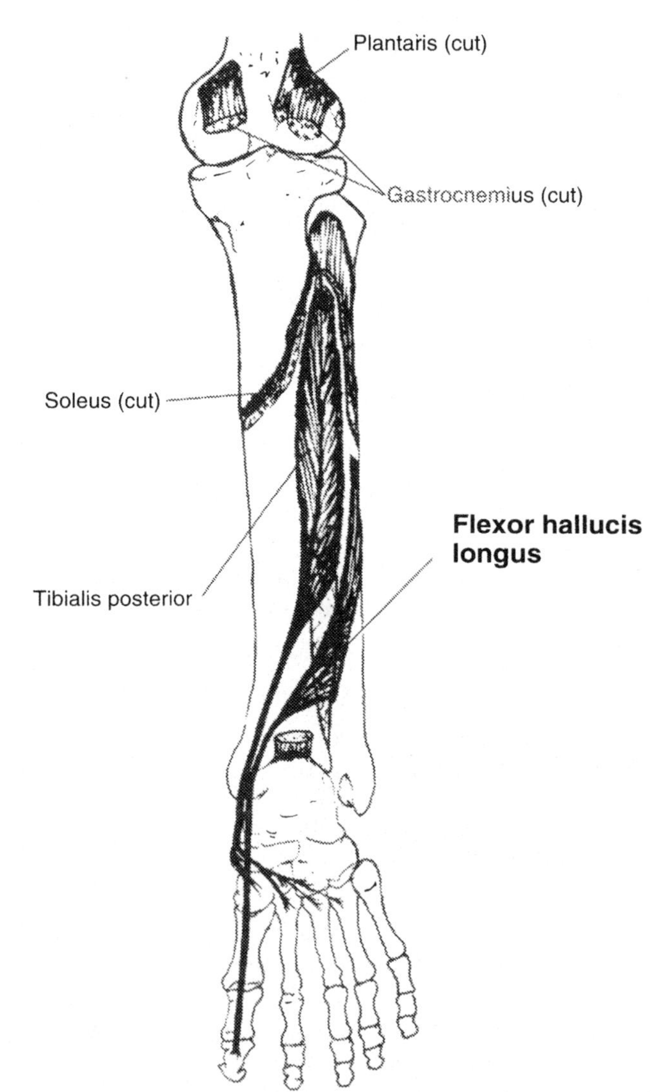

Fig. 1–36 Right leg and ankle, posterior view with the ankle plantar flexed.

Fig. 1–37 Right leg and foot, posterior view.

longus and lies deep to both muscles. It arises from the upper two thirds of the interosseous membrane, from the posterior surface of the tibia from the soleal line to about two thirds down the shaft, and from a medial line on the posterior upper two thirds of the fibula. Its tendon is crossed by the flexor digitorum tendon and passes in front of it behind the medial malleolus. The tendon passes superficial to the deltoid ligament and inserts into the tubercle of the navicular with a small slip to the sustentaculum tali. (Its other insertions are discussed later.)

Palpation of the muscle in the leg is not possible. To palpate the tendon during function, it is necessary to place the foot on an object higher than the floor and kneel, flexing the knee to more than 100°. With all the digits, including the great toe,

extended, plantar flex with inversion, and the tendon may become palpable. It is easily confused with the soleus.

Intrinsic Muscles of the Foot

Dorsal Muscles

The extensor digitorum brevis and its medial slip, the extensor hallucis brevis, arise from the superolateral surface of the calcaneus. Its tendon passes under the inferior retinaculum and attaches to the tendons of the extensor digitorum longus as they insert into digits two, three, and four. The extensor hallucis brevis inserts into the dorsum of the first phalanx of the great toe (Fig. 1–39).

Plantar Muscles

The muscles of the plantar surface are covered by the plantar aponeurosis, a strong fibrous band extending from the cal-

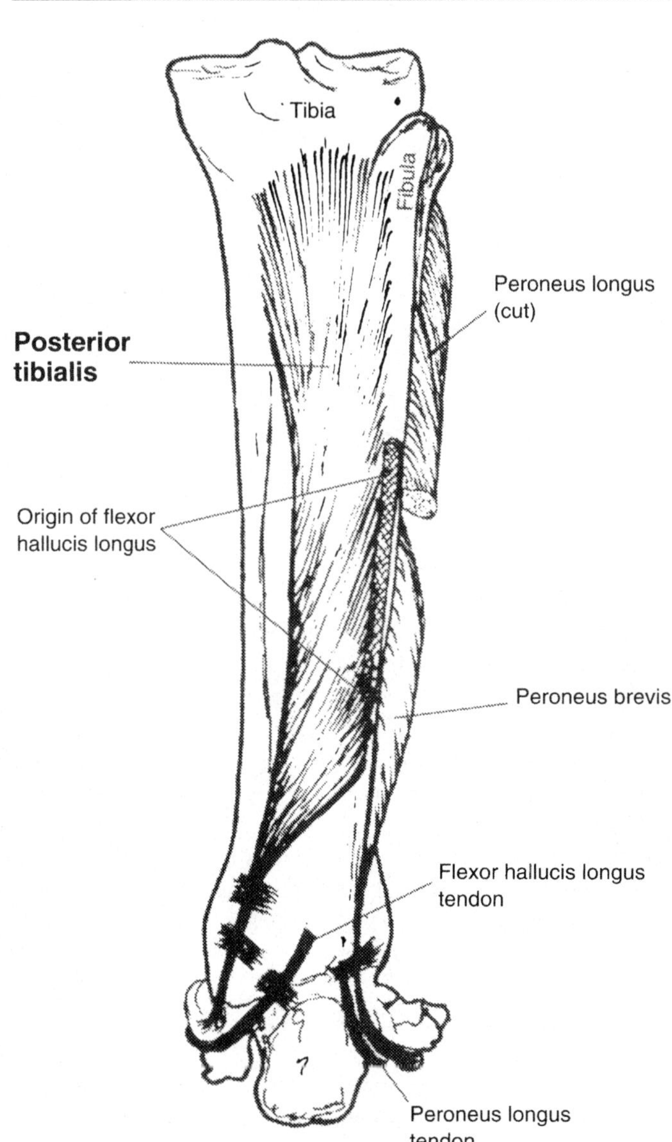

Fig. 1–38 Right leg and ankle, posterior view.

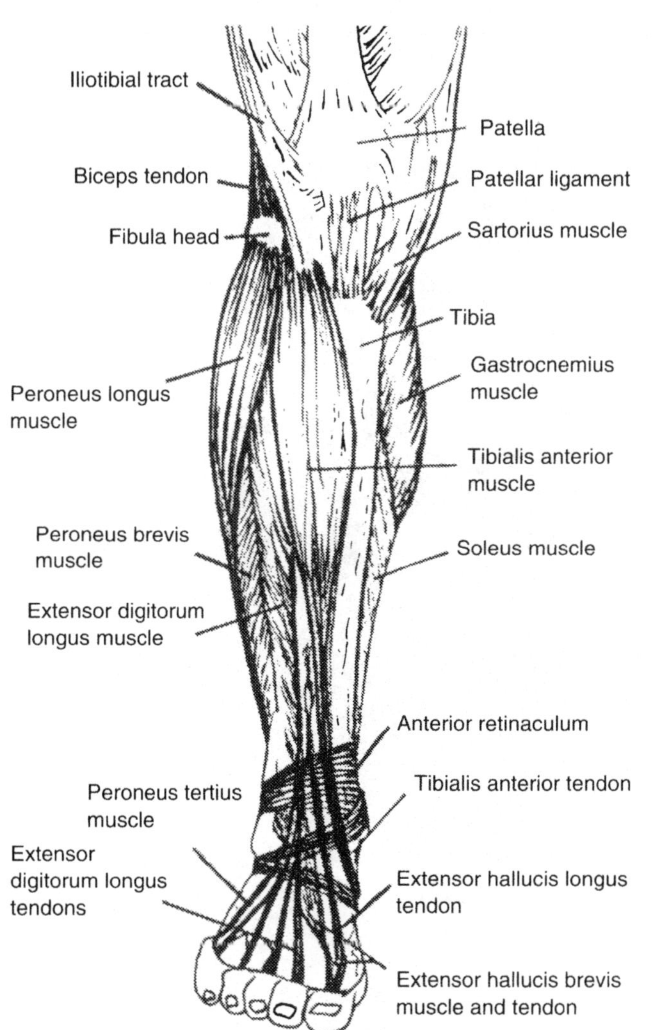

Fig. 1–39 Right leg, anterior view showing muscles and tendons.

caneus to the digits. The aponeurosis has a tensile strength of 7000 lb per square inch with only 9% stretch under a weight of 7860 lb.[3]

The flexor digitorum brevis muscle (Fig. 1–40) arises from the calcaneus and lies immediately under the aponeurosis. Its tendons divide and insert into the intermediate phalanx of the four lesser digits on either side of the flexor digitorum longus tendon.

The abductor digiti minimi muscle (Fig. 1–40) lies along the lateral side of the foot. It arises from the processes of the calcaneal tubercle and the plantar aponeurosis, gliding over a groove on the plantar surface of the fifth metatarsal. It inserts into the lateral side of the base of the first phalanx of the fifth digit.

The abductor hallucis muscle (Figs. 1–40 and 1–41) lies along the medial border of the foot, arising from the plantar aponeurosis and the medial process of the calcaneus. Its tendon inserts into the medial surface of the base of the proximal phalanx of the great toe.

The flexor hallucis brevis muscle (Fig. 1–41) arises from two heads. The lateral head originates on the plantar surface of

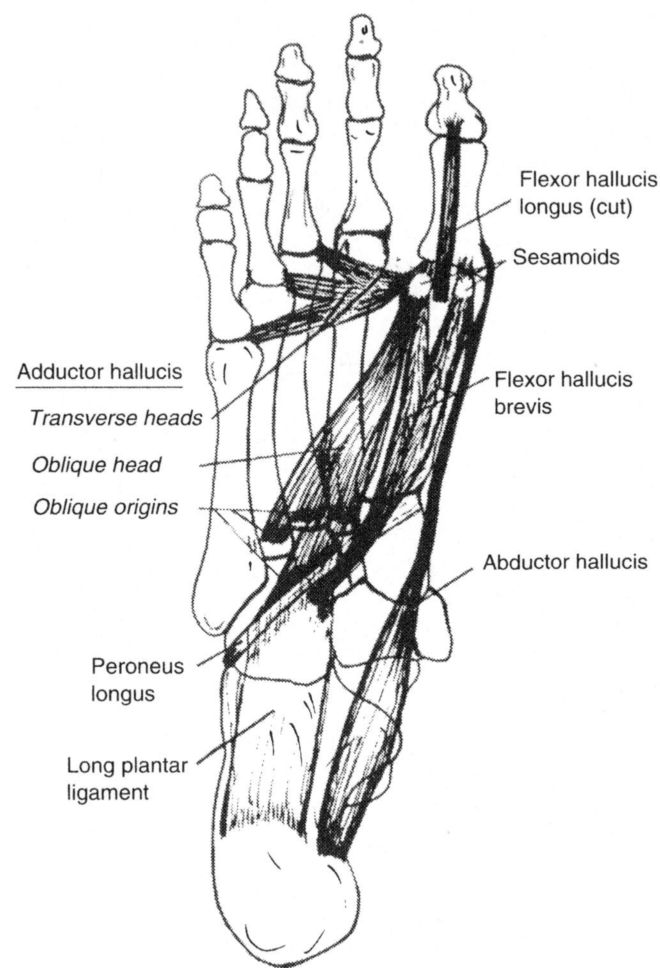

Fig. 1–41 Right foot, deep muscles of the plantar surface.

the third cuneiform. The medial head arises from the plantar surface of the cuboid posterior to the groove for the peroneus longus. The muscle divides and inserts into the medial and lateral sides of the base of the first phalanx of the great toe. A sesamoid bone occurs within each head at the insertion.

The adductor hallucis muscle (Fig. 1–41) originates by oblique and transverse heads. The oblique head arises from the bases of the second, third, and fourth metatarsals and from the tendon sheath of the peroneus longus muscle. The transverse head arises from the metatarsophalangeal ligaments of the third, fourth, and fifth toes. Both heads insert into the lateral side of the base of the first phalanx of the great toe.

Tendons of the Foot

Viewing the tendons from above (Fig. 1–42) shows the position of the tendons as they pass under the superior retinaculum of the ankle. While viewing Figure 1–42, keep in mind that the tibia faces laterally 10° to 15°. The anterior tibialis

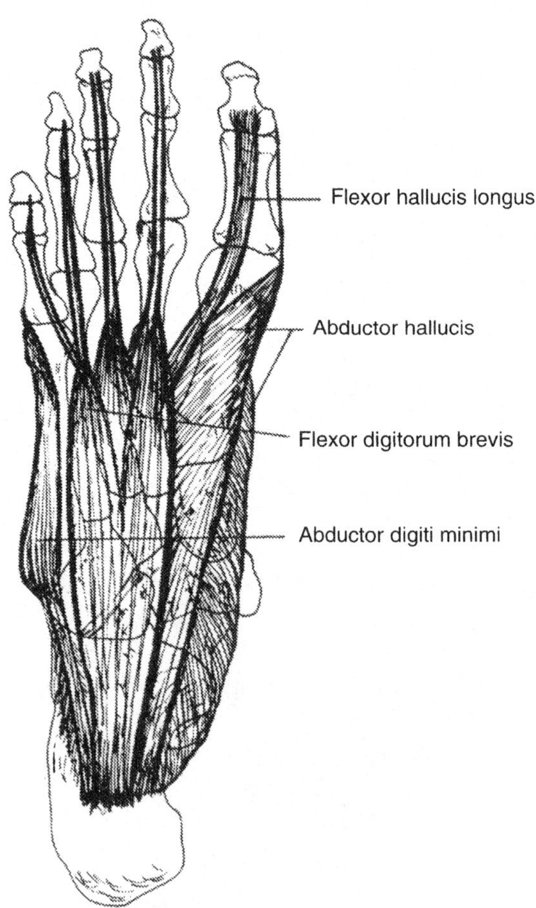

Fig. 1–40 Right foot, muscles of the plantar surface.

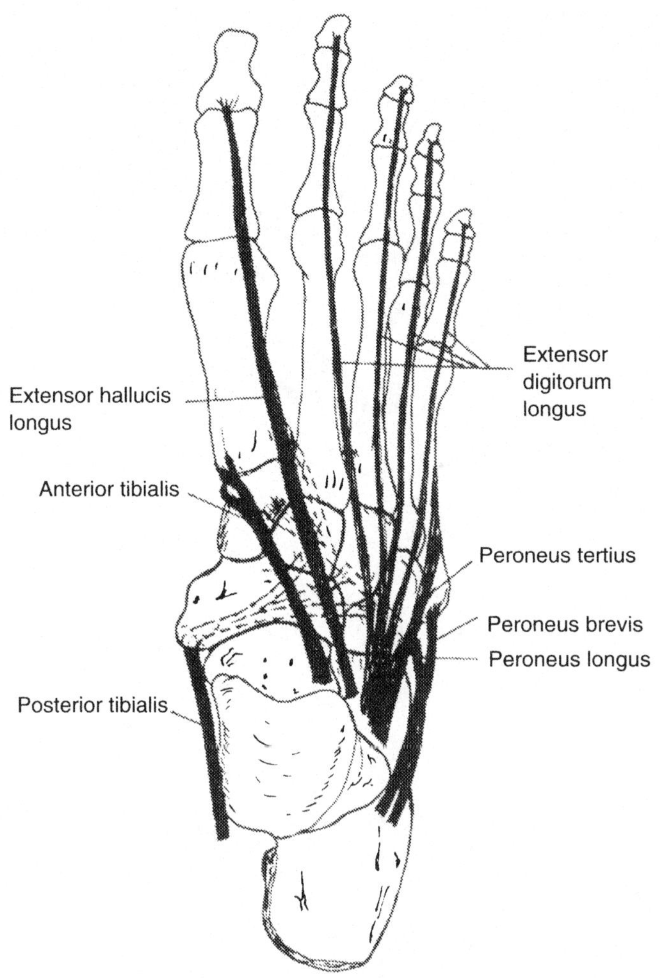

Fig. 1–42 Right foot from above showing tendons.

tendon is palpable and visible about one finger width lateral to the medial malleolus. It is the most prominent tendon visible with inversion and dorsiflexion of the foot. If differentiation is necessary, invert and dorsiflex with the great toe in plantar flexion. The tendon may be palpated to its insertion on the medial side of the first cuneiform and first metatarsal.

The next tendon laterally is the extensor hallucis longus. At the ankle, it becomes prominent by plantar flexing the foot while extending the great toe. It passes next to the anterior tibialis tendon until they pass together under the inferior retinaculum. It then passes over the medial side of the base of the first metatarsal and inserts into the distal phalanx of the great toe.

The tendons of the extensor digitorum longus and peroneus tertius muscles are easily palpated by plantar flexing the foot and great toe while extending the lesser toes. The tendons of the extensor digitorum insert into the distal phalanges of the second through fifth toes. To differentiate the peroneus tertius, maintain the above position and add abduction. The tendon

may be palpated as it inserts into the base and shaft of the fifth metatarsal.

The peroneus longus and brevis tendons (Figs. 1–42 through 1–44) may be palpated as they pass through the groove posterior to the lateral malleolus. They may also be palpated under the peroneal tubercle on the lateral side of the calcaneus. From the tubercle they go their separate ways, with the brevis inserting into the tubercle on the base of the fifth metatarsal. The peroneus longus traverses the calcaneus inferior to the brevis and passes under the cuboid within the peroneal groove, where it is retained by the long plantar ligament. The longus inserts into the lateral side of the bases of the first cuneiform and first metatarsal, directly opposing the anterior tibialis insertion.

Both tendons may be palpated while the foot is fixed and movement toward plantar flexion and eversion is attempted. Place one finger on the fifth metatarsal base and another on the proximal border of the cuboid. To identify the brevis even further, add abduction to the movement.

A medial-plantar view (Fig. 1–45) shows the relative positions and insertions of the peroneal, anterior tibialis, and extensor hallucis longus muscles. This view also shows the relative positions of the three tendons as they pass behind the medial malleolus (Fig. 1–46). The flexor hallucis longus passes under the sustentaculum tali and then crosses the flexor digitorum longus tendon on its way to the distal phalanx of the great toe (Fig. 1–47).

The flexor digitorum longus tendon, within its sheath, passes the posterior surface of the media malleolus between the hallucis longus and posterior tibialis tendons, each in their own sheaths. It then passes over the sustentaculum tali, traversing from medial to lateral, and inserts into the distal phalanges of digits two to five (Fig. 1–47).

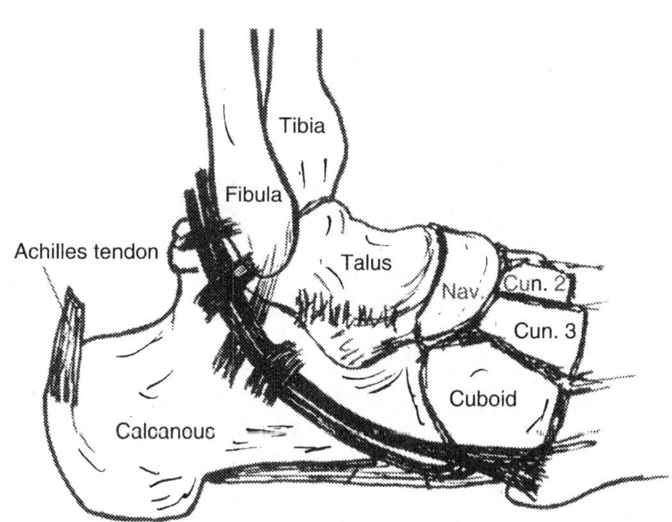

Fig. 1–43 Right foot, lateral view showing the peroneal tendons.

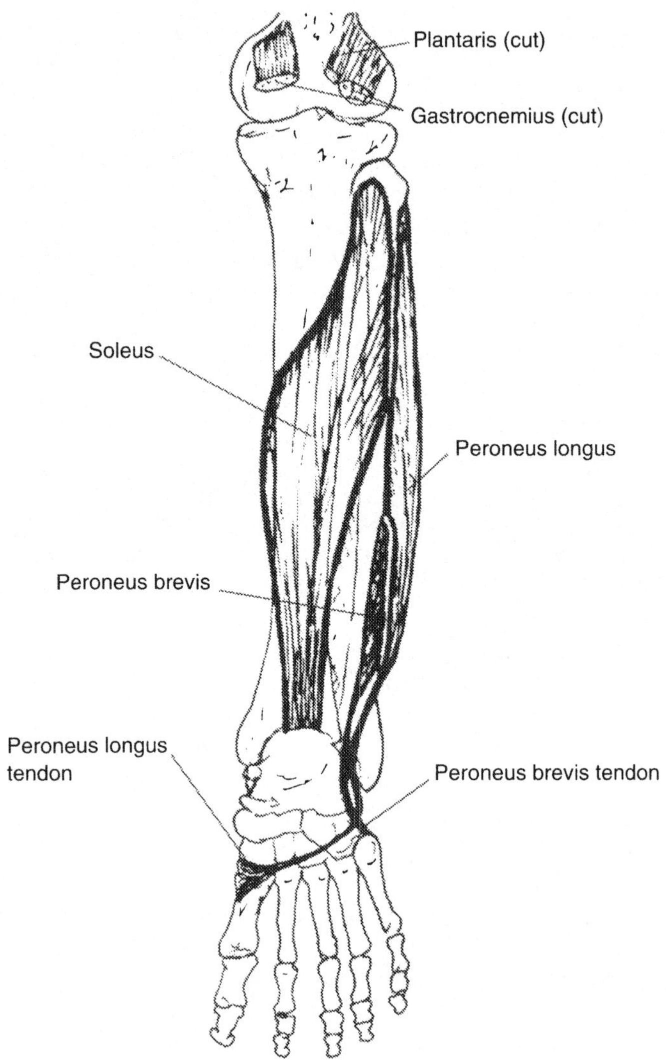

Fig. 1–44 Right leg and foot, posterior view.

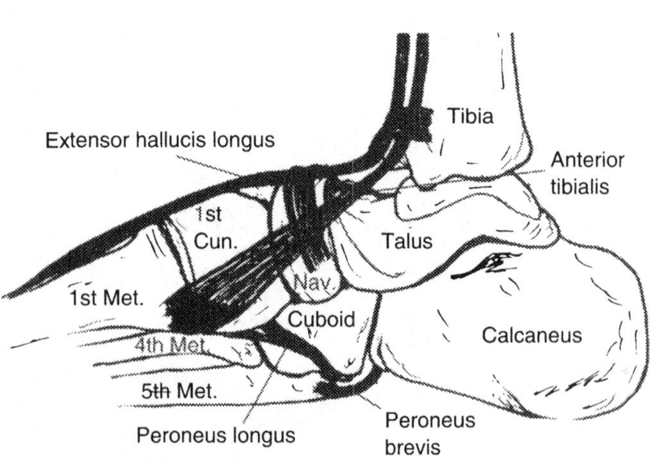

Fig. 1–45 Right ankle and foot, medial-plantar view showing tendons.

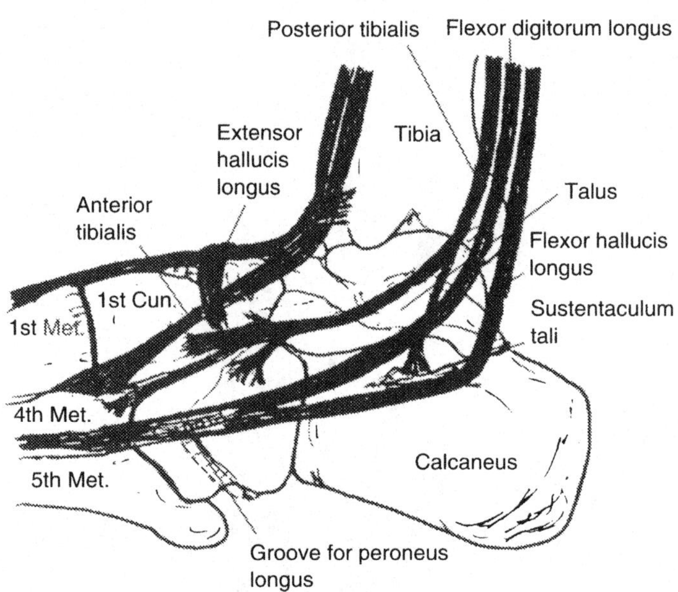

Fig. 1–46 Right ankle and foot, medial-plantar view showing tendons.

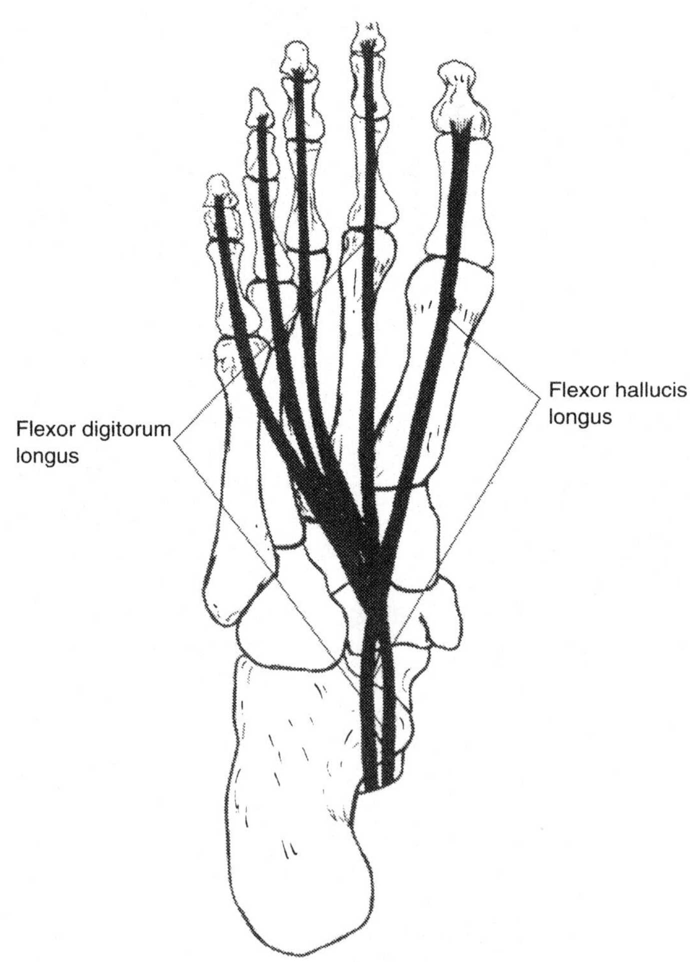

Fig. 1–47 Right foot, plantar view.

The posterior tibialis tendon, in its sheath, is the most anterior of the three as it passes in the groove on the posterior surface of the tibia. The tendon passes next to the trochlea of the
talus, giving off fibers to the sustentaculum tali. The tendon
then divides, and the larger of the two inserts into the tubercle
of the navicular (Fig. 1–48). Some fibers continue to insert
into the first cuneiform. The deeper division continues to insert into the second and third cuneiforms and sometimes the
cuboid. It also gives rise to the origin of the flexor hallucis
brevis muscle (Fig. 1–48). Palpation of the tendon is possible
behind the medial malleolus and along its course to the tubercle of the navicular. Place the heel on a stool, and have the
patient attempt adduction of the foot without plantar flexion or
dorsiflexion.

PULSES OF THE FOOT

The dorsalis pedis artery can be palpated at the ankle medial
to the extensor hallucis longus tendon, lying between it and
the anterior tibialis tendon (Fig. 1–49). The extensor hallucis
longus crosses the artery at the level of the talar head, and the
pulse may be obtained just lateral to it at the talonavicular articulation. Another point to palpate for the pulse is between
the bases of the first and second metatarsals.

The posterior tibial artery can be palpated between the tendons of the flexor digitorum longus tendon and the flexor
hallucis longus tendon (Fig. 1–50). It may also be palpated as
it crosses the tendon of the flexor hallucis longus below the
talonavicular articulation.

FUNCTIONAL ANATOMY

Hiss[3] states that feet are like faces: There are no two alike.
Shoe sizes will vary from the left foot to the right in both
length and width.

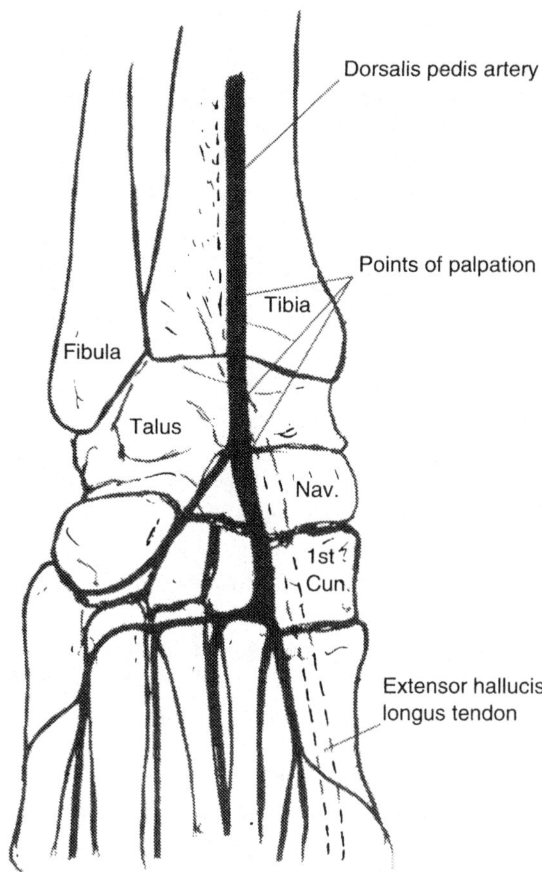

Fig. 1–49 Right foot, anterior view showing dorsalis pedis artery.

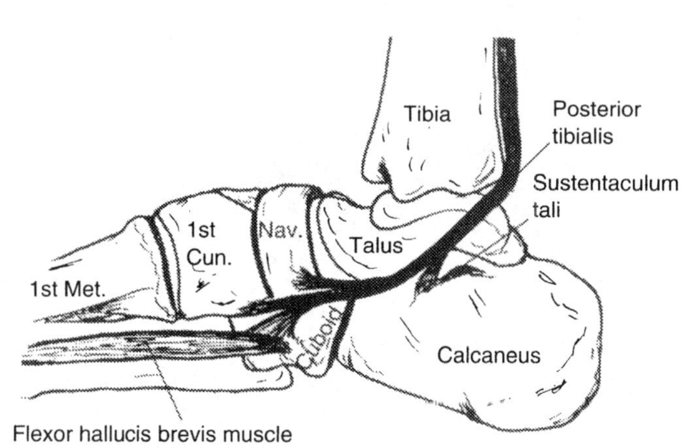

Fig. 1–48 Right ankle and foot, medial-plantar view.

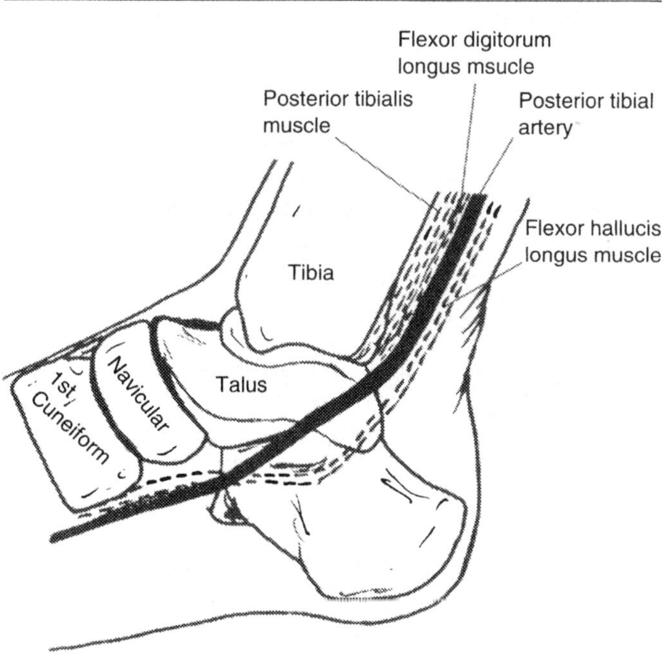

Fig. 1–50 Right foot, medial view showing posterior tibial artery.

The foot develops along with the body, adapting to the various stresses and strains placed upon it. Just looking at the general public for an hour can astound the observer. One sees great variations in body type and size, abnormalities, baffling gaits, and a variety of footwear. The observer can appreciate the abuse the feet undergo, yet many of these people experience no foot symptoms.

Many investigators have attempted to record the movements of the foot through its normal walking cycle. Most investigations (by necessity) include a limited number of normal individuals. Often the normal individuals are students within an academic setting, readily available and willing to participate. A more accurate cross-section could be obtained at Disneyland.

The cross-section that the average practitioner sees might include the obese, 45-year-old woman who has had four children and a hysterectomy and cannot figure out why her feet hurt. It might also include the 42-year-old man who still wears his favorite pair of old tennis shoes, the ones that are full of holes and worn out on the heel and allow the fifth metatarsal to participate in walking while off the sole and on the ground.

The foot must perform all its functions of support, balance, and locomotion. It must also adapt to the terrain yet still provide a rigid level for the muscles to produce the power of movement. For the foot to perform all these functions, it has to have the ability to be flexible and yet rapidly become semi-rigid. This of course requires the mobility of each articulation as well as strength in the ankle and foot.

An understanding of the movements of and stresses on the foot is necessary to help in diagnosing the causes of dysfunction and symptoms. The walking gait cycle is broken down into two phases: the stance phase, from heel strike to toe-off, and the swing phase, the movement after the foot leaves the ground. The stance phase is considered between 60% and 65% of the total gait and may be broken down further into three to five subphases. For the purposes of this text, only the stance phase is discussed and is broken down into three general subphases: heel strike, midstance, and heel rise to toe-off.

Heel Strike to Midstance

Most investigators agree that the pelvis rotates anteriorly and the lower limb rotates internally during the swing phase, leaving the tibia in internal rotation at heel strike. The ankle may be in neutral or slightly flexed. Two investigators consider the ankle plantar flexed,[14,15] and two others find it dorsiflexed[9,16] (Fig. 1–51). Still others state that it is in neutral.

Upon heel strike plantar flexion starts immediately. Heel strike is usually on the lateral side of the posterior calcaneus (Fig. 1–52), as can be noted from the normal wear and tear on the shoes. This is caused by the internal rotation of the tibia and inversion of the heel 2° to 4°. Most of the initial weight is

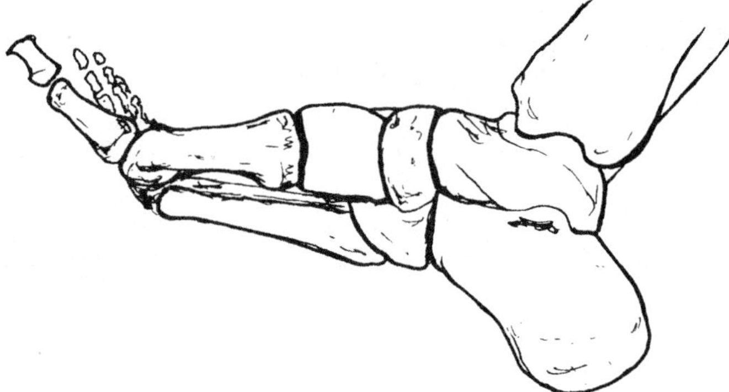

Fig. 1–51 Heel strike.

projected to the large posterior facet over the center of the calcaneus. The middle facet, directly over the sustentaculum tali, is not only distal but also at a higher elevation. This helps propel the force onto the bulk of the calcaneus. As eversion occurs, more weight is absorbed by the middle and anterior facets. Subotnick[17] states that the subtalar joint immediately goes from 2° of inversion to 4° of eversion.

The subtalar joint locks with eversion and unlocks with inversion. At heel strike the subtalar joint is unlocked, which

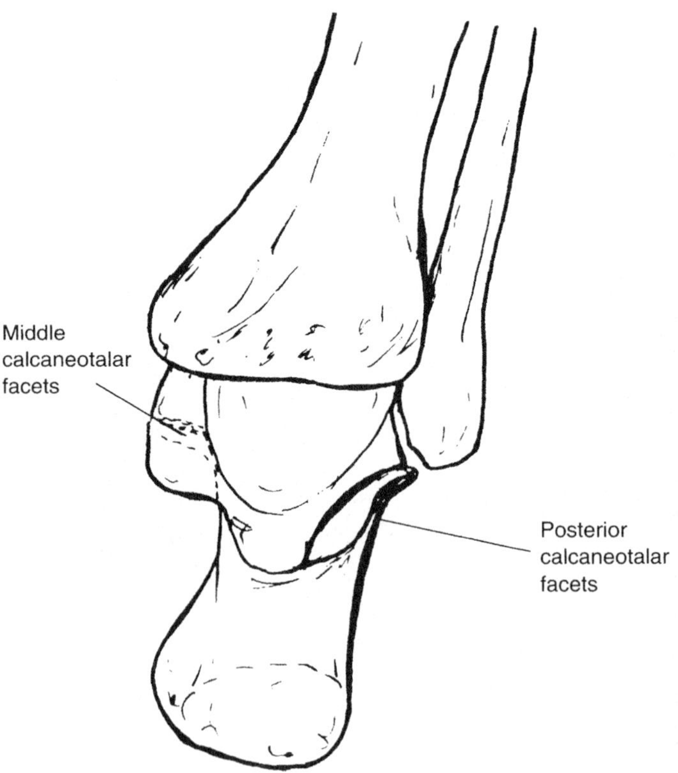

Fig. 1–52 Position of the hindfoot at heel strike.

allows the body weight to dissipate and adjust to the terrain of the ground. Once full contact is made the heel is in eversion, and the subtalar joint is locked.

The midtarsal arch and forefoot are supinated at heel strike. Supination is achieved by contraction of the anterior tibialis on the first metatarsal and first cuneiform and by the posterior tibialis action on the sustentaculum tali of the calcaneus, the cuneiforms, and, with the greatest strength, the tubercle of the navicular. Movement of the first metatarsal is dorsoplantar with some rotation. Movement of the first cuneiform on the navicular is mostly dorsoplantar. The talonavicular articulation allows a greater range of motion and becomes the primary point of movement into the supinated position at heel strike and as pronation begins.

Pronation occurs almost immediately, so that the cuboidonavicular articulation and the rest of the midtarsals assist in dissipating the stress and adapting to the terrain.

At heel strike, the extensor hallucis longus and extensor digitorum longus are either maintaining or producing dorsiflexion. The posterior tibialis is maintaining the midtarsals and, with the anterior tibialis, helps maintain the medial longitudinal arch and supination of the forefoot. The posterior tibialis also helps decelerate pronation of the subtalar joint after heel strike. The peroneal muscles help stabilize the foot.

As the phase progresses, the weight is thrust toward the outside of the foot and forward. As weight bearing begins on the base of the fifth and fourth metatarsals, the medial longitudinal arch is maintained by the anterior tibialis and posterior tibialis with help from the peroneus longus.

Midstance

The midstance, referred to by many as the flatfoot phase, is not really a flatfoot unless the medial longitudinal arch is either normally flat or broken down. As the body weight is thrust forward and laterally into what some refer to as the tripod movement, much of the weight is now distributed to the outside, weight-bearing arch and onto the fourth and fifth metatarsals (Figs. 1–53 and 1–54). The calcaneocuboid articulation, with its strong plantar ligaments, acts as the keystone, and the plantar aponeurosis provides the stability.

With the metatarsals and forefoot in supination, some of the body weight that is transmitted from the talus to the navicular, and hence the cuneiforms, is transmitted further onto the cuboid and the lateral arch. This is due to the configuration of the tarsal arch.

The angle of the cuboid–third cuneiform articulation is 45° at neutral (Fig. 1–55). At heel strike, the angle is much greater. As the weight is projected forward and the forefoot is in supination, much of the body weight is thrust downward through the navicular and cuneiforms onto the cuboid.

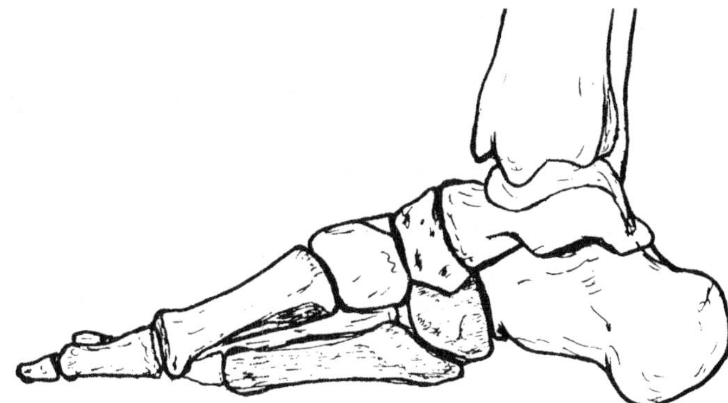

Fig. 1–53 Midstance.

The medial longitudinal arch is maintained by the anterior and posterior tibialis muscles. With most of the weight on the outside, balance is maintained by controlling the movement of the medial longitudinal arch as the forefoot strikes the ground on the fourth and fifth metatarsals and moves medially across the metatarsal heads to the first (Fig. 1–56). As the weight shifts, movement of the medial arch is decelerated by the anterior tibialis muscle. The posterior tibialis muscle assists and, with the peronei muscles, maintains stability. Metatarsal arch movement toward the medial side is produced by propulsion of the body weight forward and contraction of the flexor hallucis and flexor digitorum muscles. It is decelerated by the extensor hallucis longus and extensor digitorum longus muscles.

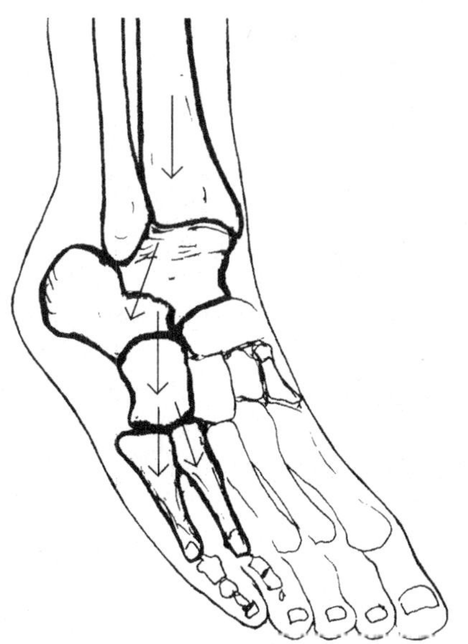

Fig. 1–54 Body weight shift to the lateral longitudinal arch.

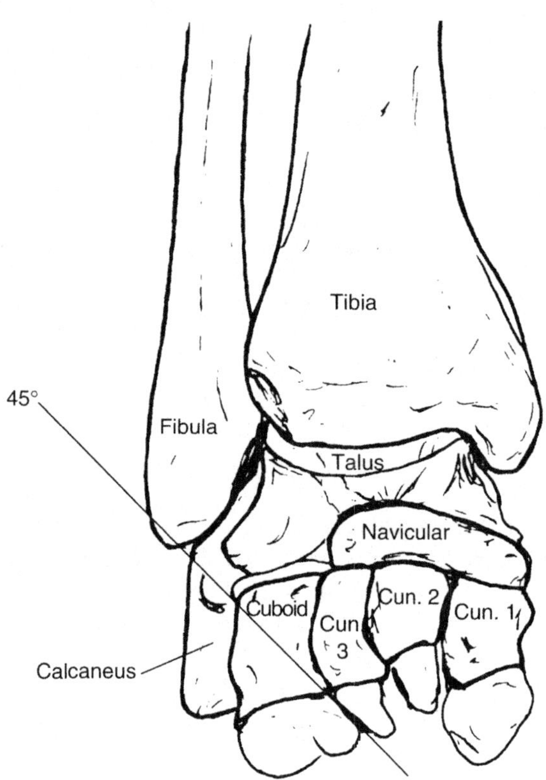

Fig. 1–55 Cross-section of the right foot with the metatarsals removed.

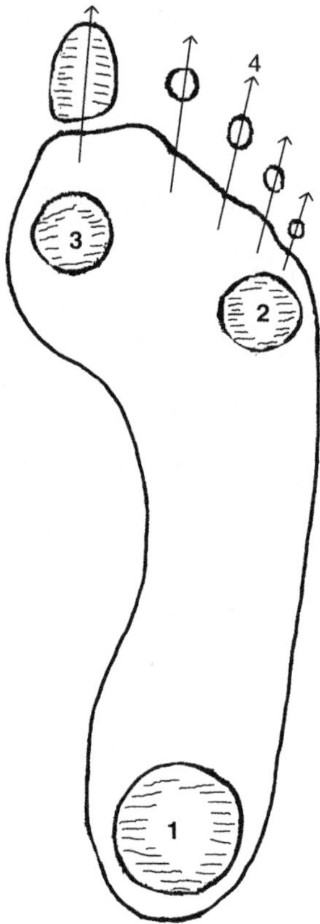

Fig. 1–56 Movement of weight bearing during gait.

Hiss[3] referred to the second phase as balancing. This phase is where balance is maintained by movement of the medial longitudinal arch. This may be demonstrated by simply standing on one foot. This does not allow the normal foot simply to depend on the ligaments for support, even though they are more than capable of doing so. Balance is maintained by the constant adaptation of the medial arch. Any disturbance in the medial arch may interfere with the ability to stand on one foot alone.

To allow the body weight to be placed onto the fifth and fourth metatarsals while the forefoot is in supination, movements of the cuboidometatarsal joints include not only dorsiflexion and plantar flexion but also rotation. The cuboidometatarsal articulations are the pivot points of movement as the weight shifts medially.[3]

The talonavicular articulation, with its greater range of motion, becomes the primary adjusting point for maintaining balance.

Heel Rise to Toe-Off

As the body weight shifts further forward, the medial arch drops inferiorly (with pronation), becoming more stable. At heel rise (Fig. 1–57), as the weight shifts onto the digits, the triceps surae contracts. The tibialis muscles maintain stability. The posterior tibialis inverts the calcaneus, and the anterior tibialis contracts, helping provide controlled movement onto all the digits. The peronei muscles contract, helping maintain stability. The flexor hallucis is stretched and then begins con-

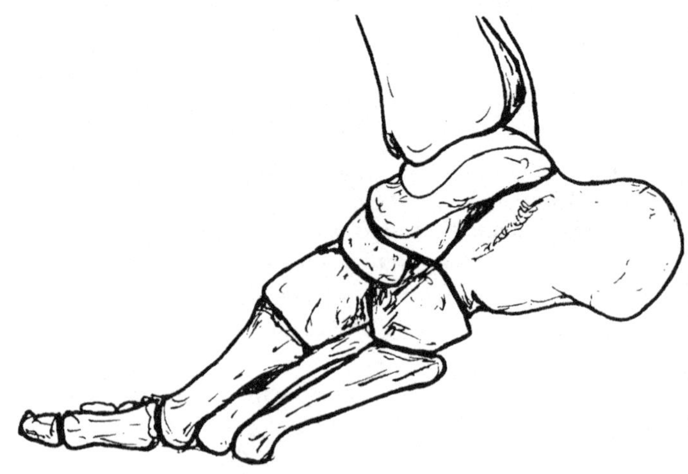

Fig. 1–57 Heel rise.

tracting during extension of the great toe. Its tendon location under the sustentaculum tali and the tibialis posterior with its attachment on the sustentaculum tali produce inversion of the calcaneus immediately after heel-off.

As the heel lifts off the ground, the plantar aponeurosis is stretched tighter and, with the other ligaments, forms a rigid lever to assist the musculature in propelling the body weight forward (Fig. 1–58). As the weight is thrust forward, the metatarsals become flat on the ground and splayed at first. Then most of the weight is placed on the first three with little or no function of the fifth digit at lift off. At this point the triceps surae is contracting as the major player in propulsion. With the digits extended, further power is added by the flexor digitorum longus, the flexor hallucis longus, the peronei muscles, and all the plantar intrinsic muscles. They provide not only the power for toe-off but stabilization as well.

Swing Phase

The swinging limb provides the motion of gait, and the stance phase of the opposite limb provides the stability.

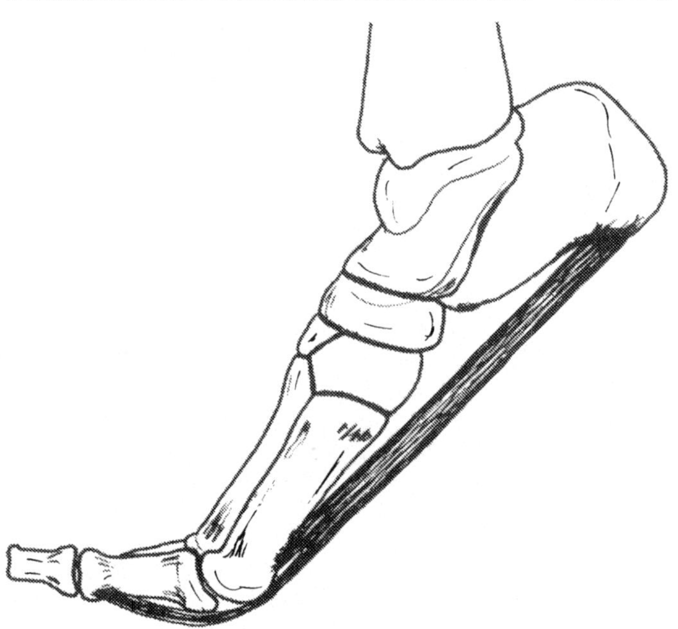

Fig. 1–58 Stretching of the plantar aponeurosis.

Shifting of the body weight changes at heel contact and at heel-off. The pelvis is forward, and the limb is in internal rotation at heel contact. At lift-off, the limb is in external rotation.

Conditions that produce a laterally rotated limb (anatomic short leg, fixation, etc) cause a toeing-out gait. This produces a greater pressure on the medial longitudinal arch. The reverse is true with a pronated foot: The femur will rotate internally, affecting the entire posture.

Summary

Gait is a coordinated effort involving most of the body. Fixations, instabilities, and other dysfunctions produce alterations in the young, developing foot and, in the adult, dysfunction.

THE FOOT DURING RUNNING

Running greatly alters function, depending upon the type of running gait (eg, the heel striker, forefront striker, or midfoot striker). Foot function is further altered by the type and function of the body the foot is carrying. Jahss[16] reports many studies that show that increased rates of ambulation cause progressively less plantar flexion after heel contact. During jogging at a rate of 5 min/mile, there is no plantar flexion after heel contact; rather, the foot progresses immediately into dorsiflexion.[16] In running the calcaneus is typically in 4.9° of supination at heel contact with maximum pronation of 11.7°.[16]

CONCLUSION

It is necessary to have an understanding of the normal range of motion, with and without weight bearing, to determine the presence of dysfunction. It is also necessary to have the ability to motion palpate each articulation of the ankle and foot to find the cause of, or the result of, dysfunction.

The examiner must keep in mind that restricted mobility (fixation) of any articulation of the ankle and foot may produce major symptoms not only in the foot but elsewhere in the body. A fixation in the foot may be symptom free yet be the cause of back problems. One must also keep in mind that fixations of the foot may be caused by dysfunction elsewhere, causing persistent symptoms in the foot but no symptoms at the causal site.

REFERENCES

1. Shands AR, Raney RB. *Handbook of Orthopedic Surgery.* St Louis, Mo: Mosby; 1967.

2. Mennell J. *Foot Pain.* Boston, Mass: Little, Brown; 1969.

3. Hiss J. *Functional Food Disorders.* New York, NY: Oxford University Press; 1949.

4. Schultz A. The feet. *Digest of Chirop Econ.* January/February 1970; 12 (4):12–14.

5. D'Ambrosia R. *Musculoskeletal Disorders.* Philadelphia, Pa: Lippincott; 1986.

6. Calliet R. *Foot and Ankle Pain.* Philadelphia, Pa: Davis; 1968.

7. Scholl W. *The Human Foot.* Chicago, Ill: Foot Specialist; 1920.

8. Netter FH. *Atlas of Human Anatomy.* Summit, NJ: CIBA-GEIGY Corp.; 1989.

9. Kapandji IA. *The Physiology of the Joints.* New York, NY: Churchill Livingstone; 1970;2.

10. *Dorland's Illustrated Medical Dictionary* (24th ed). Philadelphia, Pa: Saunders; 1957.

11. Warwick R, Williams P. *Gray's Anatomy* (35th Br ed). Philadelphia, Pa: Saunders; 1973.

12. Kessler R, Hertling D. *Management of Common Musculoskeletal Disorders.* New York, NY: Harper & Row; 1983.

13. Michaud T. Pedal biomechanics as related to orthotic therapies. *Digest Chirop Econ.* November/December 1986;29:12–14.

14. Greenawalt M. *The Foot, Gait and Chiropractic* (research bulletin 699). Roanoke, Va: Foot Levelers, Inc.; 1990.

15. Czerniecki J. Foot and ankle biomechanics in walking and running. *Am J Phys Med Rehabil.* 1988;67:246–252.

16. Jahss M. *Disorders of the Foot.* Philadelphia, Pa: Saunders; 1982.

17. Subotnick S. Biomechanics of the subtalar and midtarsal joints. *J Am Podiatr Assoc.* August 1975;65:756–764.

Chapter 2

Examination

Examination should begin with observation of the patient's gait, if possible, as he or she enters the examination room and sits down.

HISTORY

Solicit a complete history of the symptoms, their onset, and, if an injury, the exact circumstances involved. Whether or not the symptoms are associated with an injury, previous problems with the ankle and foot and all other biomechanical problems in the past must be considered. The correlation of examination findings with the history is important in arriving at a proper treatment program.

Occupations that involve unusual use of the ankle and foot must be considered, including cement masonry, carpet laying, or those requiring the use of ladders. Recreational activities may be involved, such as skiing, playing catcher on a baseball team, or running.

A complete history includes detailed information concerning the onset of symptoms. One's line of questioning should lead to a clear picture of the patient's complaint and its origin. Was the onset gradual or sudden? When did the symptoms first appear? When did the symptoms increase sufficiently for the patient to seek help? Was there a change in activity before the onset of symptoms? Were other symptoms present before the onset of these symptoms? If it was an injury, exactly how did it occur? Was there immediate disability? Was there immediate pain? Was there swelling? When did it appear?

OBSERVATION

Not only should the observation begin when the patient walks into the examination room and sits down, it should continue during and after the history taking. Note any abnormal posture or movement not only of the foot but of other parts of the body as well.

For the purpose of this text, the examination procedures are based on the ambulatory patient. Examination of the nonambulatory patient would, of course, begin immediately in a non–weight-bearing position.

STANDING EXAMINATION

In my examination of every ambulatory patient, I begin with the patient standing comfortably. Whether the patient's complaints are related to the spine, the upper extremity, or the feet, I begin my examination with the patient standing. Simply looking at the feet without examining the entire body is an error made by many physicians. The following procedure can reveal significant information.

With the patient gowned or undressed sufficiently to observe the entire body, begin the examination in the erect posture. Instruct the patient to stand with his or her feet even but not touching, making sure the knees do not touch. (Some obese patients with extreme valgus knees or patients with overdeveloped thigh muscles may find it necessary to stand with the feet wider apart.) With this instruction, the patient will usually assume the foot placement that habit patterns allow. Any unilateral rotation of the foot should be noted as a part of the patient's habit pattern. If unilateral rotation is found, have the patient correct the stance with each foot within the normal 5° to 10° of lateral rotation.

Toeing Out

Toeing out (Fig. 2–1) is common with anatomic short leg, hip problems (including lateral rotation from prone sleeping), and other postural faults. Patients who automatically stand toeing out may resist placing the feet in the correct position. Whether this is a result of or the cause of other postural faults has yet to be determined. The patient usually feels uncomfortable when instructed to place the feet correctly. This would indicate that the patient's body has compensated for the abnormality and automatically assumes the position best suited to respond to the command to stand erect. Correction of the foot placement reveals the true distortion pattern, if one exists. Continuing the examination without correcting the foot placement would be a mistake. This also applies to positioning for standing radiographs. By insisting upon the correct position,

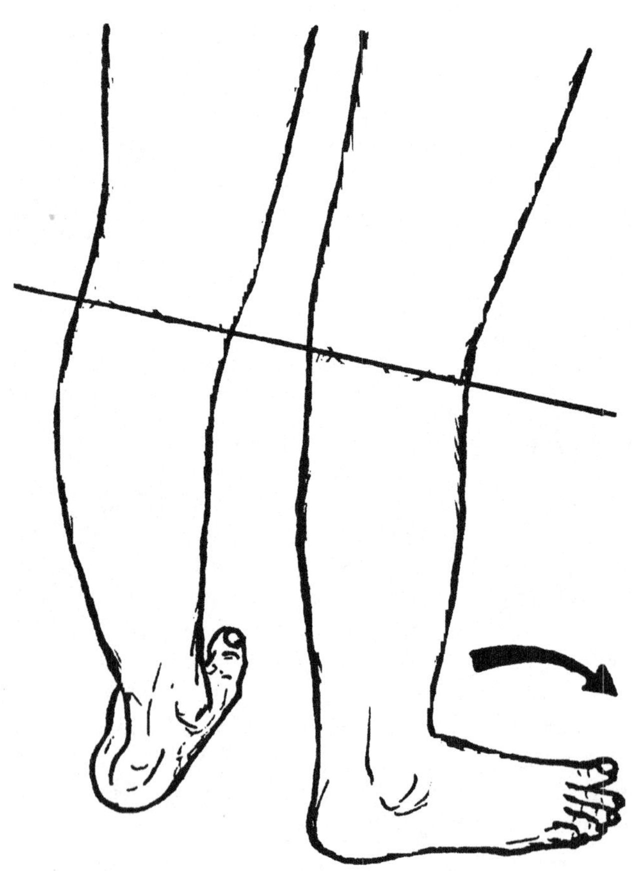

Fig. 2–1 Right foot toed out.

the observer has the opportunity to see the true distortions from the feet up.

On radiographs of the standing lumbosacral spine, the alteration of the lesser and greater trochanter–to–femoral head distance will give a clue to correct foot placement. If the femur is laterally rotated, the lesser trochanter will appear more prominent as it is moved from its posteromedial position compared with the opposite side.

If possible, the patient should maintain the erect posture for at least 1 full minute. It takes approximately 1 minute for the postural muscles to allow the normal posture to be assumed. During the interval any movement of the body to adapt to the position should be noted.

Asking about a patient's sleeping posture is vital to diagnose biomechanical problems. It is one that is frequently overlooked. Some people sleep on their side, some sleep on their back, and some move around all night with little or no problem. Patients who sleep prone, however, can have unique problems. As a result of remaining in position for 5 to 8 hours or more, muscle strain and imbalance are produced. This will either cause or contribute to symptoms in many areas of the body, including the foot. In the prone position the head is turned to one side, stretching one group of cervical muscles while allowing the opposite group to contract, the origin being held closer to the insertion. By the patient's remaining in this position for several hours, problems must be expected. If the head is turned to the right, the right femur must rotate laterally with the foot out to the right and the knee flexed. The left foot rotates medially. To remain in this position, the entire pelvis must rotate anteriorly, increasing the lumbar curve.

The prone sleeper will display a functional long leg on the right when examined in the supine position. The same patient will usually walk with the right foot toed out. Every step places abnormal stress on the medial longitudinal arch, and upon lift-off all the weight is on the great toe.

POSTERIOR EXAMINATION

With the patient maintaining the proper stance, begin observing the posterior aspect, starting with the feet. The feet are the base of the structure and as such are the first area to examine, even if the symptoms are in a remote location. During the examination, patients will have a tendency to turn around to answer a question and must be reminded to remain looking straight ahead. Postural faults, such as a tilted head, high shoulder, or spinal distortions, may be either contributing to or caused by a lower extremity problem.

Ask the patient to relate where he or she feels the body weight on the feet as the posture is maintained. In the normal body with a normal foot, the patient should not be able to relate any specific area where the weight is felt. If the weight is felt specifically on an area, such as "under my big toe," it usually indicates a fixation or other disturbance in the foot itself.

Postural distortions produce abnormal pressure on the foot. One example is weight felt forward on both feet, which may indicate bilaterally weak gluteus maximus muscles or bilaterally hypertonic psoas muscles pulling the body weight forward. Wearing a bra may alter the posture sufficiently to produce weight forward on the feet. Another example, weight being felt on the inside of both feet, may indicate bilateral pronation due to obesity and the inability to walk straight.

Hindfoot Pronation

Observe the Achilles tendon for abnormal curvature. If the hindfoot is pronated, the Achilles tendon will usually curve with the apex medial (Fig. 2–2). The normal hindfoot position during weight bearing is neutral with a relatively straight Achilles tendon. A curved tendon may indicate hindfoot pronation alone or in combination with forefoot pronation and must be identified.

Palpation of the Medial Arch

Whether or not the Achilles tendon is straight, compare with the asymptomatic side. Place the fingers under the medial arch of each foot to check for a dropping of the medial arch (Fig. 2–3). If unilateral and on the symptomatic side, the loss of height should be identified (the navicular, first cuneiform, or first metatarsal) and compared with the non–weight-bearing side.

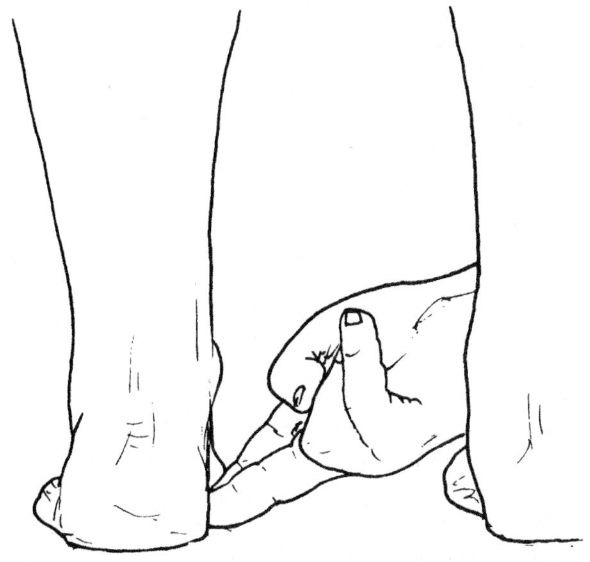

Fig. 2–3 Palpation of the medial arch while standing.

Heel Inversion with Elevation

Have the patient rise up on the toes while keeping the knees extended (Fig. 2–4). Upon rising the calcaneus should immediately invert, as demonstrated by the left foot in Figure 2–4. Failure to do so indicates possible rupture or severe strain of the posterior tibialis muscle. The posterior tibialis muscle assists in plantar flexion, and its major attachment is to the tubercle of the navicular with an insertion on the sustentaculum tali of the calcaneus. If functioning normally, its action immediately inverts the heel.

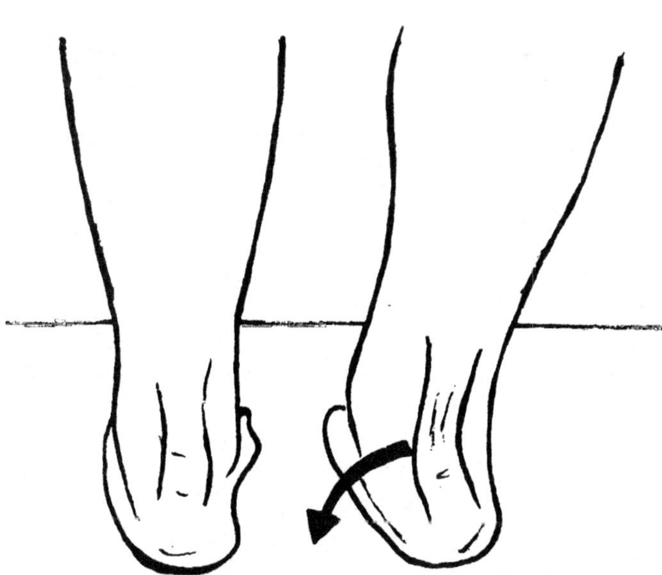

Fig. 2–2 Hindfoot pronation with curved Achilles tendon.

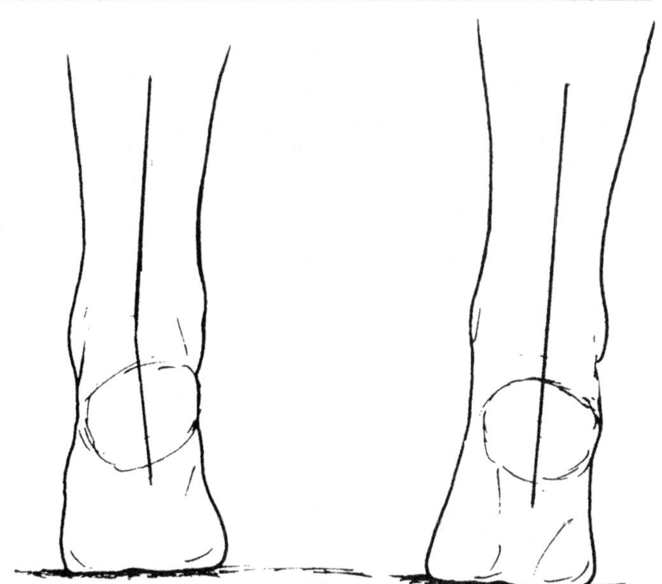

Fig. 2–4 Lack of inversion of the right foot on elevation of the hindfoot.

Comparison of Knee Fold Height

Compare the knee fold height (Fig. 2–5). A low knee fold may indicate a short tibia and an anatomic short leg, which will affect foot function.

Comparison of Flexion-Extension of the Knees

Compare the flexion-extension posture of the knees, looking for hyperextension or flexion in one or both knees (Fig. 2–6). Unilateral flexion may indicate an anatomically long leg. To level the pelvis, it is necessary to flex the knee. This could indicate the inability to bear weight without pain. If so, cease the examination in the erect posture. Noting distortions produced by pain is a waste of time. Unilateral flexion could also be the result of a knee problem that needs to be evaluated and corrected first. Unilateral hyperextension of the knee may indicate damaged ligaments, a pelvic distortion, or possibly gallbladder dysfunction[1] (See Appendix A).

ANTERIOR EXAMINATION

Valgus Knee

A valgus condition of the knees (knock knees) places great strain on the medial arch of the feet. If unilateral (Fig. 2–7), it

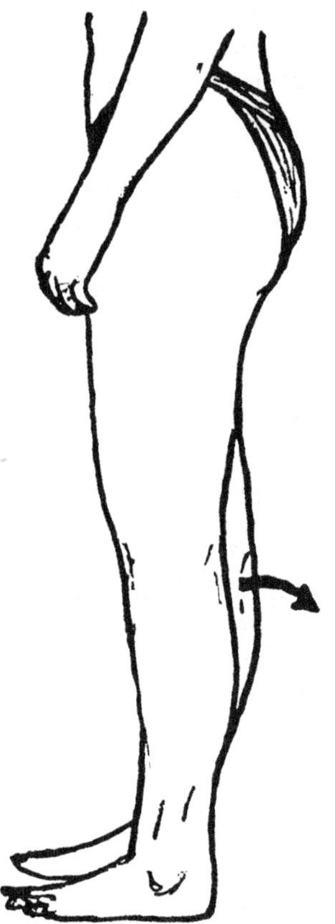

Fig. 2–6 Hyperextended right knee.

usually is accompanied by a laterally rotated tibia, which places even greater stress on the medial arch and interferes with normal mechanics of the foot. This is a common condition seen more often in women than in men. It is often associated with postural distortions after childbirth when the proper exercises were not included in prenatal care or the wrong exercises were instituted after delivery.[1]

Hallux Valgus

Another common distortion is hallux valgus (Fig. 2–8), usually associated with pronation. The great toe is pulled toward, and sometimes onto, the second digit with what appears as an enlargement of first metatarsophalangeal articulation. Have the patient take a few normal steps and report any discomfort. Determine its location and the part or parts of the step in which it was felt. If no discomfort is felt, have the patient repeat with longer strides and at a faster pace. An understanding of normal functional anatomy during gait is necessary to diagnose the patient's problem.

Observe the feet for any obvious stress. Look for disturbances in the forefoot–hindfoot relationship compared with the asymptomatic foot and the findings posteriorly.

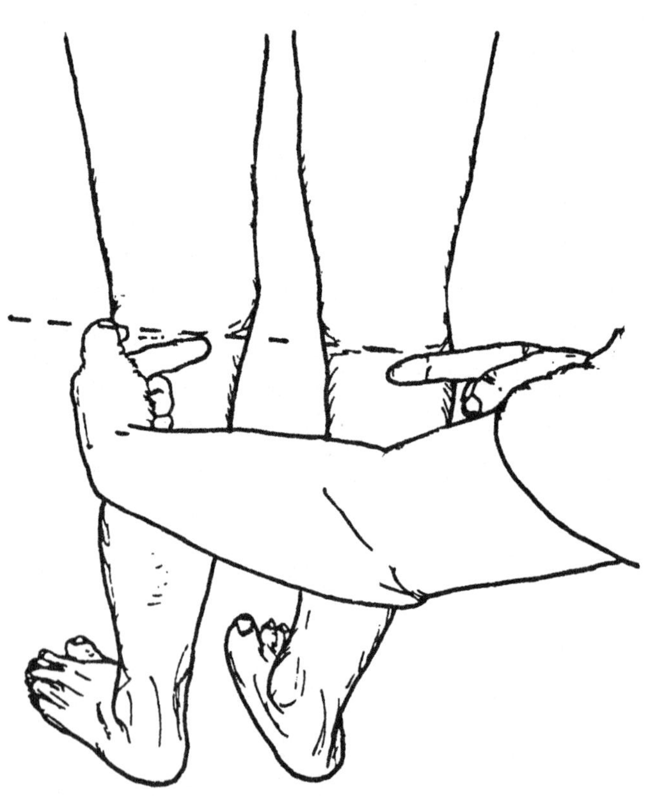

Fig. 2–5 Comparison of knee fold height.

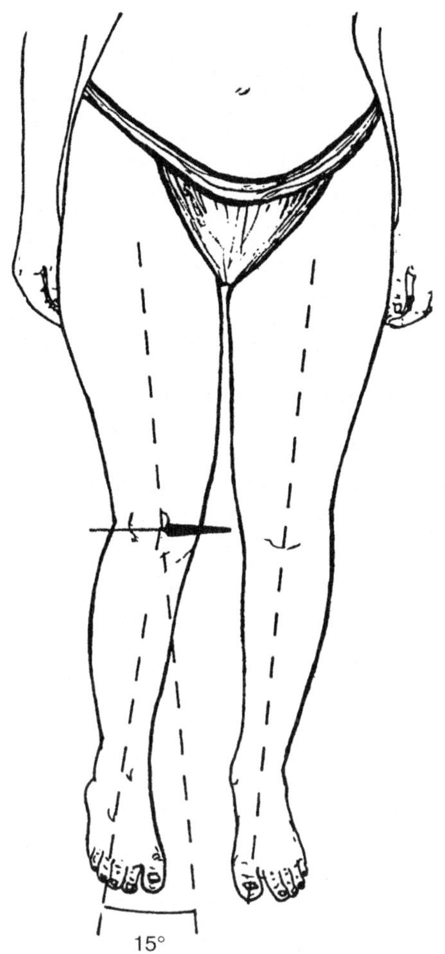

Fig. 2–7 Valgus right knee.

If the Achilles tendon appears normal yet the forefoot appears pronated (Fig. 2–9), it may indicate a weakness of the anterior tibialis muscle (inserting into the first cuneiform and first metatarsal). A normal, strong posterior tibialis muscle (inserting into the sustentaculum tali of the calcaneus and the tubercle of the navicular) maintains the calcaneal position. Obvious gripping of the toes and whiteness are signs of a disturbance in weight bearing.

FUNCTIONAL EXAMINATION

Talonavicular Articulation

Use the index and middle fingers to palpate the talonavicular articulation (Fig. 2–10). It is just anterior and about two finger widths inferior to the medial malleolus. The medial side of the talar head is palpated as a rather sharp ridge, and the navicular tubercle, just anterior, is prominent. To help in locating the articulation, restrain the calcaneus and ask the patient to adduct the foot. The navicular becomes immediately prominent. (This also helps in palpation of the posterior tibialis tendon as it attaches to the navicular tubercle.)

While palpating the articulation, have the patient remove the body weight (Fig. 2–11). The talar head and navicular should retract laterally as the calcaneus is lifted from the floor. As weight is reapplied (Fig. 2–12), the talar head and navicular should move medially. The navicular should move slightly farther with some inferior movement (rotation). The application of weight causes a shifting of the talus with greater stress over the sustentaculum tali. Its medial movement is limited by the calcaneonavicular ligament.

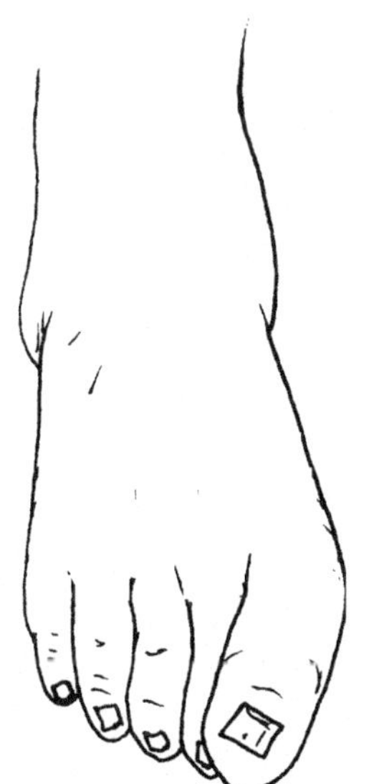

Fig. 2–8 Hallux valgus (bunion).

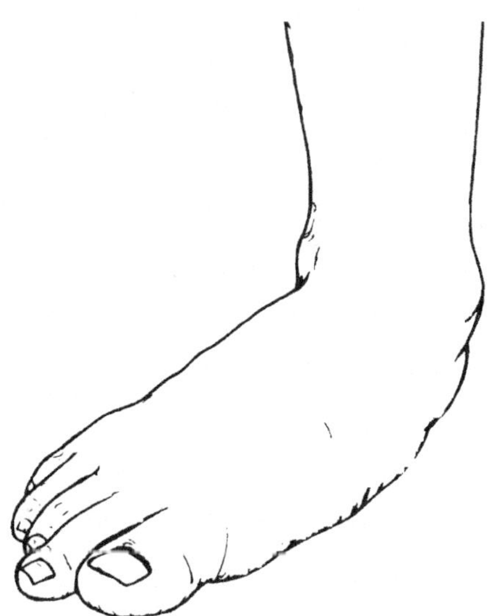

Fig. 2–9 Extreme pronation of the right foot.

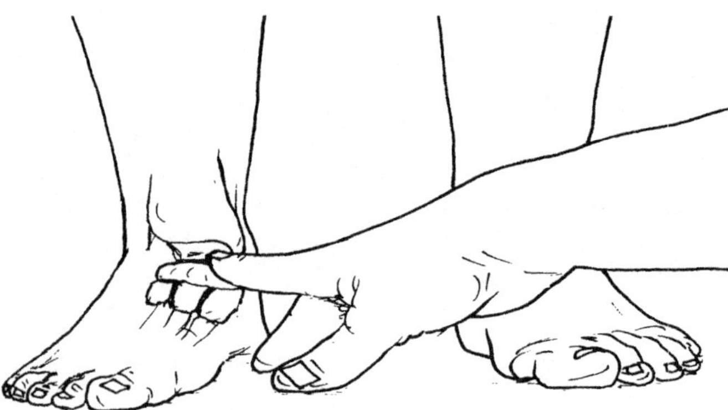

Fig. 2–10 Palpation of the talonavicular articulation.

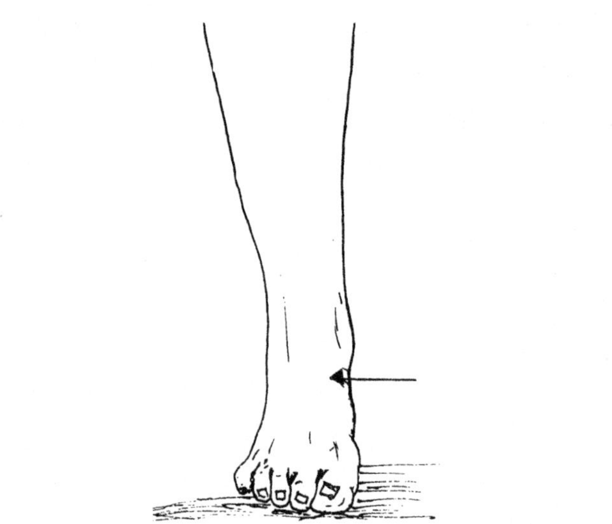

Fig. 2–11 Talonavicular articulation, right foot, non–weight-bearing.

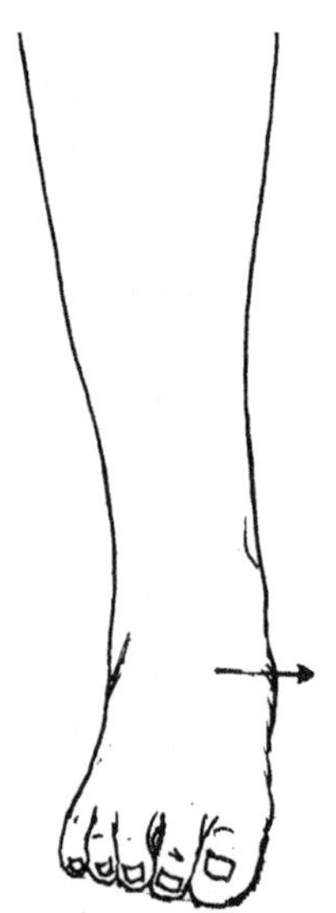

Fig. 2–12 Talonavicular articulation, right foot, weight-bearing.

Toe-Heel Walk

Have the patient toe-walk to evaluate the S-1 nerve root (Fig. 2–13). Observe not only the attempt to toe-walk but the patient's posture as well. Often, a telltale sign of malfunction will be observed if a patient moves irregularly in attempting to perform a task. Ask whether pain is present during the attempt. Many patients will not report pain unless asked. If pain is present, have the patient relate exactly where the pain is.

Have the patient heel-walk (Fig. 2–14) to eliminate L-4 and L-5 nerve root problems. Note the attempt to walk, paying particular attention to body posture during the attempt. If the ankle is truly dorsiflexed, the body posture should be relatively normal.

With restricted ability to dorsiflex the ankle, the patient must lean forward at the hips and project the buttocks posterior to walk only on the heels (Fig. 2–15). Performance with this posture indicates the inability to dorsiflex the ankle as a result of shortened triceps surae muscles, a problem with the dorsiflexor muscles, or a problem of innervation. Ask the patient whether any pain is present and, if so, to point out the exact location.

Balancing on One Foot

Have the patient stand and balance on the asymptomatic foot and then on the symptomatic one. Standing on one foot tests the ability of the foot and its muscles to adapt while maintaining balance (if there are no vestibular disturbances). Note the constant rotation of the medial arch to maintain balance. Fixations, weakness, or other disturbances may affect the ability of the foot to adapt and therefore will make it difficult to remain standing on one foot (Fig. 2–16).

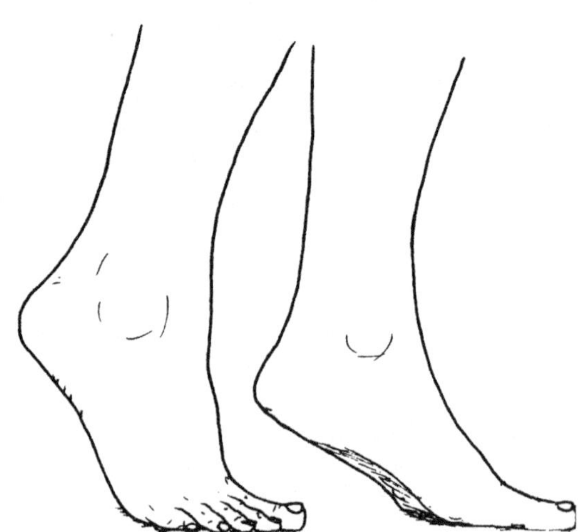

Fig. 2–13 Toe walk.

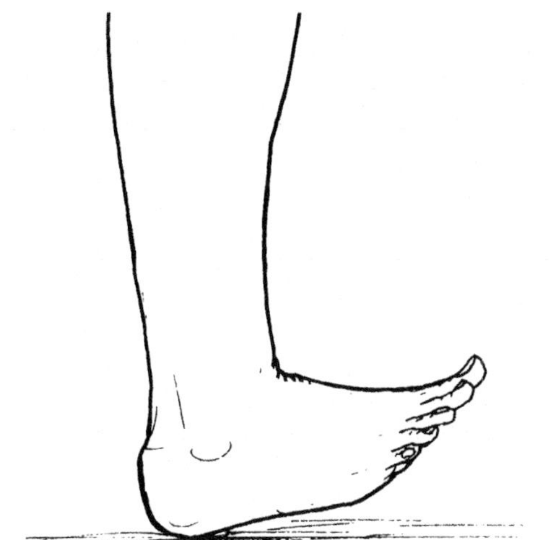

Fig. 2–14 Heel walk.

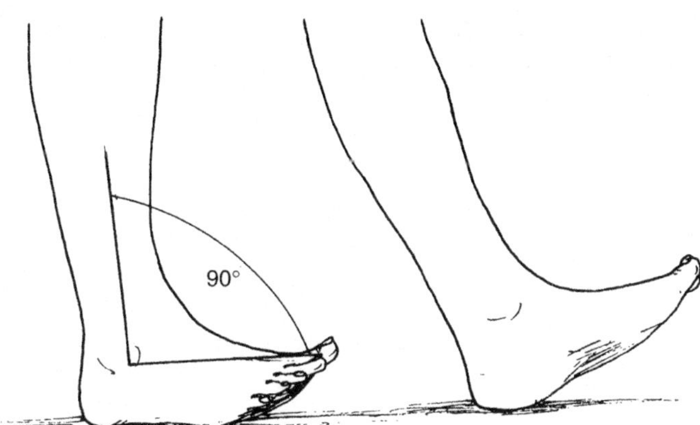

Fig. 2–15 Heel walk with restricted dorsiflexion.

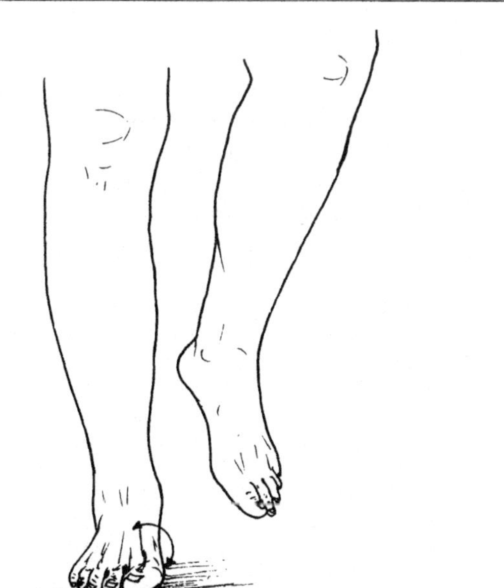

Fig. 2–16 Medial arch adaptation while balancing on one foot.

SUPINE EXAMINATION

Observe and palpate both feet at the same time, comparing the general appearance, condition of the toenails, texture of the skin, and skin temperature. Also look for the presence of a callus, corns, plantar warts, and fungal infection (athlete's foot). The presence of edema in both extremities indicates the possibility of a systemic problem; if edema is present only on the symptomatic side, a more localized problem would be expected.

Vascular diseases are a common cause of problems of the feet. Palpation of the posterior tibial artery is possible (Figs. 2–17 and 2–18) behind the medial malleolus between the tendons of the flexor digitorum longus and flexor hallucis longus muscles. It may also be palpated as it crosses the tendon of the flexor hallucis longus below the talonavicular articulation.

The dorsalis pedis artery (Fig. 2–19) may be palpated at the ankle medial to the extensor hallucis longus tendon, lying between it and the anterior tibialis tendon. The pulse may also be obtained just lateral to the tendon of the extensor hallucis longus after it crosses the artery at the talonavicular articulation. Another point to palpate for the pulse is between the bases of the first and second metatarsals.

It cannot be emphasized too much that palpation as well as observation of both feet is important. It helps greatly to run the hands over both ankles and feet simultaneously, comparing flexibility, sensitivity to palpation, temperature, and any differences in structure. Palpation should include each of the muscles pertaining to the foot simultaneously. Any contrac-

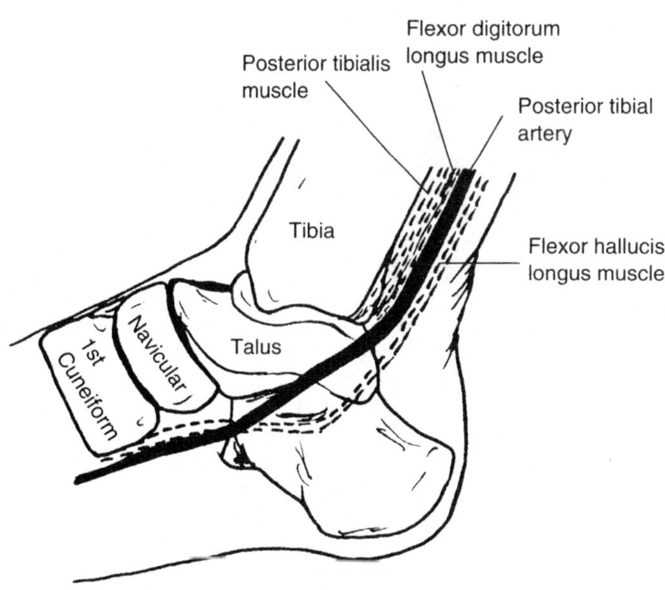

Fig. 2–17 Right foot, medial view showing location of posterior tibial artery.

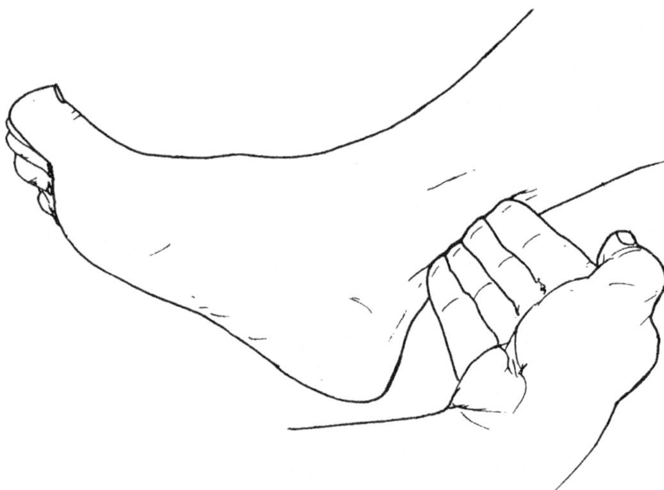

Fig. 2–18 Palpation of the posterior tibialis artery, right ankle.

tions, nodules, laxity, edema, and reported sensitivity should be noted.

Observe both feet for their resting position on the table. If one foot is laterally rotated (Fig. 2–20), it may indicate that the

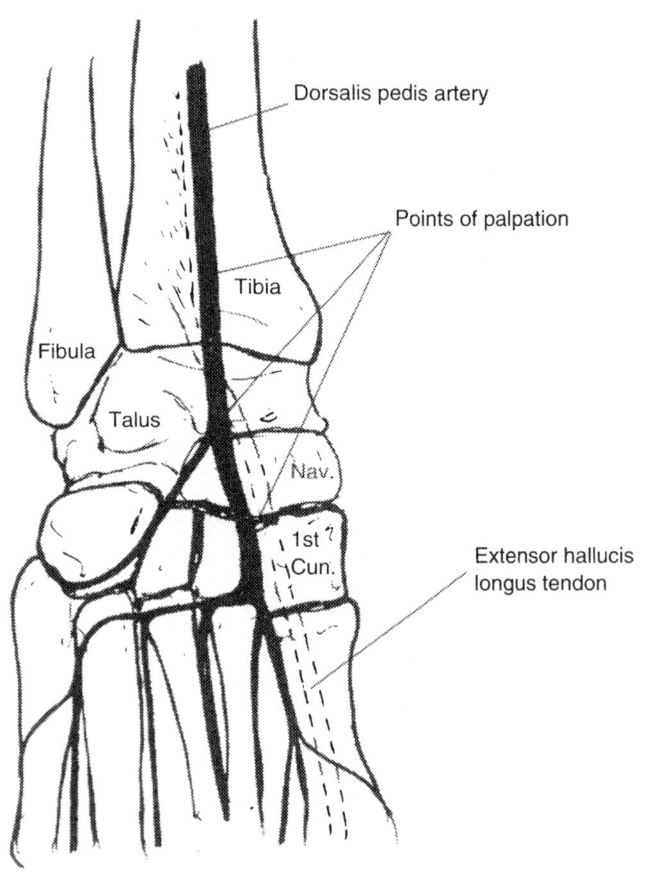

Fig. 2–19 Right foot, anterior view showing location of dorsalis pedis artery.

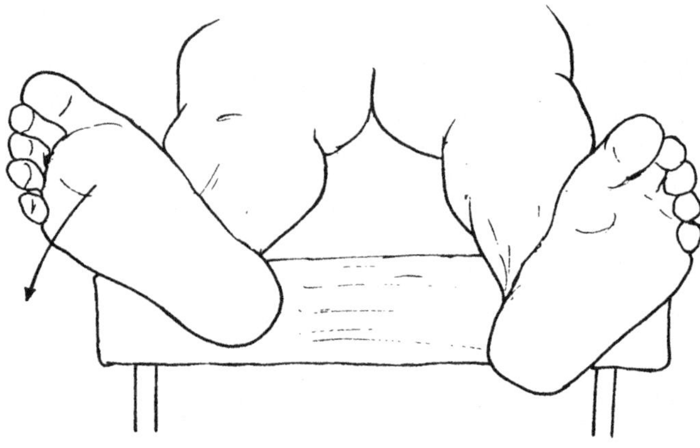

Fig. 2–20 Right foot laterally rotated.

piriformis or a portion of the gluteus maximus muscles are contracted or that a weakness of the medial rotators of the hip exists. It could indicate a laterally rotated tibia on the femur.

The patient may be a prone sleeper. If so, in the supine position with the iliac crest and the anterosuperior iliac spine level, the affected leg will palpate longer at each area of palpation (ie, the distal medial condyle of the femur, the medial malleolus, and the bottom of the heel). Also, the hip flexors on that side will test weak, and a laterally rotated femur fixation usually will be present. This will affect foot function. Breaking the prone sleeping habit and correcting the imbalances and habit patterns caused by it are necessary. Otherwise, therapy on the foot may be futile.

Observing the foot slightly plantar flexed and inverted (Fig. 2–21) may reveal that the everters and dorsiflexors of the foot are either stretched or weak. Compare with the opposite foot and with the inverters of the same foot. One must keep in mind, however, that the attachment of the everters and dorsiflexors (peroneus tertius and extensor digitorum longus) as well as of the peroneus brevis, which aids in eversion, all originate on the fibula. All too often, I have found this situation, tested the affected muscles, and assumed that they were at fault only to discover upon further investigation that the real problem was a weak (for whatever reason) biceps femoris (lateral hamstring). The biceps is the only muscle moving the fibula superiorly and securing the fibula to allow the above mentioned foot muscles to function properly. In the resting position, a weak biceps may, and often does, allow the above foot distortion to occur in the supine resting position.

A medially rotated foot (Fig. 2–22) is not a common occurrence in the adult. In children it occurs often with weakness of the lateral rotators of the hip (piriformis and a portion of the gluteus maximus). In the adult, it may occur with an injury to the lateral rotators severe enough to cause tissue damage. The patient probably would not come into the office complaining about the feet but rather about pelvic or low back pain.

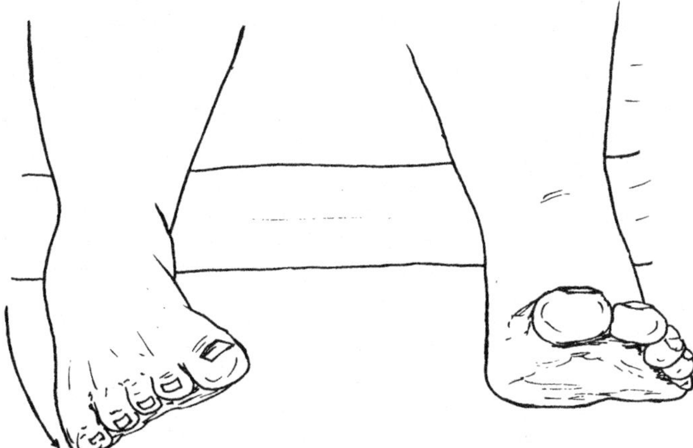

Fig. 2–21 Right foot plantar flexed and slightly inverted.

In an adult with a chronic weakness of the piriformis and a portion of the gluteus maximus (as found in the typical lordotic lumbar syndrome, Fig. 2–23), medial rotation of the foot is usually not found. Even though the femur is rotated medially, the tibia usually rotates laterally in compensation. As an example, consider the female patient with three children whose abdominal muscles have been stretched or interfered with by surgery. This allows the pelvis to rotate anteriorly. The femur rotates medially with the knee being forced into valgus position, increasing the Q angle (valgus angle of the knee). The medial rotation of the femur and the increased Q angle force the patella laterally, and the tibia rotates laterally to make up for it.[1]

RANGE OF MOTION

Before testing for passive range of motion (produced by the examiner), have the patient go through the active range of

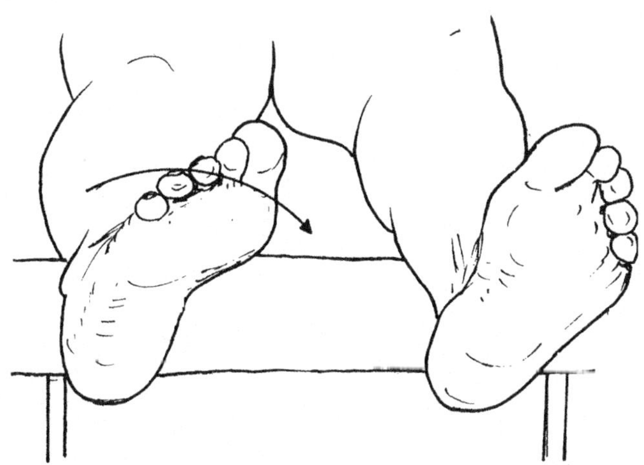

Fig. 2–22 Right foot rotated medially.

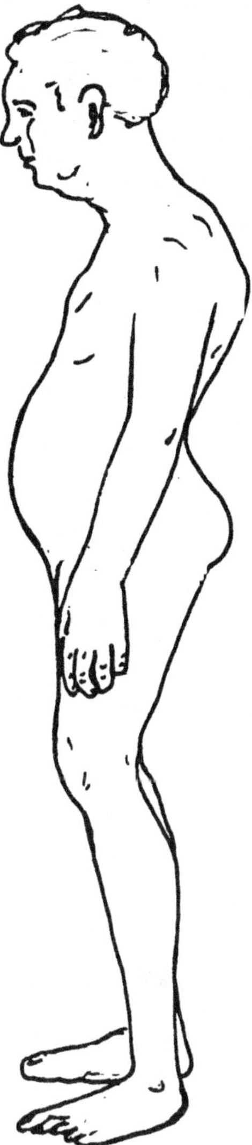

Fig. 2–23 Lumbar lordosis and associated posture.

motion for comparison. If trauma is involved and ligamental damage is suspected, care must be exercised throughout the range of motion tests.

Normal plantar flexion (toward the sole) involving the ankle and foot may range from 30° to 50° (Fig. 2–24).[2] It is limited by the dorsiflexors and encroachment of the posterior process of the talus on the calcaneus. Normal dorsiflexion (backward bending) is 20° (Fig. 2–24). It is limited by the triceps surae and the encroachment of the talus neck on the tibia. Always compare with the asymptomatic limb.

Plantar Flexor Test (Triceps Surae)

Most of the strength of plantar flexion is derived from the gastrocnemius and soleus with some help from the plantaris, posterior tibialis, and peroneus longus.

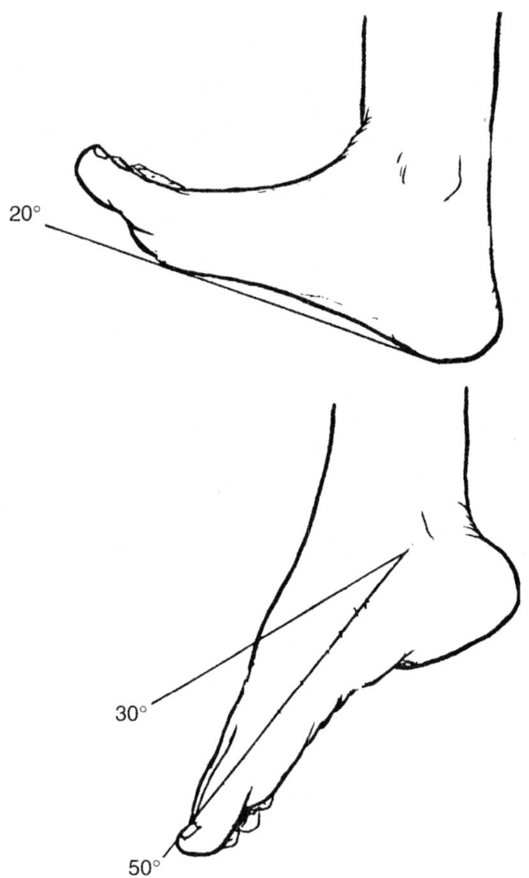

Fig. 2–24 Normal dorsiflexion and plantar flexion of the foot.

Test with the leg straight and the patient plantar flexing the foot. Grasp the heel and place the forefoot on the volar surface of your forearm (Fig. 2–25). Apply dorsiflexion pressure by maintaining a firm grasp of the heel and stepping forward. To help in isolating the soleus, some of the function of the gastrocnemius may be removed by repeating the test with the knee bent (Fig. 2–26).

Dorsiflexor Test

The dorsiflexors (anterior tibialis, extensor digitorum longus, extensor hallucis longus, and peroneus tertius) may be tested by having the patient dorsiflex and resist plantar pressure (Fig. 2–27A). Isolate and test the everter/dorsiflexor muscles (extensor digitorum longus, the peroneus tertius, and, to some degree, the peroneus brevis; Fig. 2–27B). Isolate and test the inverter/dorsiflexor muscles (anterior tibialis and extensor hallucis longus; Fig. 2–27C).

The normal range of dorsiflexion is 20° (Fig. 2–28).[2] Reduced range fof motion is a common finding. Many chronic problems of the feet and back are caused by restricted dorsiflexion and a shortened triceps surae. Symptoms include

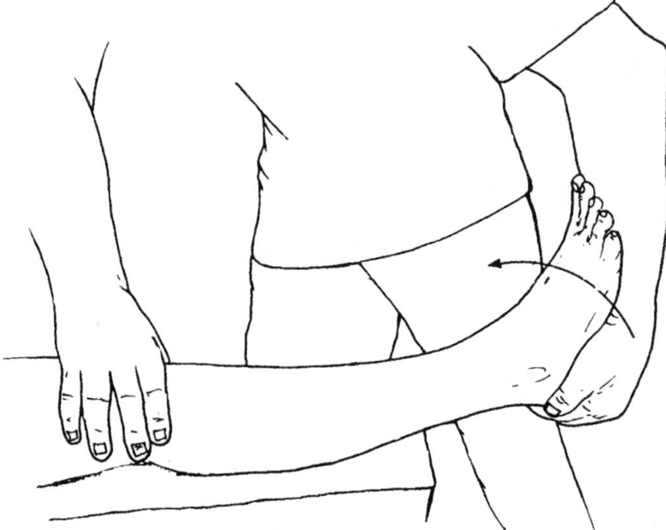

Fig. 2–25 Plantar flexor muscle test.

problems in the midthoracics, low back, foot, and ankle and produce a guarded, restricted gait.

I use a small incline board (13 × 13 in rising to 5½ in in the front) to demonstrate to the patient the restriction and to show a part of the solution (Fig. 2–29). With restricted dorsiflexion, standing in this position may not be possible, and if possible the stance is extremely distorted and/or it is felt severely in the calf of the legs. The solution is to stretch the triceps surae. This may be accomplished by standing on the board several times per day for several minutes over a period of several weeks. Gradually, the muscles will elongate.

Gait is affected greatly with a short triceps surae, often causing symptoms in the midthoracics. During a long stride,

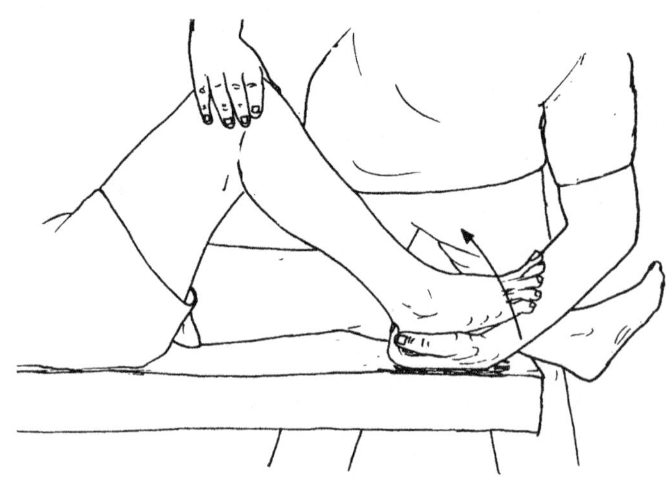

Fig. 2–26 Soleus test.

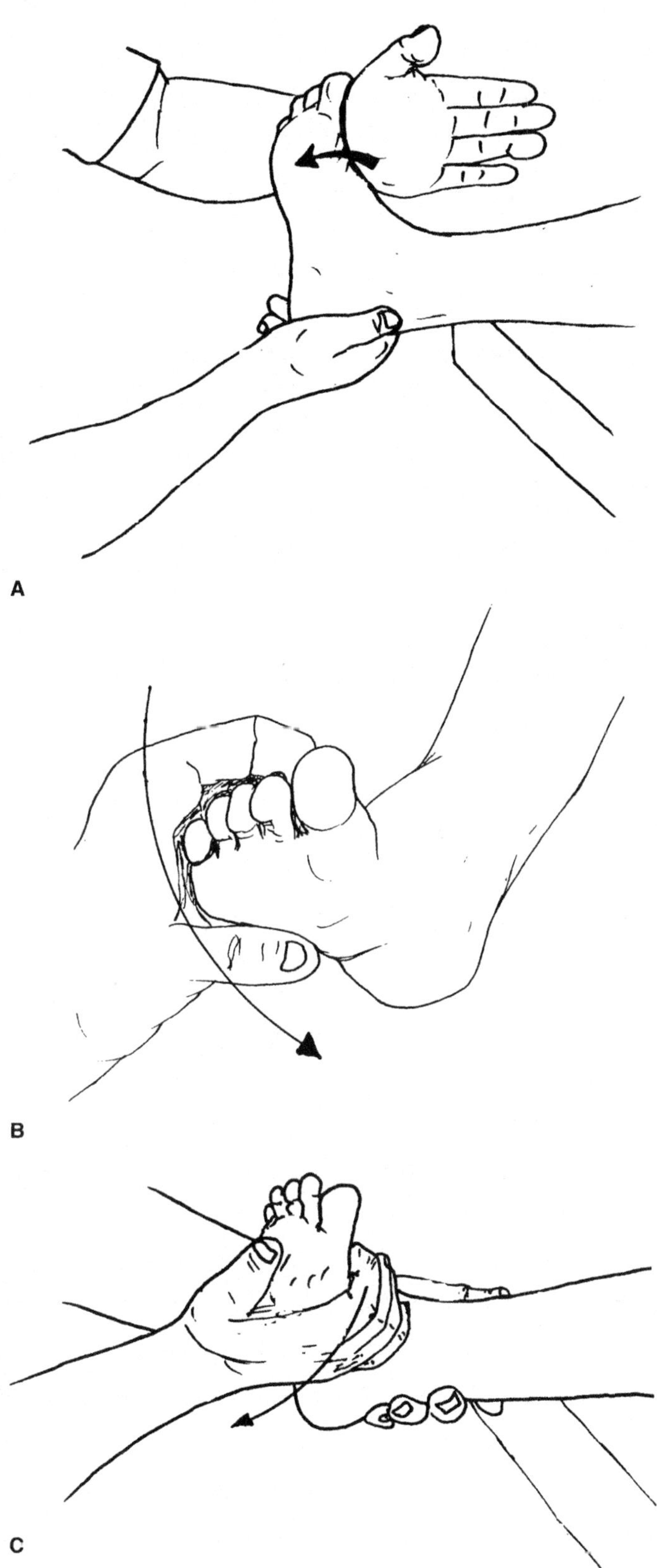

Fig. 2–27 (A) Dorsiflexor muscle test. **(B)** Extensor digitorum longus and peroneus tertius test. **(C)** Anterior tibialis test.

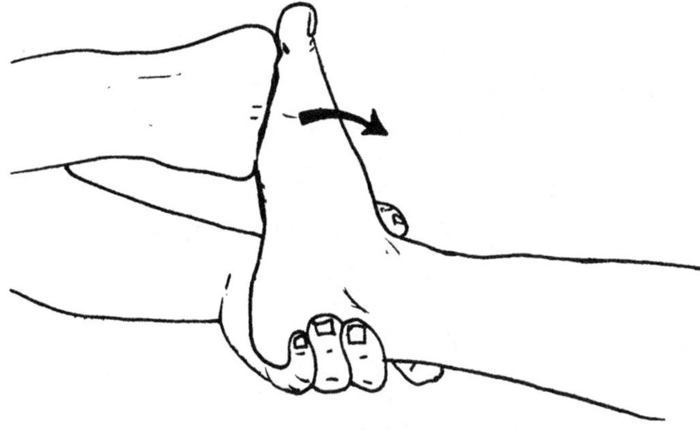

Fig. 2–28 Test for passive dorsiflexion.

the normal triceps surae allows the body to move well beyond the foot before it is necessary to elevate the heel from the ground (Fig. 2–30). When the triceps surae is shortened, it will not allow dorsiflexion past the neutral 90° (Fig. 2–31). This is a common finding. As the body weight approaches the half-

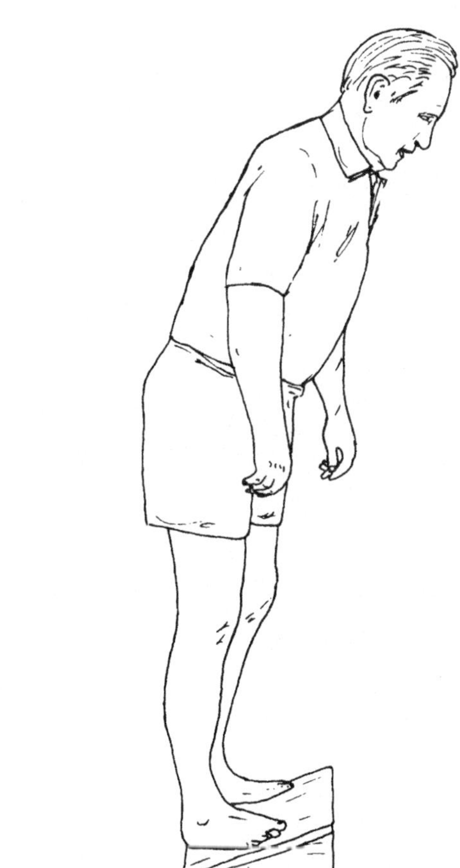

Fig. 2–29 Posture while standing on the incline board with restricted dorsiflexion.

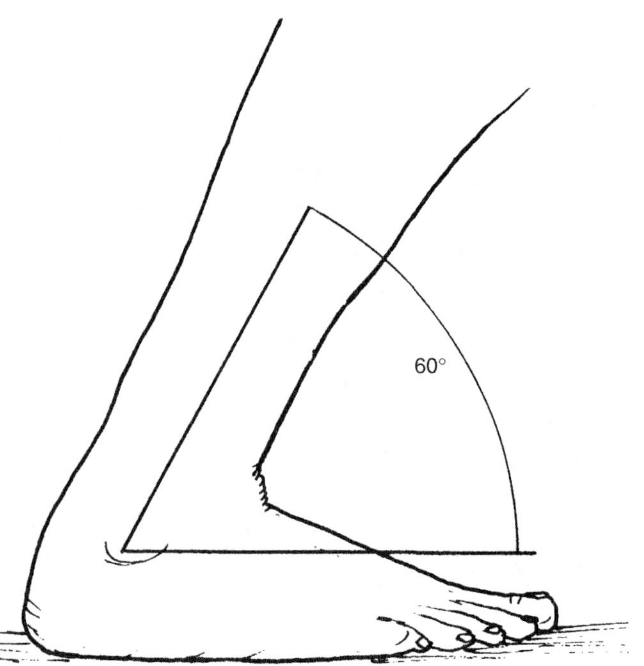

Fig. 2–30 Dorsiflexion of the ankle during long stride.

way point directly over the foot, the triceps surae must give. If not, either the knee must bend, giving the patient a shuffling gait, or the heel must immediately elevate from the ground (or both). With the heel-off occurring too soon, the entire normal function of the foot is interrupted, and great strain is placed upon the foot.

It is not uncommon to find patients with no dorsiflexion and many more with some degree of limitation. In my opinion, the degree of stress and strain on the foot is directly related to the degree of restricted dorsiflexion.

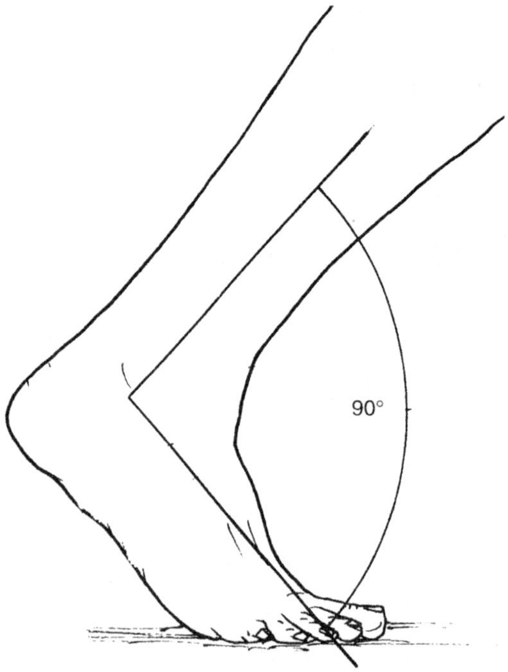

Adduction of the Forefoot

To test adduction of the forefoot, the hindfoot must be stabilized. Secure the heel with the fingers, and place the thumb pad (for patient comfort) on the medial side of the talar head. Maneuver the forefoot medially without inversion (Fig. 2–32). Lack of adduction indicates possible fixations of the transverse tarsal arch. Rarely, there may be hypertonic everter muscles. Excessive adduction may indicate a strain or weakness of the peronei muscles.

Abduction of the Forefoot

To test forefoot abduction, support the heel and place the thumb pad on the lateral surface of the anterior calcaneus. Apply abduction without eversion (Fig. 2–33). Restriction may indicate fixations of the transverse tarsal arch and/or a hypertonic posterior tibialis muscle. Excessive abduction may indicate a stretched or weakened posterior tibialis with involvement of the flexor hallucis longus as well.

Fig. 2–31 Lack of dorsiflexion of the ankle during long stride.

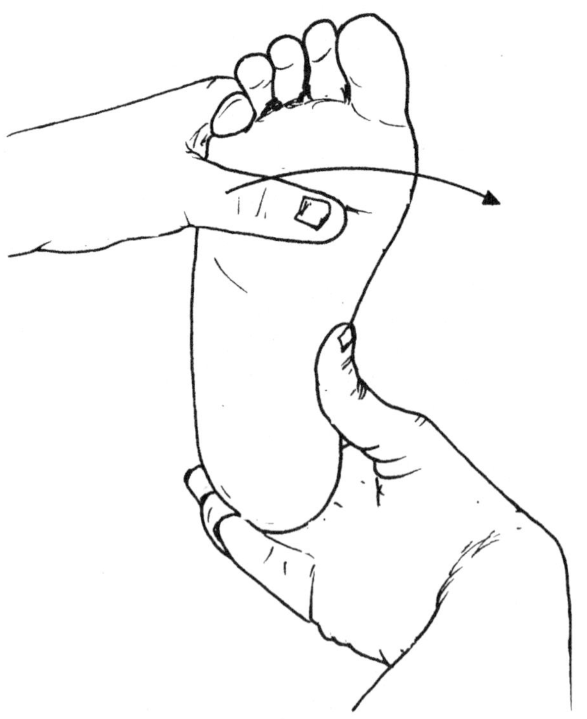

Fig. 2–32 Adduction of the forefoot.

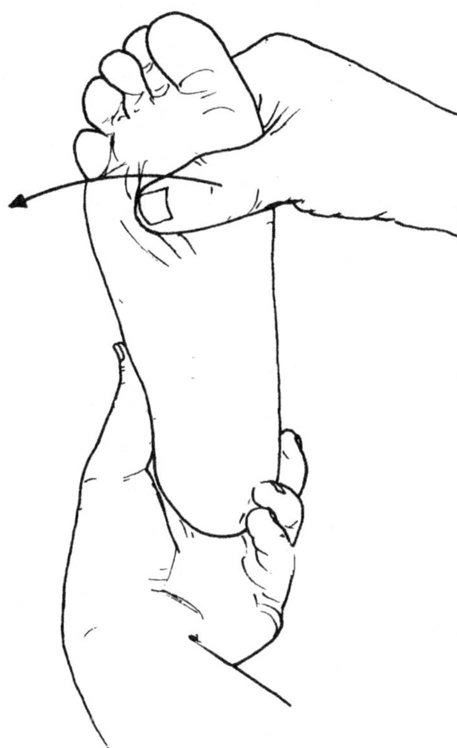

Fig. 2–33 Abduction of the forefoot.

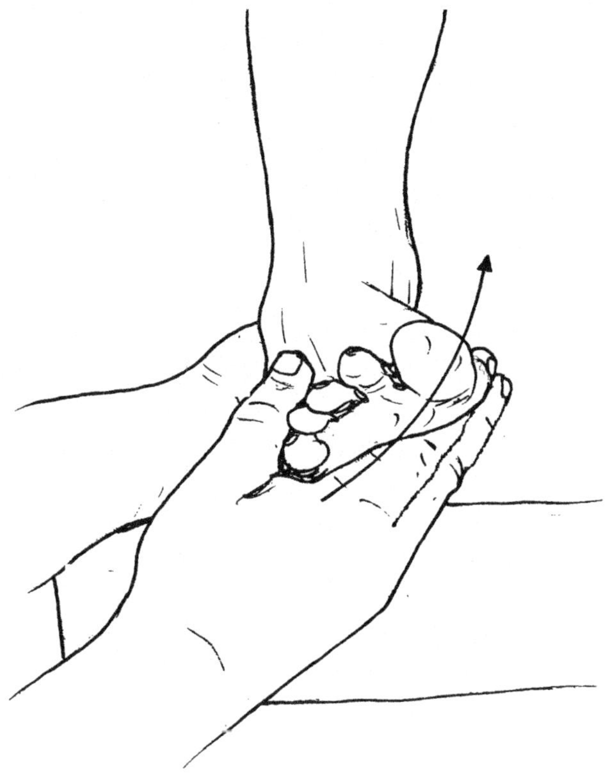

Fig. 2–34 Supination of the forefoot on the stationary hindfoot.

Supination of the Forefoot on the Stationary Hindfoot

Supination of the forefoot also requires securing the heel. Supinate the forefoot (Fig. 2–34). Supination should be approximately twice that of pronation.

Pronation of the Forefoot on the Stationary Hindfoot

To test for forefoot pronation, secure the heel while pronating the forefoot (Fig. 2–35).

Inversion of the Foot and Ankle

Inversion is a combination of adduction and supination and, when executed by the patient, usually some plantar flexion (Fig. 2–36). The range of supination is 52°.[2]

Eversion of the Foot and Ankle

Eversion is a combination of pronation, abduction, and usually some dorsiflexion (Fig. 2–37).

Adduction of the Hindfoot

To test hindfoot adduction, use the inside hand to grasp the tarsal arch and the forefoot. Adduct the heel with the outside hand (Fig. 2–38).

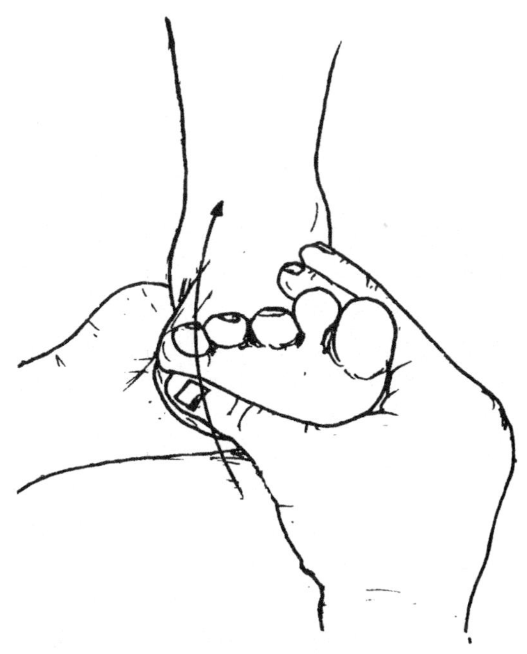

Fig. 2–35 Pronation of the forefoot on the stationary hindfoot.

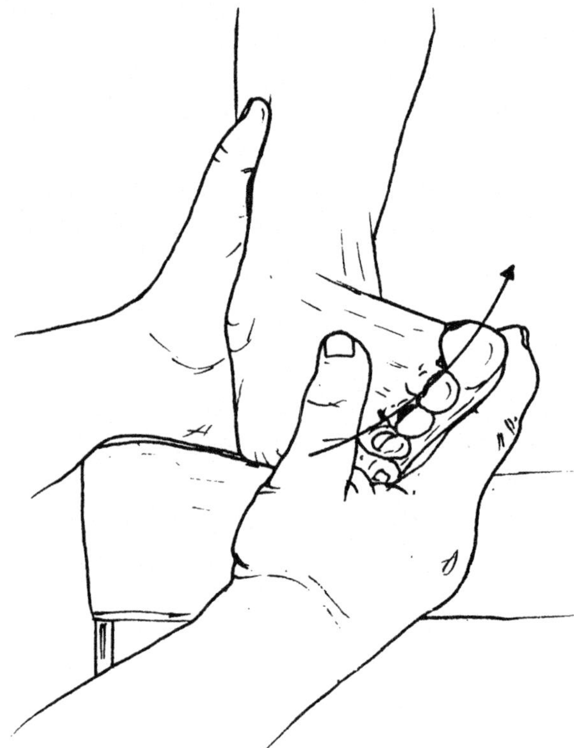

Fig. 2–36 Inversion of the foot and ankle.

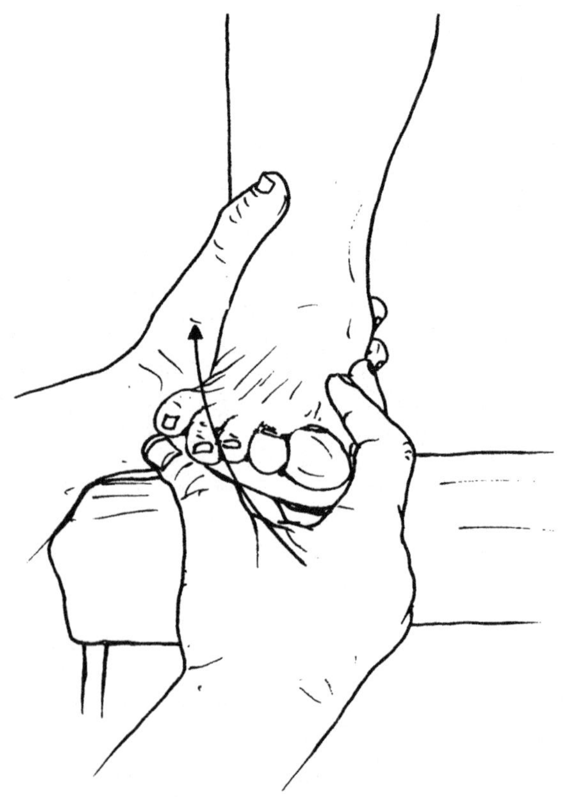

Fig. 2–37 Eversion of the foot and ankle.

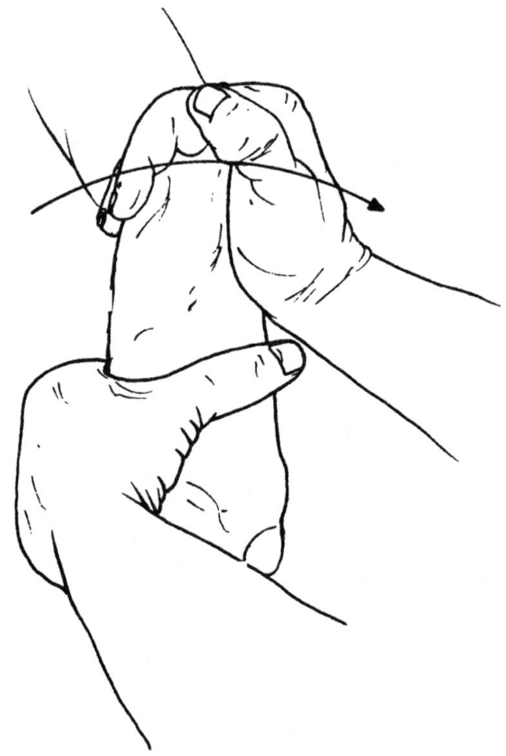

Fig. 2–38 Adduction of the hindfoot.

Abduction of the Hindfoot

Test for abduction of the hindfoot with the inside hand grasping the tarsal arch and the forefoot. Abduct the heel with the outside hand (Fig. 2–39).

Pronation-Supination of the Hindfoot

With the patient in the prone position and the leg fixed on the table, pronation and supination of the hindfoot are easily accomplished (Fig. 2–40). If an injury has occurred and a sprain is suspected, care must be used in testing abduction, adduction, eversion, and inversion of the foot itself. If a sprain is a consideration in the ankle joint and edema is present, there may be interference with normal testing. An accurate assessment may be made after the edema is reduced.

Pronation of the hindfoot is usually about half the movement of supination. Grasp the calcaneus with the outside hand and evert the heel. If pain is present and/or ligamental damage is suspected, testing with an emphasis on the posterior and anterior fibers may be performed to determine the exact tissue that is injured.

Drawer Test

The drawer test at the ankle is performed by placing resistance against the tibia and fibula and then drawing the hindfoot

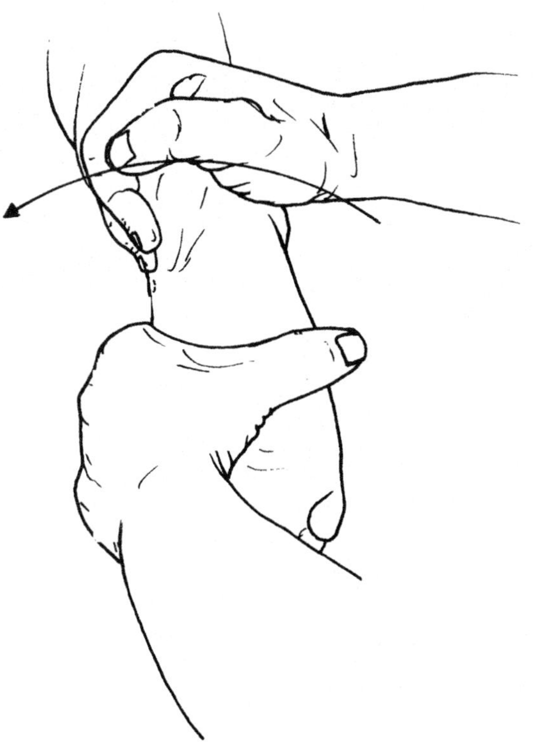

Fig. 2–39 Abduction of the hindfoot.

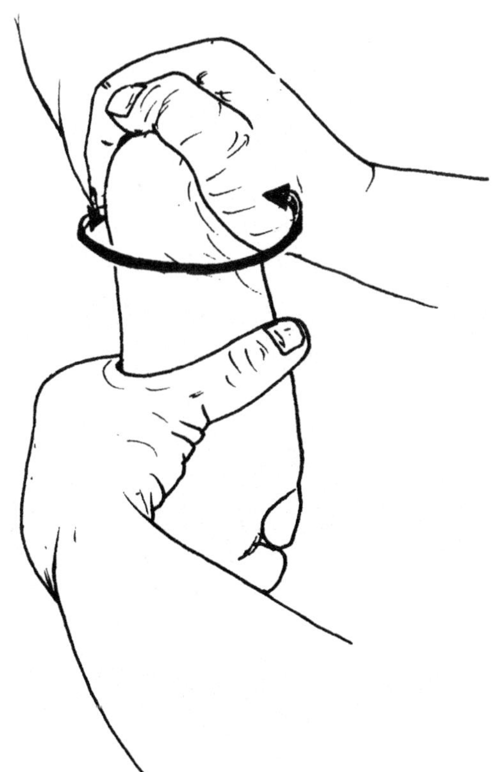

Fig. 2–40 Pronation-supination of the hindfoot.

forward (Fig. 2–41). Movement greater than 3 mm is considered positive for anterior ligamental damage. To be more specific, further testing may be done to differentiate the anterior and posterior ligaments medially and laterally.

Test for the Anteromedial Ligaments

Test for anteromedial ligaments (Fig. 2–42) with the patient in the supine position and the heel off the end of the table (fix the tibia). Grasp the heel with the inside hand. Place the outside hand over the tarsal arch and contact the calcaneus below the sustentaculum tali with the thumb (Fig. 2–43). Pressure may be exerted to pronate the calcaneus, placing stress on the tibiocalcaneal portions of the deltoid ligament (medial collateral ligament, MCL).[2] By altering the pressure toward the forefoot, stress may be placed on the tibionavicular and the anterior tibiotalar ligaments as well.

Test for the Posteromedial Ligaments

To test for the posteromedial ligaments, grasp the heel with the inside hand. With the outside hand over the tarsal arch, contact the talus and tibia posteriorly with the thumb (Fig. 2–44). Pressure may be applied to induce pronation of the calcaneus and to stress the posterior tibiocalcaneal ligament (PTL) and the medial and posterior talocalcaneal ligaments as well.

Test of the Posterolateral Ligaments

To test the posterolateral ligaments (Fig. 2–45), grasp the heel with the outside hand. Place the inside hand over the tar-

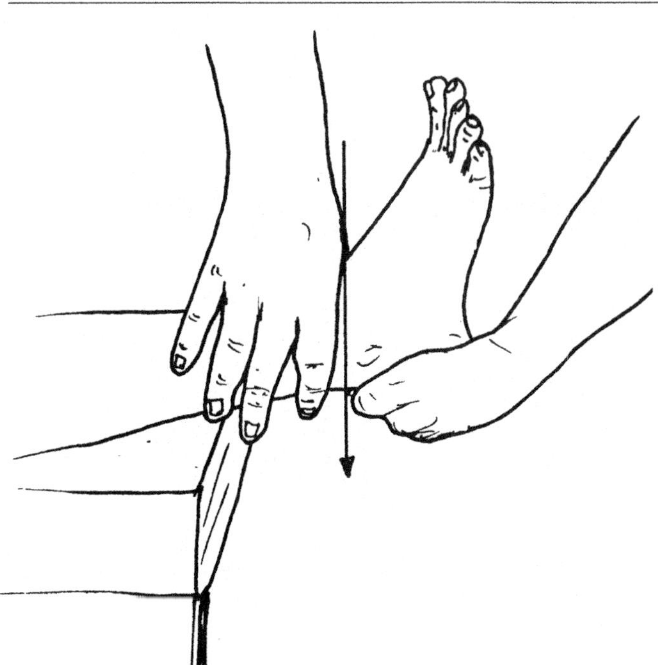

Fig. 2–41 Drawer test.

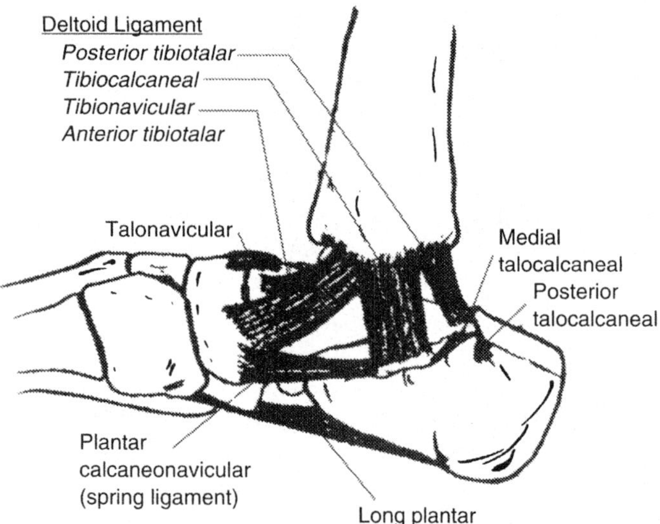

Fig. 2–42 Right ankle and foot, medial view showing ligaments.

sal arch with the thumb posterior on the fibula (Fig. 2–46). Pressure may be applied to produce supination of the calcaneus, stressing the calcaneofibular ligaments.

Test for the Cervical Ligament

Test the cervical ligament. With the thumb of the outside hand, secure the fibula and tibia and grasp the talus head with

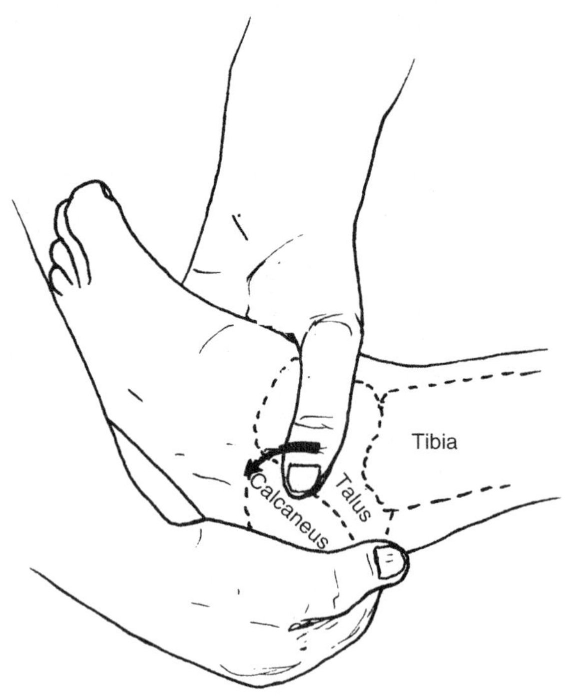

Fig. 2–43 Anteromedial ligament test.

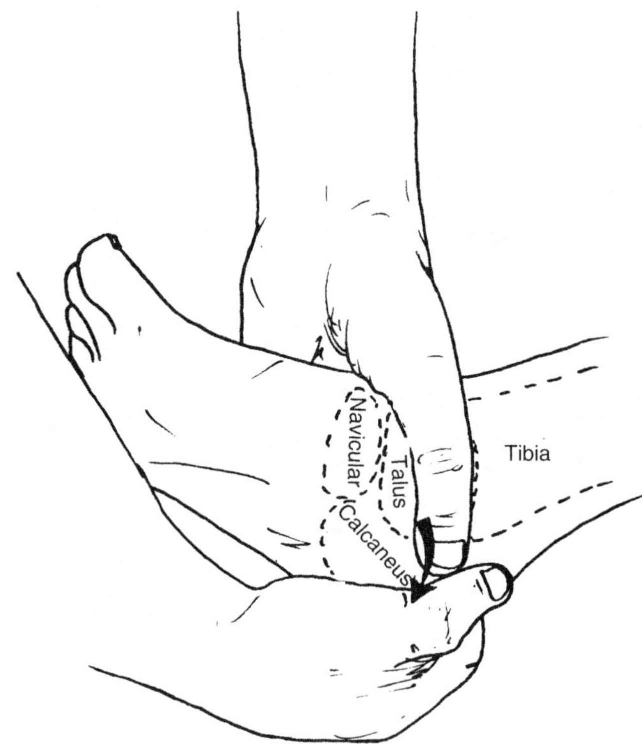

Fig. 2–44 Posteromedial ligament test.

the middle finger (Fig. 2–47A). Place the inside hand over the foot with the thumb pad on the superior surface of the calcaneus and apply plantar and anterior pressure, placing stress on the cervical ligament (Fig. 2–47B).

Test for the Anterior Talofibular Ligament

Test the anterior talofibular ligament. With the outside hand, support the heel and secure the fibula posteriorly with

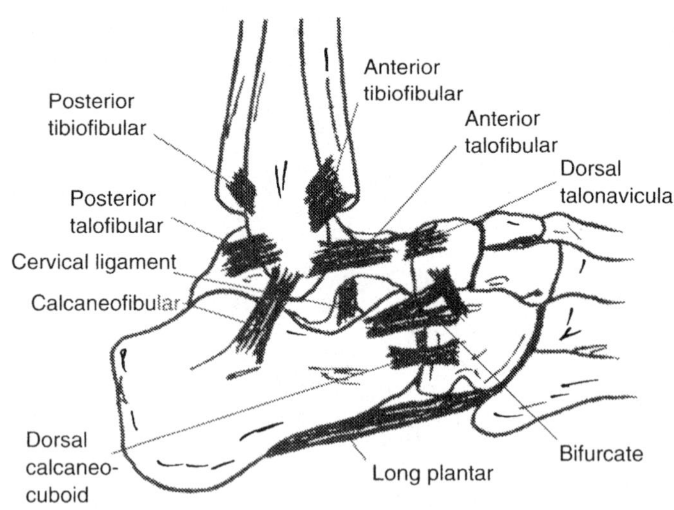

Fig. 2–45 Right ankle and foot, lateral view showing ligaments.

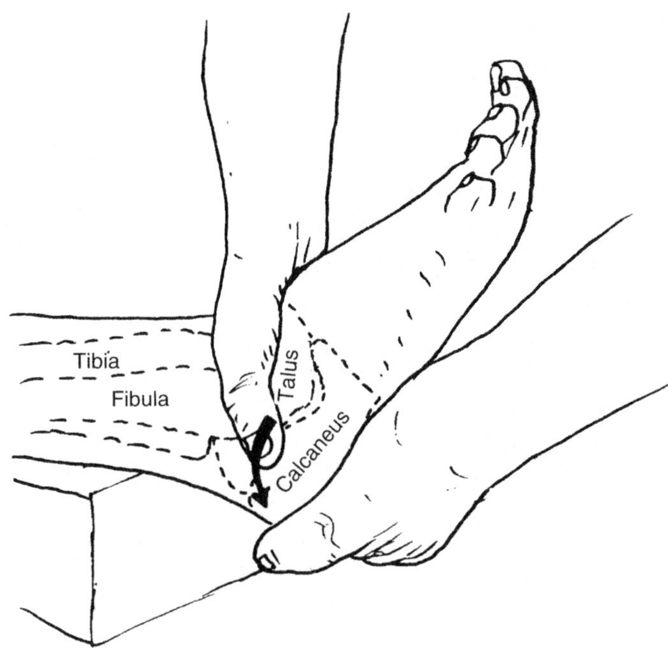

Fig. 2–46 Posterolateral ligament test.

---

the thumb. Hook the thumb of the inside hand over the talar head and apply pressure anteriorly and medially, placing stress on the anterior talofibular ligament (Fig. 2–48).

Test for Abduction Sprain

To test for possible anterior tibiofibular ligament damage (abduction sprain of the ankle), support the tibia and fibula with the inside hand and palpate the anterior articulation (Fig. 2–49A). With the outside hand, hook the thumb over the talonavicular articulation and the index finger along the lateral surface of the calcaneus (Fig. 2–49B). Apply pressure to produce abduction of the foot on the tibia. Only minimal separation movement should be felt, if any. With ligamental tearing, movement would be greater and accompanied by pain.

Test for Flexion of the Lateral Longitudinal Arch

To test for flexion of the lateral longitudinal arch, use the outside hand to support the heel, placing the thumb pad under the cuboid bone. With the fingers of the inside hand, flex the fourth and fifth metatarsals (Fig. 2–50). The movement should be smooth and unrestricted and with no pain. If restrictions are felt, more specific palpation will be necessary to determine exactly which articulation is fixed.

Test for Extension of the Lateral Longitudinal Arch

To test extension of the lateral longitudinal arch, use the outside hand over the heel, placing the thumb pad over the

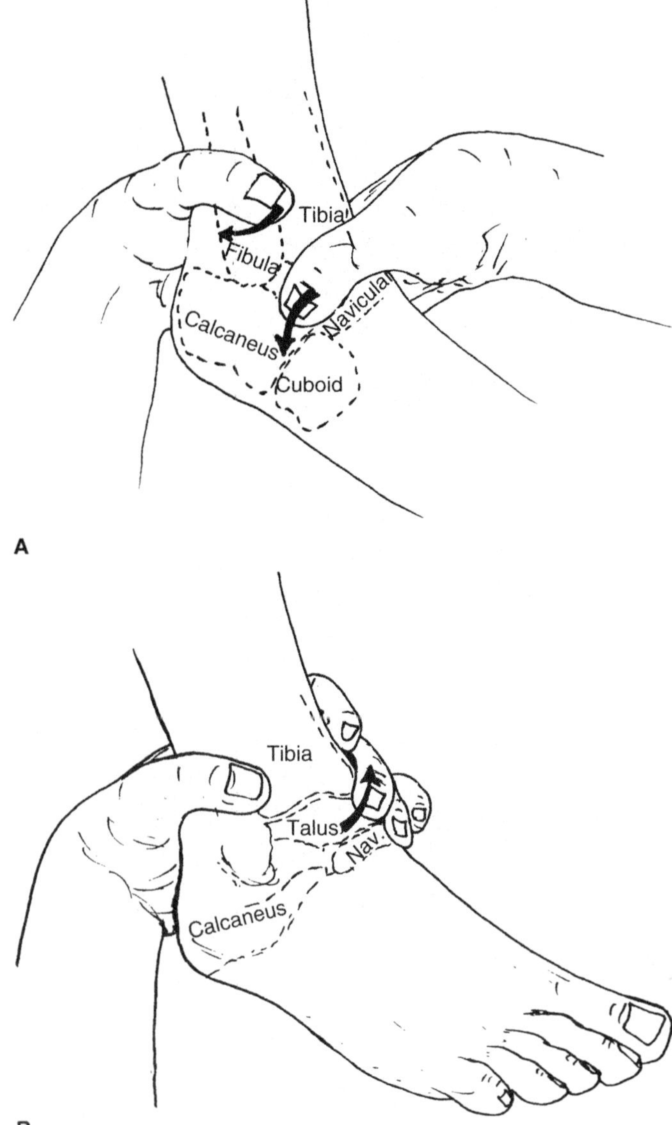

Fig. 2–47 **(A)** Cervical ligament test. **(B)** Contact to secure the talus for cervical ligament test.

---

cuboid bone. With the thumb of the inside hand, extend the lateral arch (Fig. 2–51). Because the ligaments are already stretched, minimal extension takes place. There should be a firm yet pliant end feel. If excessive extension occurs, careful analysis of each articulation must be done to eliminate ligamental damage. If the end feel becomes rigid or is restricted, specific palpation will be necessary to determine exactly which articulation is fixed.

Test for Flexion of the Medial Longitudinal Arch

To test flexion of the medial longitudinal arch, support the heel with the outside hand, placing the thumb on the plantar

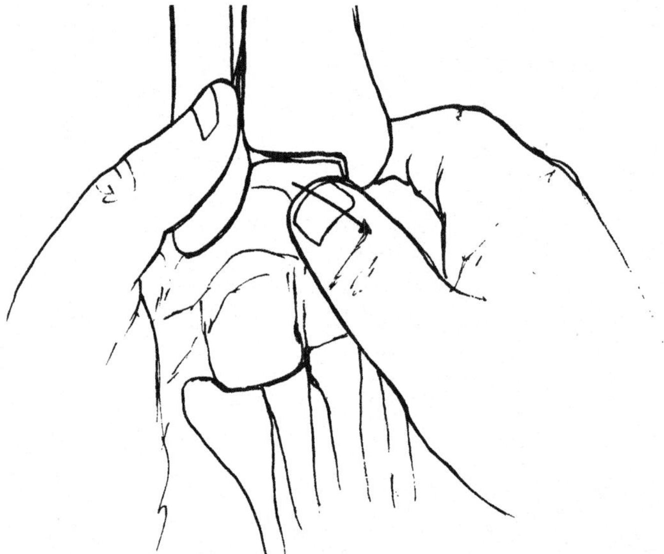

Fig. 2–48 Test for anterior talofibular ligament.

surface of the calcaneus and talus. With the inside hand, apply flexion stress on the medial arch, testing for flexibility or restriction of movement (Fig. 2–52). If some restriction is felt, the thumb contact may be moved progressively under the na-

vicular and first cuneiform to determine the location of the restriction (Fig. 2–53). As with the lateral arch, the movement should be smooth and not excessive and should have a comfortable end feel. Any interruption of the above requires further investigation to determine the specific articulation that is fixed or unstable.

Test for Extension of the Medial Longitudinal Arch

By hooking the thumb of the inside hand over the articulations (Fig. 2–54), testing for extension of the medial longitudinal arch may be performed. As with the lateral arch, extension is minimal and should have a normal end feel. If not, further investigation is called for.

If testing for flexion and extension of the lateral and medial arches reveals normal flexibility with no discomfort, pain, or restrictions, the time-consuming motion palpation of each articulation (described later) is not necessary.

Test for Rotation of the Medial Arch on the Talus

Test rotation of the medial arch on the talus. With the inside hand, grasp the heel and secure the talus with the thumb. With the outside hand, grasp the foot as near the navicular as pos-

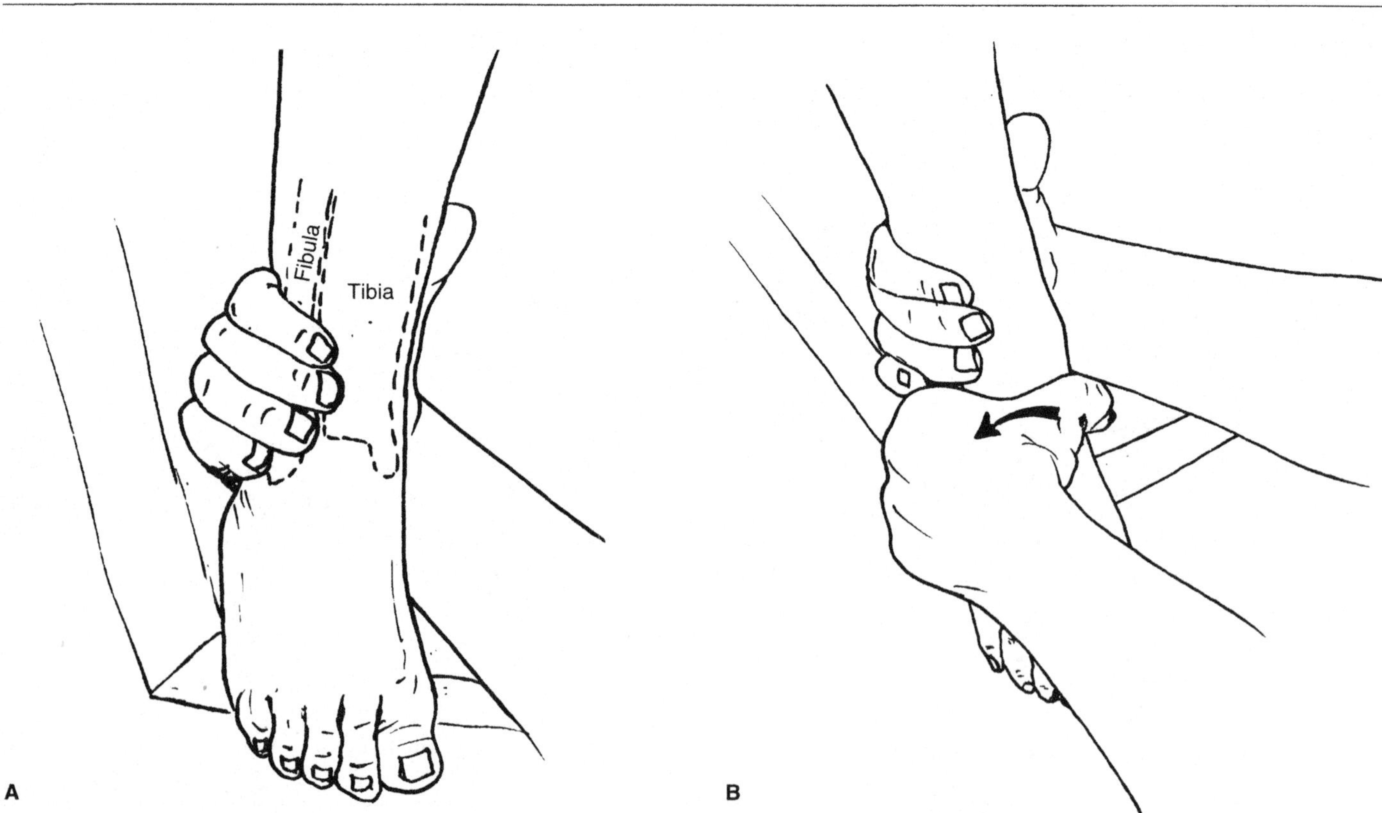

Fig. 2–49 **(A)** Support contact for tibiofibular ligament test. **(B)** Test for tibiofibular ligament damage.

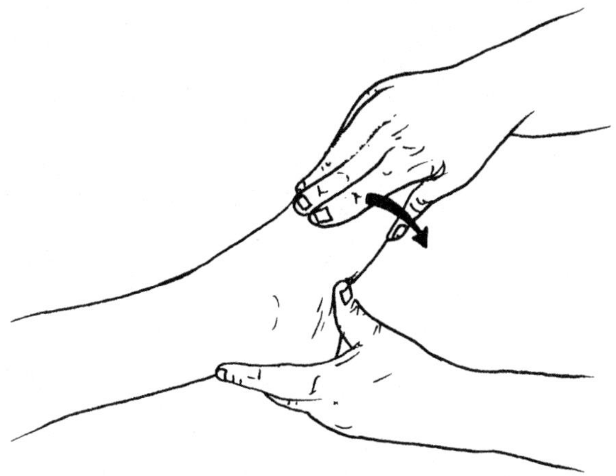

Fig. 2–50 Test for flexion of the longitudinal arch.

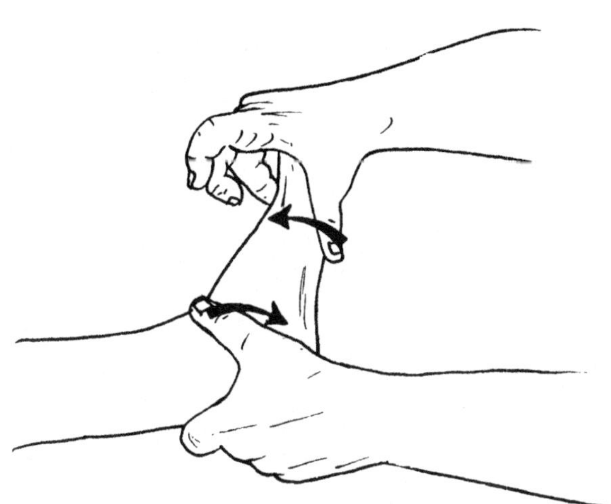

Fig. 2–51 Test for extension of the lateral longitudinal arch.

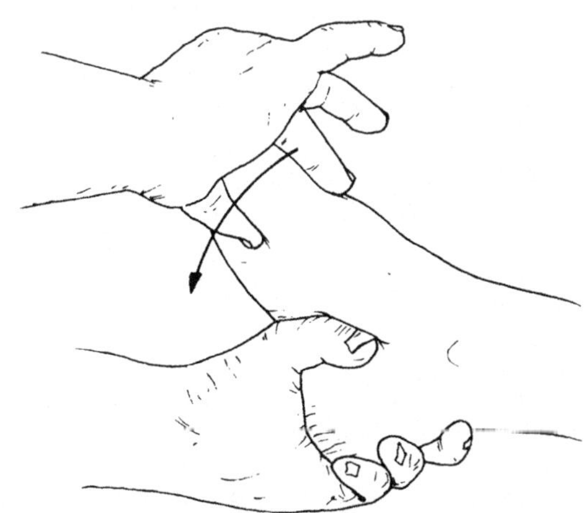

Fig. 2–52 Test for flexion of the medial longitudinal arch.

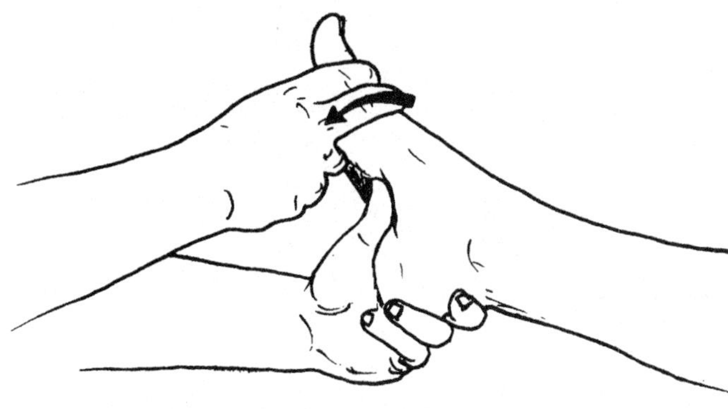

Fig. 2–53 Medial arch flexion with support hand on the navicular and first cuneiform.

sible and rotate (Fig. 2–55). Movement should be smooth and painless and should have a normal end feel.

Rotation of the Fourth and Fifth Metatarsals

To test rotation of the fourth and fifth metatarsals, secure the cuboid bone with the outside hand and test for rotation of the fifth and then the fourth metatarsal (Fig. 2–56).

Metatarsalgia

Questioning of the patient may reveal a symptom of feeling pain and the sensation of a pebble in the shoe. The patient may

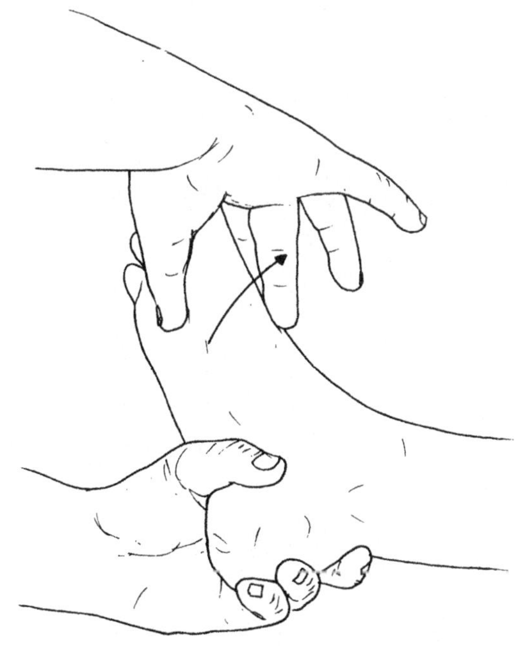

Fig. 2–54 Test for extension of the medial longitudinal arch.

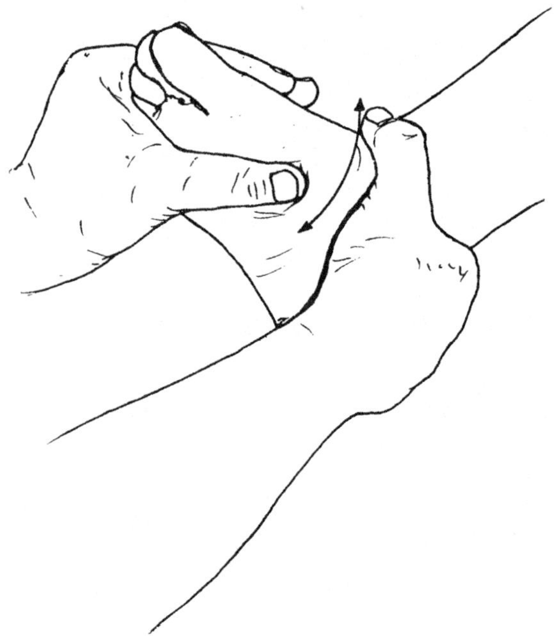

Fig. 2–55 Test for rotation of the medial arch on the talus.

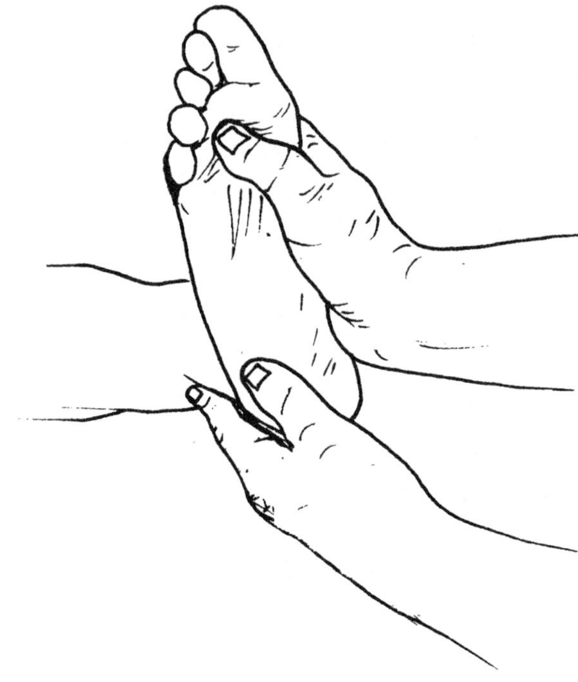

A

have pain walking barefoot on a hard surface that is relieved by wearing soft crepe-soled shoes.

With symptoms in the forefoot, examination should include careful palpation of each metatarsal and its phalangeal joint. Palpate for tenderness of the metatarsal heads (Fig. 2–57A). Palpate not only the plantar surface of the head but also the distal end (Fig. 2–57B).

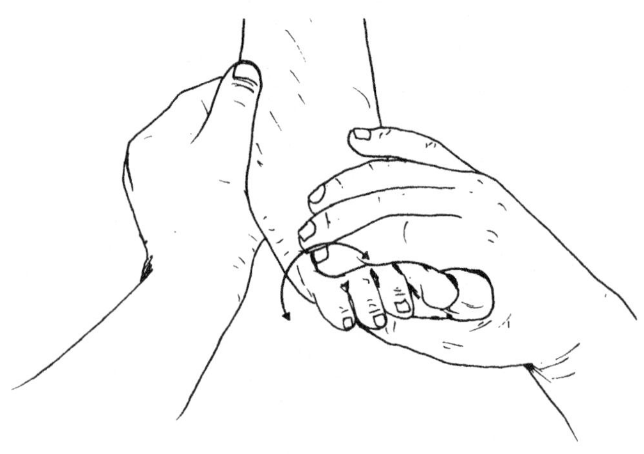

Fig. 2–56 Rotation of the fourth and fifth metatarsals.

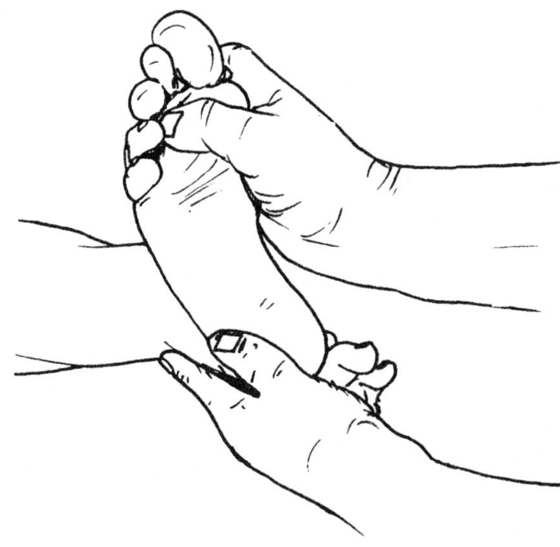

B

Fig. 2–57 **(A)** Palpation of the metatarsal heads. **(B)** Palpation of the distal ends of the metatarsals.

Synovitis and Edema

Edema due to synovitis of the metatarsophalangeal joints is easily recognized on comparison with the opposite non-symptomatic side (Fig. 2–58). Pain accompanies its presence and may be more acute on the dorsal surface than on the plantar surface.

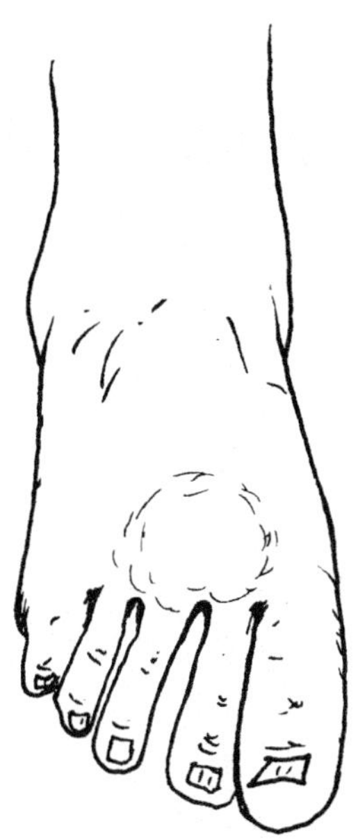

Fig. 2–58 Edema due to synovitis of the metatarsophalangeal joints.

Intermetatarsal Palpation

If the application of intermetatarsal pressure (Fig. 2–59) produces pain, two conditions must be ruled out. Interdigital neuroma is the first. The term is a misnomer. The entrapment of the common digital nerve causes degeneration of the nerve fibers with extensive perineural fibrosis.[3] The other is a strain-sprain of the intermetatarsal fascia and the interosseous muscles.

In the presence of nerve damage, squeezing of the metatarsals will increase the pain and, in extreme cases, will cause paresthesias into the toes (Fig. 2–60). If the condition is due to a simple strain-sprain, the symptoms will ease with support of the metatarsal arch.

The Great Toe

Flexion

Flexion of the great toe should be tested with the ankle in neutral (Fig. 2–61). With the ankle plantar flexed, the great toe may not be flexed because of extensor hallucis longus muscle tightness.

Extension

Extension of the first metatarsophalangeal joint is approximately 70° (Fig. 2–62). Extension is necessary for toe-off, requiring at least 35° to 40°. As the body weight is thrust forward and the heel rises, extension places a stretch on the plantar aponeurosis and the flexor hallucis longus muscle before the latter contracts to project the body weight forward.

Hallux Rigidus

If extension is reduced or is in the process of being fused (hallux rigidus), the gait is altered greatly (Fig. 2–63). Either

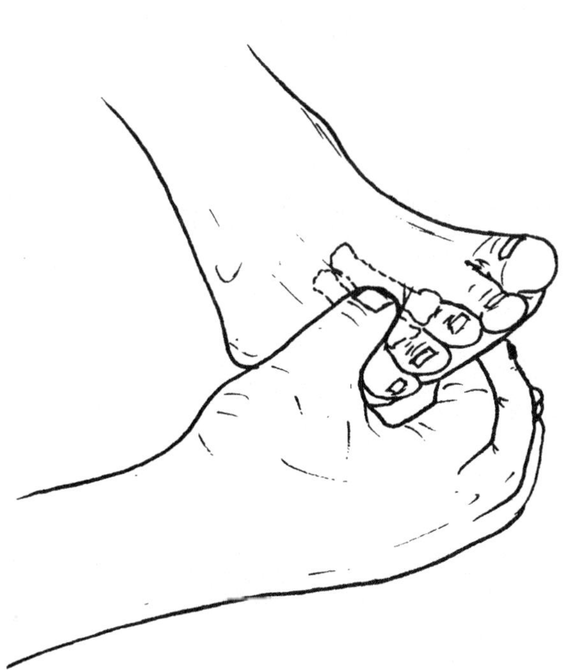

Fig. 2–59 Intermetatarsal pressure.

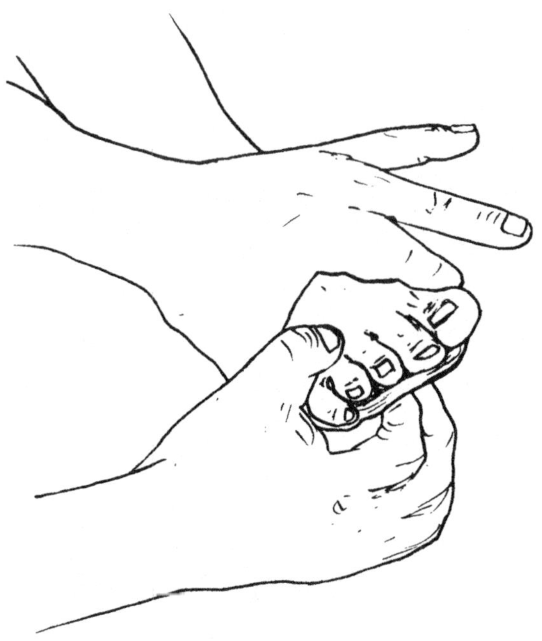

Fig. 2–60 Intermetatarsal pressure with metatarsal arch support.

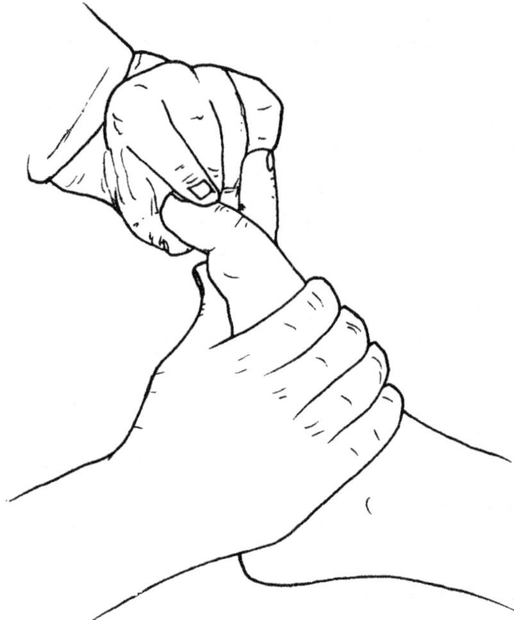

Fig. 2–61 Flexion of the great toe with the ankle in neutral.

the weight shifts to the lesser toes, altering foot function, or the gait is halted at 0°, making a shuffling motion instead of the normal push-off.

Rotation

With the outside hand, grasp the forefoot to include the first metatarsal. Grasp the great toe with the thumb and finger on the proximal phalanx and rotate (Fig. 2–64).

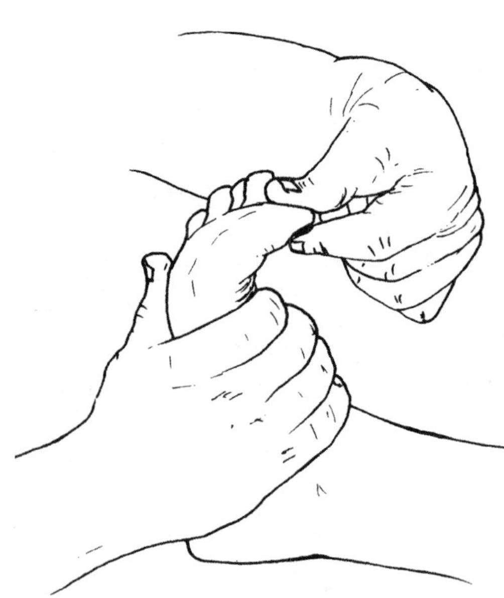

Fig. 2–62 Extension of the great toe.

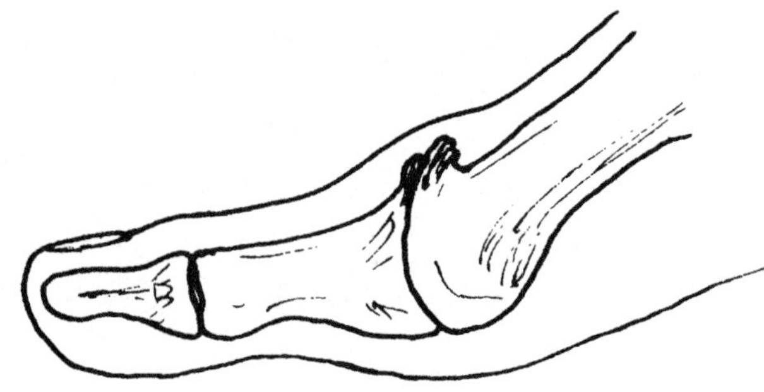

Fig. 2–63 Degeneration of the first metatarsophalangeal joint preventing extension (hallux rigidus).

Heel Pain

With patient complaints of heel pain, several conditions must be ruled out: Achilles tendinitis, retrocalcaneal bursitis, and plantar fascitis.

Achilles Tendinitis

Palpate the Achilles tendon for tears and/or inflammation (Fig. 2–65). If inflammation exists only on one side, further investigation is necessary into possible muscular problems with the gastrocnemius muscle on the opposite side. (The tendon twists on itself 180° to its insertion.) Pain is usually found proximal to the insertion itself.

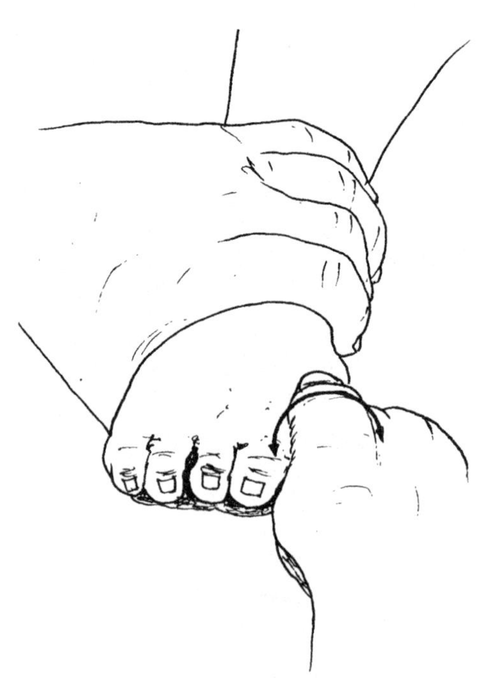

Fig. 2–64 Test for rotation of the first metatarsophalangeal joint.

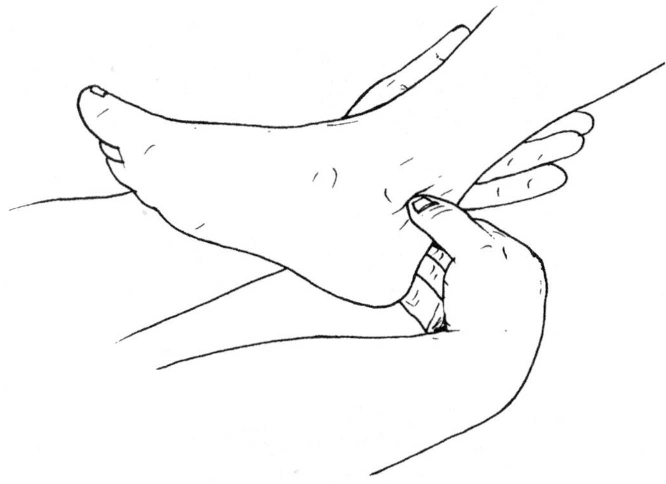

Fig. 2–65 Palpation of the Achilles tendon.

Retrocalcaneal Bursitis

The inflamed bursa may be palpated at the insertion of the Achilles tendon (Fig. 2–66). Palpation will reveal not only pain but edema. Some pain may extend slightly up the Achilles tendon but will be restricted to the bursa area. If pain should be present more than 2 to 3 cm superiorly, Achilles tendinitis should be suspected.

Plantar Fasciitis

The plantar aponeurosis originates on the medial tubercle of the calcaneus and anchors into the metatarsophalangeal joint

complex, with the thickest part extending to the great toe (Fig. 2–67). Tenderness should not be mistaken for generalized tenderness of the plantar surface due to congestion or pain over the intrinsic muscles. If in doubt, extend the toes, which will increase the pain in fascial involvement.

Heel Squeeze Test

To test for possible stress fracture of the calcaneus, squeeze the heel with both hands (Fig. 2–68). This should not aggravate symptoms other than those of a stress fracture of the calcaneus.

The Thompson Squeeze Test

The Thompson squeeze test is used to test for the integrity of the Achilles tendon. On squeezing of the belly of the gastrocnemius and soleus muscles, the foot should plantar flex (Fig. 2–69).

Tendinitis

The presence of tendinitis may be determined by careful palpation along the course of the tendon in question.

The anterior tibialis tendon is palpable and visible about one finger width lateral to the medial malleolus (Fig. 2–70). It is the most prominent tendon visible with inversion and

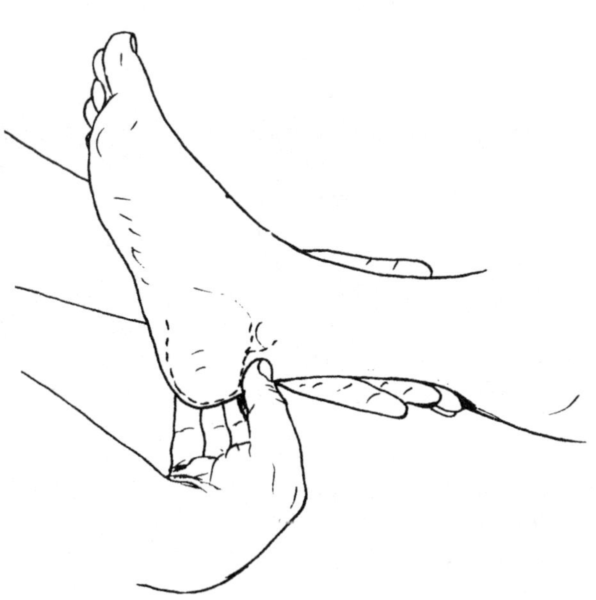

Fig. 2–66 Palpation of the retrocalcaneal bursa.

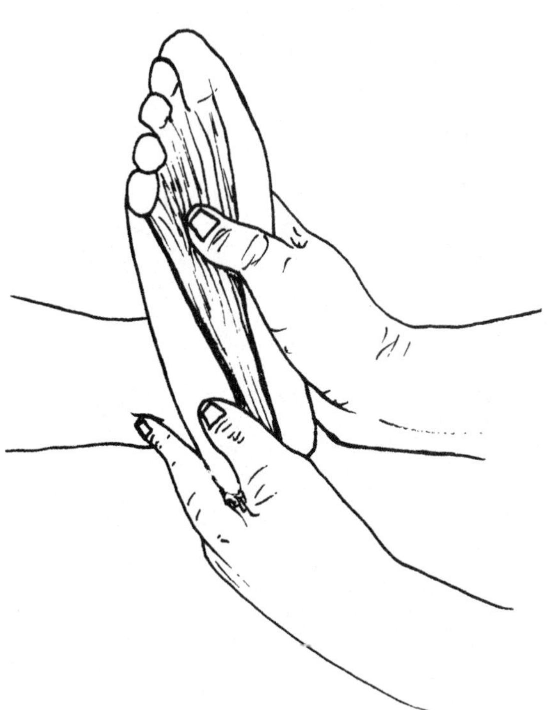

Fig. 2–67 Palpation of the plantar aponeurosis.

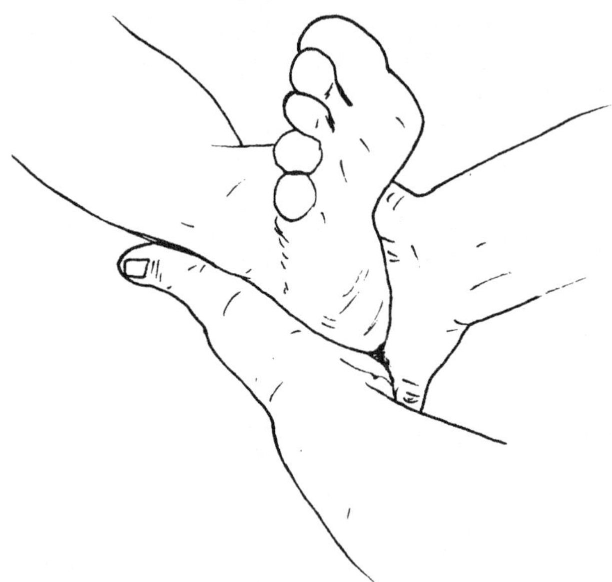

Fig. 2–68 Heel squeeze test for possible stress fracture of the calcaneus.

dorsiflexion of the foot. If differentiation is necessary, invert and dorsiflex with the great toe in plantar flexion. The tendon may be palpated to its insertion on the medial side of the first cuneiform and the first metatarsal.

The next tendon laterally is the extensor hallucis longus (Fig. 2–70). At the ankle, it becomes prominent while plantar flexing the foot and extending the great toe. It passes next to the anterior tibialis tendon, until they pass together under the inferior retinaculum. Then it passes over the medial side of the base of the first metatarsal and inserts into the distal phalanx of the great toe.

The tendons of the extensor digitorum longus and peroneus tertius muscles (Fig. 2–70) are easily palpated by plantar flex-

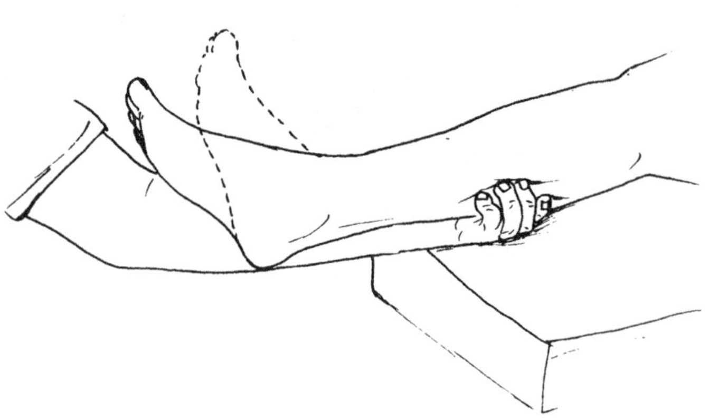

Fig. 2–69 Thompson's squeeze test for integrity of the Achilles tendon.

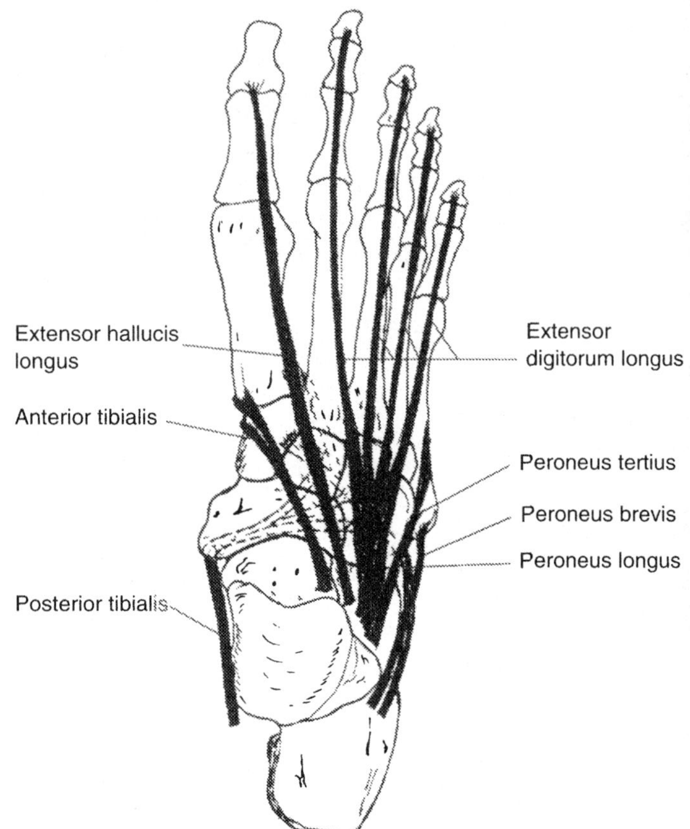

Fig. 2–70 Right foot from above showing tendons.

ing the foot and great toe while extending the lesser toes. The tendons of the extensor digitorum insert into the distal phalanges of the second through fifth toes. To differentiate the peroneus tertius, maintain the above position and add abduction to it. The tendon may be palpated as it inserts into the base and shaft of the fifth metatarsal.

The peroneus longus and brevis tendons may be palpated as they pass through the groove posterior to the lateral malleolus and under the peroneal tubercle on the lateral side of the calcaneus (Fig. 2–71). Rupture of the ligaments may allow dislocation of the tendons from behind the fibula. Palpation is possible by having the patient evert and dorsiflex the foot. Rupture is also possible at the peroneal tubercle, which will allow the tendons to dislocate superiorly. From the tubercle the tendons go their separate ways, with the brevis inserting into the tubercle on the base of the fifth metatarsal. The peroneus longus traverses the calcaneus inferior to the brevis and passes under the cuboid within the peroneal groove, where it is retained by the long plantar ligament. The longus inserts into the lateral side of the bases of the first cuneiform and first metatarsal (Fig. 2–72). Both tendons may be palpated while the foot is fixed and movement toward plantar flexion and eversion is attempted. Place one finger on the fifth metatarsal

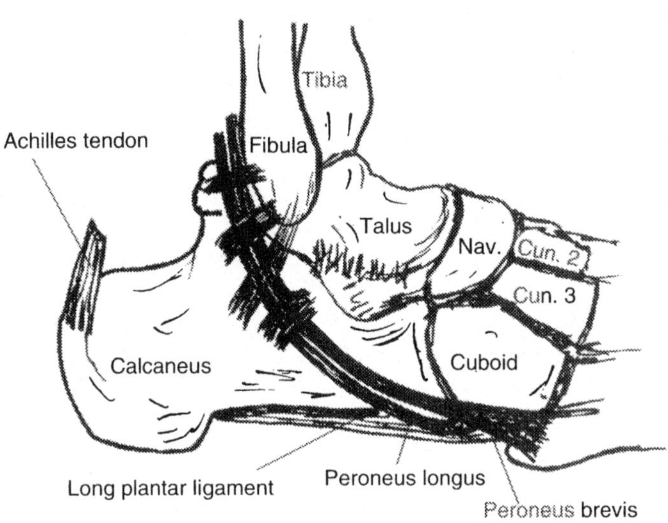

Fig. 2–71 Right foot, lateral view showing peroneal tendons.

base and the other on the proximal border of the cuboid. To identify the brevis even further, add abduction to the movement.

Figure 2–73 shows the relative positions and insertions of the peroneal, anterior tibialis, and extensor hallucis longus

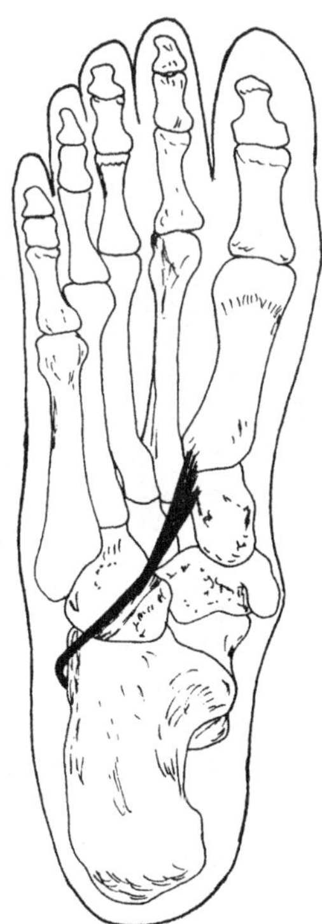

Fig. 2–72 Peroneus longus tendon.

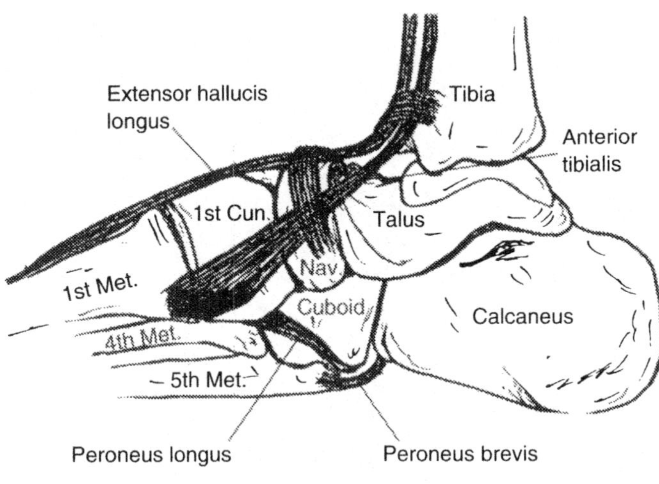

Fig. 2–73 Right ankle and foot, medial-plantar view showing tendons.

muscles. Figure 2–74 shows the relative positions of the three tendons as they pass behind the medial malleolus.

The flexor hallucis longus passes under the sustentaculum tali and then crosses the flexor digitorum longus tendon on its way to the distal phalanx of the great toe (Fig. 2–75).

The flexor digitorum longus tendon, within its sheath, passes the posterior surface of the medial malleolus between the hallucis longus and posterior tibialis tendons in their sheaths. It then passes over the sustentaculum tali, traversing

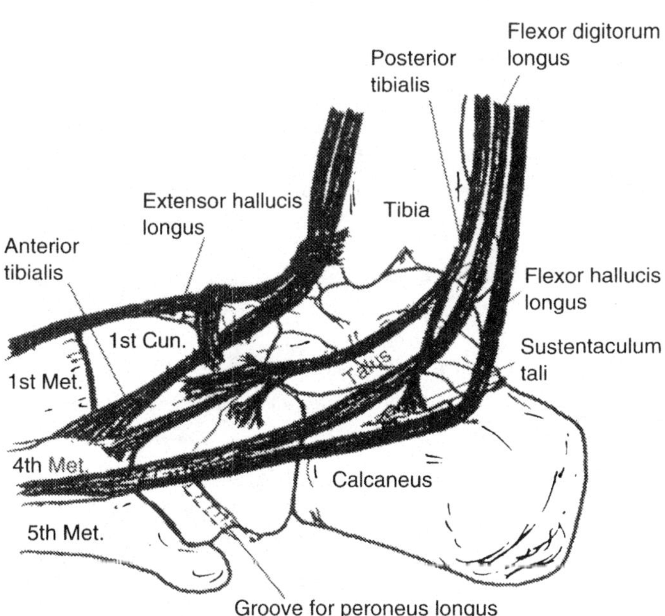

Fig. 2–74 Right ankle and foot, medial-plantar view showing tendons.

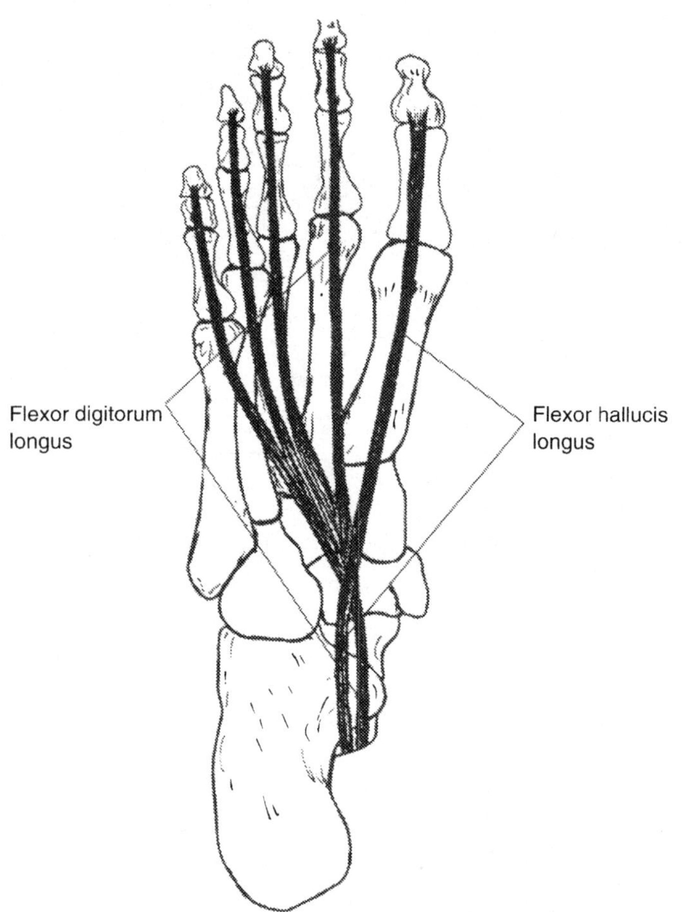

Fig. 2–75 Right foot, plantar view showing tendons.

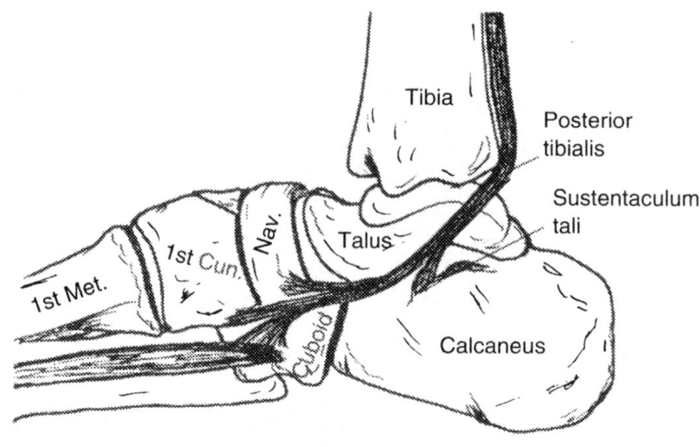

Fig. 2–76 Right ankle and foot, medial-plantar view showing tendons.

from medial to lateral, and inserts into the distal phalanges of digits two to five (Fig. 2–75).

The posterior tibialis tendon, in its sheath, is the most anterior of the three as it passes in the groove on the posterior surface of the tibia (Fig. 2–76). The tendon passes next to the trochlea of the talus, giving off fibers to the sustentaculum tali. The tendon then divides, the larger portion inserting into the tubercle of the navicular with fibers continuing to insert into the first cuneiform. The smaller, deeper division continues and inserts into the second and third cuneiforms and sometimes the cuboid. It also gives rise to the origin of the flexor hallucis brevis muscle. Palpation of the tendon is possible behind the medial malleolus and its course to the tubercle of the navicular. Place the heel on a stool, and have the patient attempt adduction of the foot without plantar flexion or dorsiflexion.

Palpation for Fracture, Ligamental Damage, or Anomaly

If, after the above general examination, fracture, ligamental damage, or anomaly is suspected, careful evaluation with the use of passive motion palpation will allow the examiner to pinpoint the exact location of the site. By pinpointing the articulation that does not move, produces pain, or is hypermobile, it will be possible to obtain more accurate radiographic positioning. This is covered completely in Chapter 5.

REFERENCES

1. Logan AL. *The Knee.* Gaithersburg, Md: Aspen; 1993.
2. Kapandji IA. *The Physiology of the Joints.* New York, NY: Churchill Livingstone; 1970; 2.
3. Alexander I. *The Foot, Examination and Diagnosis.* New York, NY: Churchill Livingstone; 1990.

Chapter 3

Muscle Testing

Muscle testing is essential in the examination of all musculoskeletal problems. A muscle imbalance becomes an important objective finding when it verifies subjective complaints, observation of functional tests, and findings on palpation. Muscle weakness, when found to be a causative factor, becomes important in implementing the correct treatment program.

Testing of an individual muscle is difficult, if not impossible. By isolating a primary muscle, the test must also include the stabilizers and the secondary support muscles.

Muscle testing is the continuation of an active movement by the patient, with the examiner using his or her skill to provide resistance. Resistance should be from a position, and in a direction, to elicit the greatest response by the primary muscle. The skilled examiner will observe the patient's effort and his or her body's reaction during the attempt.

The movement of an articulation requires primary and secondary movers, joint stabilizers, and secondary support muscles stabilizing the bone structures on which the movers originate. A lack of normal strength in muscles other than the prime mover may result in evidence of compensation, adaptation, or abnormal recruitment for stabilization.

Testing of the primary mover may seem normal yet may be accompanied by shifting of body position to give the secondary muscles greater advantage, abnormal muscle reaction by the patient, a shaking of the muscle being tested, or overzealous attempts to secure the rest of the body to support the tested muscle. The prime mover may test weak when a weakness of a secondary muscle does not secure the origin, thus interfering with the normal response. For example, testing of the hip flexors (psoas and iliacus) in the presence of a weak iliocostalis lumborum muscle on the opposite side will result in what tests as weak hip flexors. It will be accompanied by abnormal abdominal movement during the test.

The patient must understand the test being made. Place the patient in a position in which the muscle being tested will have its greatest advantage and have the patient hold the position. Using an open hand (where possible), indicate the direction in which pressure is to be applied. Do not grasp the limb. Grasping makes it difficult for the patient to understand the correct direction. Apply slight pressure, and instruct the patient to resist the movement unless it is painful to do so. Do not pounce on it. Gradually increase pressure to maximum so that the patient has the opportunity to react. Both extremities should be tested and the affected limb compared with the opposite one.

The object of the test is not to determine whether the muscle may be overpowered. It is to determine whether the response corresponds with normal expectations from a patient of the same size, age, and build. A judgment must be made about whether the patient is making the effort called for. This of course is difficult without experience. It is helpful to test other muscles away from the area of complaint first to experience the patient's effort and strength for comparison.

Comparing muscle strength from one side to the other is relatively easy in the normal person. When testing an unusually strong person, such as a body builder, a greater amount of pressure must be applied. If the limb is positioned properly and the pressure is applied in the correct direction, any muscle or group of muscles may be evaluated, even by a small examiner. Comparison with the opposite side while watching for signs of imbalance and muscle tone is essential to obtaining the correct diagnosis. Muscle balance is the key to comfort, not strength.

Muscle tests must not be prejudged by the examiner. If the foot appears to bear more weight on the outside, do not assume that the everters are weak. The examiner must keep an open mind, free to test and observe objectively.

Pain during any part of the test negates the test. It is important to observe the patient closely for reaction and to question the patient. Some patients will not report pain unless asked and will simply make the effort because they were asked to. If pain is present, it is important to know at what part of the test it hurt and the exact location of the pain. If the muscle tests strong yet there is pain, locating the pain may be helpful in identifying a small muscle tear, tendinitis, or bursitis. Pain away from the primary joint being tested might indicate a problem in the support structure.

Recruitment of other muscles may be necessary for the patient to perform the test. Most movements of the body are carried out smoothly with ease and strength and against varying resistance. In the presence of pain, joint dysfunction, or muscle weakness, the body cannot function efficiently. It is forced to use alternative methods to achieve movement when commanded to do so.

Normal movement is replaced with whatever is necessary and possible for the patient to carry out the command. Shifting of the body or unusual movements of other musculature may occur to provide greater leverage to muscles recruited for the function. For want of a better term, I refer to these unusual movements as cheating.

The normally smooth movement may now be supplanted by abnormal direction or hesitation during the course of the movement. Subtle alterations of direction by the patient must be detected and corrected by the examiner. Only with a knowledge of what normal movement is can an examiner detect abnormal movement.

To aid in determining whether a secondary muscle is at fault, give manual assistance to the muscle, or do the job of stabilizing the structure while retesting the primary muscle. If in doubt, retest. A single effort is representative of the patient's ability to perform only once and does not represent the ability to perform the action repeatedly. In injury cases where muscle weaknesses have been demonstrated, I have found that the muscle test should be performed four times consecutively. The fourth test should be normal before the patient is released to return to normal work. If one does otherwise, depending upon only one test, the patient may return to work, perform normally for a short time, and then exacerbate the condition with repeated activity.

Several instruments have been developed in the attempt accurately to test, record, and place a numeric grade on muscle tests. Although interesting, each apparatus I have tested is still dependent upon the skill of the operator, and each of the fac-

tors mentioned above must still be considered. Comparison studies with manual muscle testing tend to conclude that the apparatus eliminates the potential for unwanted bias that could be present when determining muscular strength by manual methods.

One study by Oberg et al[1] used a Cybex isokinetic dynamometer to measure strength at the ankle during plantar flexion and dorsiflexion. The investigators found that they could not evaluate individual muscles but could develop standardization in the testing of muscle groups as functional units. They concluded that this type of evaluation could be helpful in athletic training.

In evaluating a patient, there is much more information to be obtained by objective, manual muscle testing. For instance, in the foot eversion with plantar flexion is performed by the peroneus longus assisted by the brevis (which also abducts the foot). Eversion with dorsiflexion is performed by the extensor digitorum longus and peroneus tertius. Each of these may be isolated by manual testing methods. Testing of eversion with an instrument would by definition include only dorsiflexion. It involves the extensor digitorum longus and peroneus tertius but not the peroneus longus and brevis. The findings could not be expected to be the same. I am not aware of any apparatus that can isolate muscle function as efficiently as manual testing.

When muscle testing reveals a muscle that is weaker than expected, goad the origin and insertion of the muscle and retest. Goading is applying a quick, deep, oscillating pressure by finger or thumb pad without allowing the contact to slide over the skin. If a muscle has had a mild stretch and is just not functioning up to par, it may respond to goading, and that may be all that is necessary. If a muscle is truly weak, goading the origin and insertion may cause a temporary response, with the muscle weakening after several retests.

When a muscle tests weak, there are a number of causes that need to be considered to make a diagnosis. A muscle that tests weak may be mildly stretched as a result of a loss of habit pattern and use. For example, consider the postpartum abdominal muscles. Stretching during pregnancy alters the habit pattern of use and, if not restored, may result in chronic weakness.

A muscle may be stretched sufficiently to inhibit normal function. Prolonged stretching of the popliteus muscles while sitting with the heels resting on a foot stool and the knees extended without support can create a weakness. A muscle may simply be weak from lack of use. It may test weaker than its opposite or its antagonist. It can also test weak if there is a loss of fulcrum in the joint. A lateral fixation of the patella can weaken the quadriceps.

Muscle function can be inhibited by fixations. Fixations (see Appendix A) are articulations that have no movement without necessarily being out of alignment or subluxated. Certain fixation patterns can affect specific muscles. Two examples that have been shown clinically are an anterior atlas fixation with the occiput affecting the dorsiflexors of the ankle and causing a weakness, and an L-5 fixation causing weakness of the gluteus maximus.

Organic problems (see Appendix A) also can affect muscle strength. Hypertonic muscles can test weak. A good example is finding a hypertonic psoas, proved by the Thomas test, weak upon testing.

Trauma can obviously cause variable degrees of damage and loss of function. Minimal stretching, without fiber damage, can inhibit normal function and may only require light exercise to remind the muscle to return to work. Mild trauma can cause a reaction even without any damage. A knuckle blow to the deltoid may cause no damage other than a slight bruising but may create a weakness that can linger.

A mild strain, with a few fibers torn, may test at 80% of normal without significant pain. There may even be no palpable evidence of a lesion. A moderate strain will have damage sufficient enough to be palpable. Testing produces pain and little functional response. Severe injuries can cause large tears with palpable depressions in the contour of the muscle. Surgical repair may be necessary.

Tears may occur within the bulk of the muscle, at the junction of the muscle and tendon, or from the muscle's origin or insertion. The tendon itself can tear or separate from its bony attachment, or the periosteum can be torn from the underlying bone.

Although the examiner must keep in mind the many things that may influence a test, the ability to test the muscle and to determine whether it is normal is important. If a muscle fails to respond normally, the examiner has to investigate all possibilities to reach a proper diagnosis and to treat successfully.

Normal dorsiflexion (Fig. 3–1) is 20°. Before testing the individual muscles of dorsiflexion (peroneus tertius, extensor digitorum longus, extensor hallucis longus, and anterior tibialis), test the group as a whole (Fig. 3–2). Use the forearm placed proximal to the toes to test. The dorsiflexors should be strong enough for you to pull the patient footward on the table without any give in the muscle. Clinically it has been shown that if an anterior fixation of the atlas (with the occiput) is present the dorsiflexors, as a group, may test weak even though individually they may test strong. This should be evaluated and corrected before one proceeds with the evaluation.

The anterior tibialis muscle (Fig. 3–3) is a strong dorsiflexor and inverter of the foot as well as one of the strong supporters of the medial longitudinal arch. The tendon is easily recognized as the patient inverts and dorsiflexes the foot. To test (Fig. 3–4), place the foot into dorsiflexion and inversion and have the patient flex the great toe to remove the extensor hallucis longus as a factor in the test (Fig. 3–3). The anterior tibialis is innervated by L-4 with some L-5 fibers. Individuals with an extreme weakness will display a drop-foot

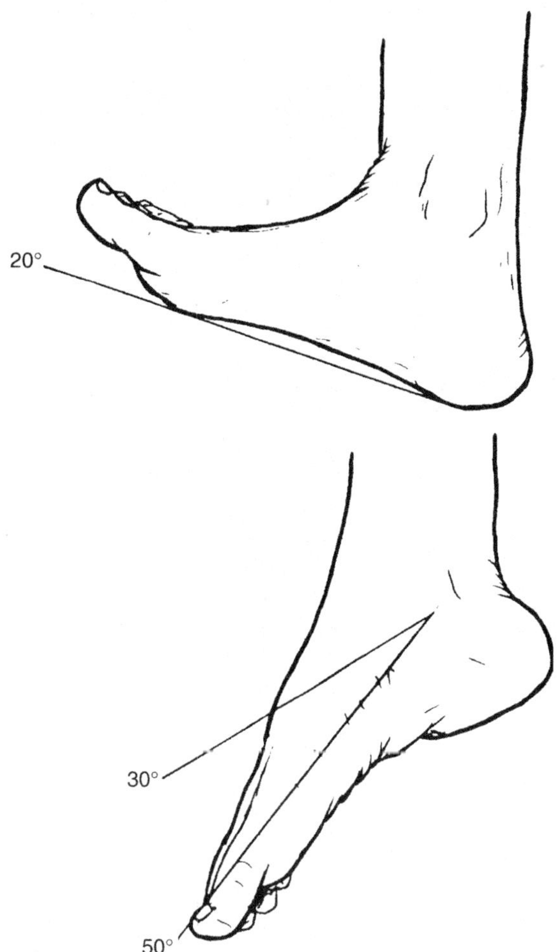

Fig. 3–1 Range of motion in dorsiflexion and plantar flexion.

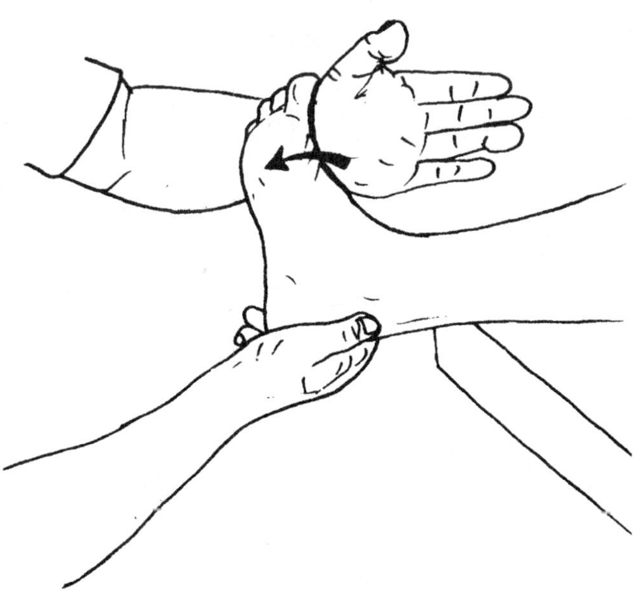

Fig. 3–2 Dorsiflexor test.

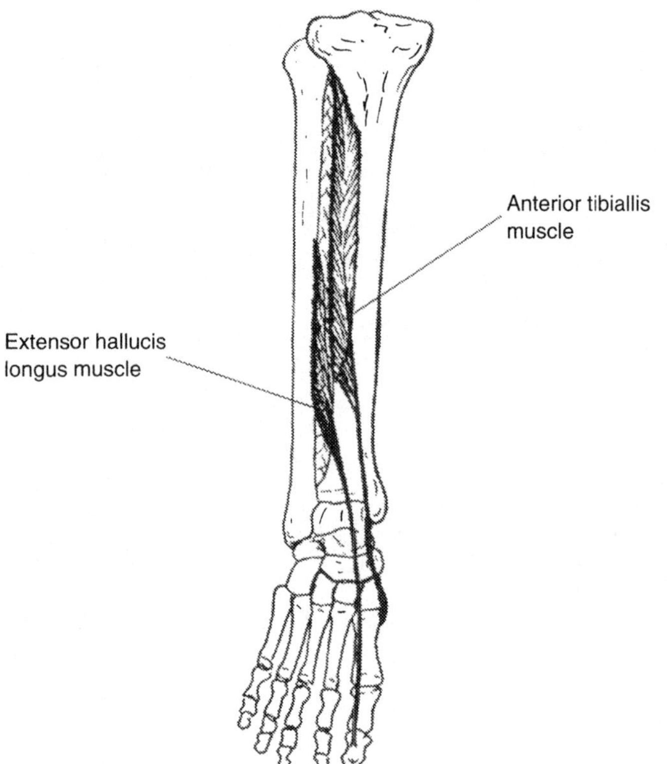

Fig. 3–3 Right leg and foot, anterior view.

gait. Anterior tibialis weakness may also be associated with urethral problems and is a common finding in patients with incontinence (see Appendix A).

Test the extensor hallucis longus with the support hand on the plantar surface of the foot, instructing the patient to keep the foot rigid (Fig. 3–5). Place the great toe into extension and use the pads of two fingers, one on each phalanx, to test the muscle. The extensor hallucis longus is innervated by the deep peroneal nerves (L-5 and S-1).

The peroneus tertius (Fig. 3–6) may be considered merely an extension of the extensor digitorum longus, originating just

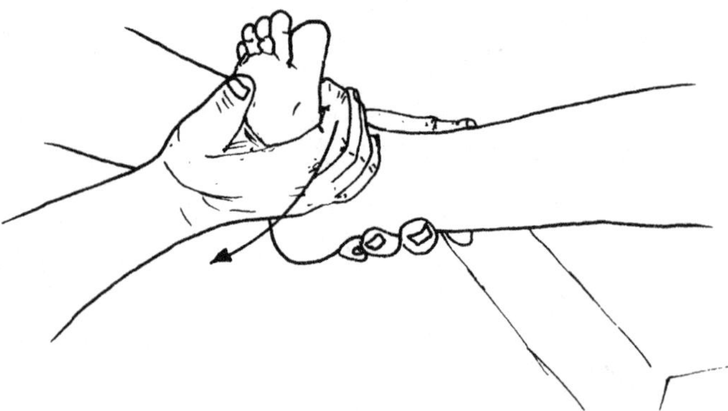

Fig. 3–4 Anterior tibialis test.

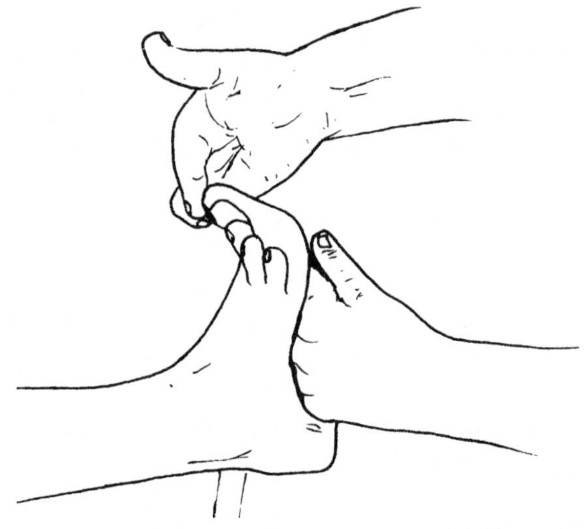

Fig. 3–5 Extensor hallucis longus test.

below it on the fibula. Their tendons join under the superior retinaculum, and their innervation is the same (L-5 and S-1).

To test the extensor digitorum longus, place the hand over the four metatarsals and digits (Fig. 3–7) and place the foot into dorsiflexion and eversion. Although isolation of the peroneus tertius tendon is possible for identification, isolation for testing is not.

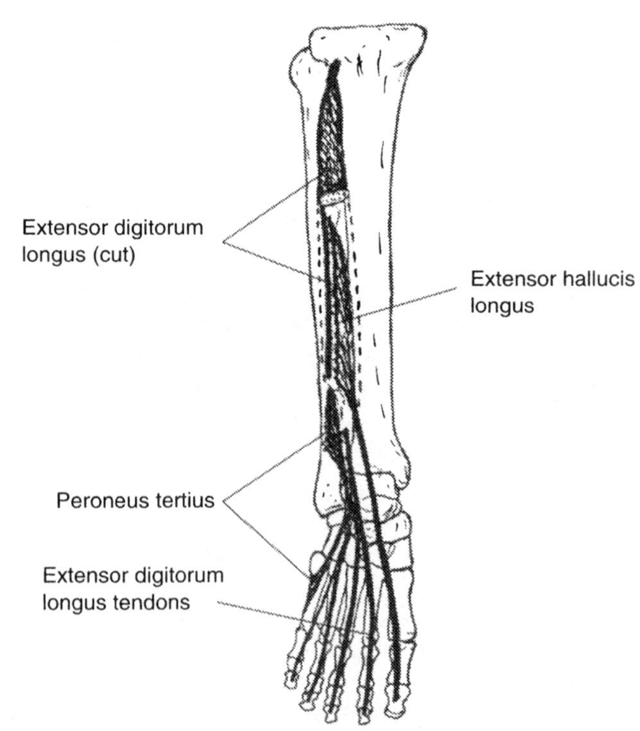

Fig. 3–6 Extensor muscles of the right leg and foot, anterior view.

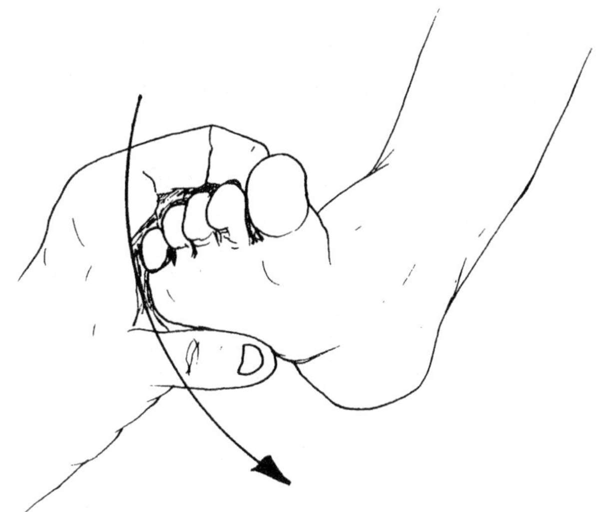

Fig. 3–7 Extensor digitorum longus and peroneus tertius test.

Weakness of the dorsiflexor-everters may be associated with bladder problems (see Appendix A). An apparent weakness may be the result of a weak biceps femoris muscle not supporting the fibula and affecting the origin of the muscles being tested. This should be ruled out in the evaluation.

Test the flexor hallucis longus (Fig. 3–8) with the support hand securing the forefoot. Do not allow the patient to flex the

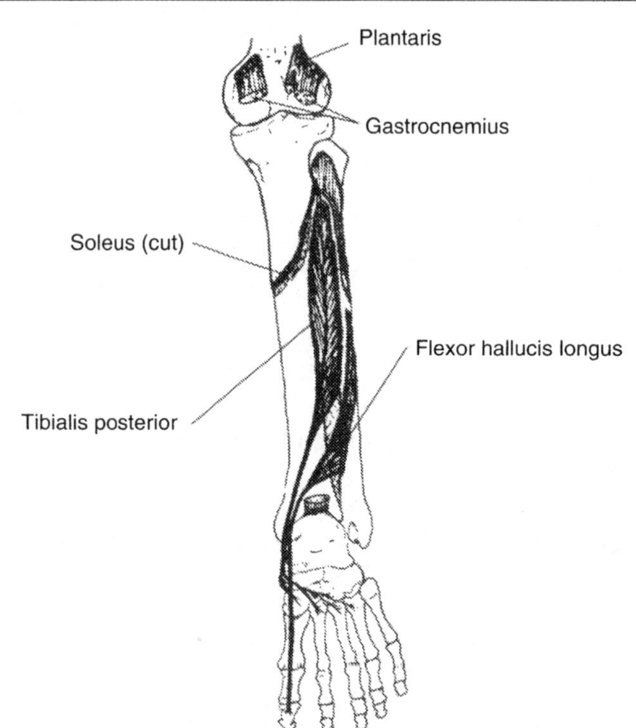

Fig. 3–8 Right leg and foot, posterior view.

foot. Place the great toe into flexion and test (Fig. 3–9). A weak flexor hallucis longus will affect the gait because it provides the power for toe-off.

The peroneus longus muscle (Fig. 3–10) is the direct opposite of the anterior tibialis; it functions in eversion and plantar flexion. To test, place the foot into plantar flexion and eversion and apply pressure in the opposite direction (Fig. 3–11).

The peroneus brevis is primarily an abductor-everter, assisting the longus. Test by placing the foot into abduction, and have the patient resist pressure in the opposite direction (Fig. 3–12).

Test the flexor digitorum longus with the support hand securing the foot. Make sure that the patient does not flex the foot. Have the patient flex the four lesser toes and test (Fig. 3–13).

The posterior tibialis muscle is a strong adductor of the foot as well as an inverter and plantar flexor. Recall from Chapter 1 that it has a complex insertion on several tarsal bones (Fig. 3–14). It is the main support of the tarsal arch and, with the anterior tibialis, maintains the medial arch during standing and balancing and throughout the stance phase of the gait. When testing, eliminate as much of the gastrocnemius muscle function as possible. The knee should be flexed to 100° or more. Place the foot into inversion and plantar flexion. Instruct the patient to extend the large toe to remove the flexor hallucis longus as a factor. Grasp the forefoot and, with the patient's resistance, apply pressure into dorsiflexion and eversion with the emphasis on eversion (Fig. 3–15). This muscle is hard to isolate because of the strong triceps surae. The anterior tibialis is also a factor, but it is a dorsiflexor.

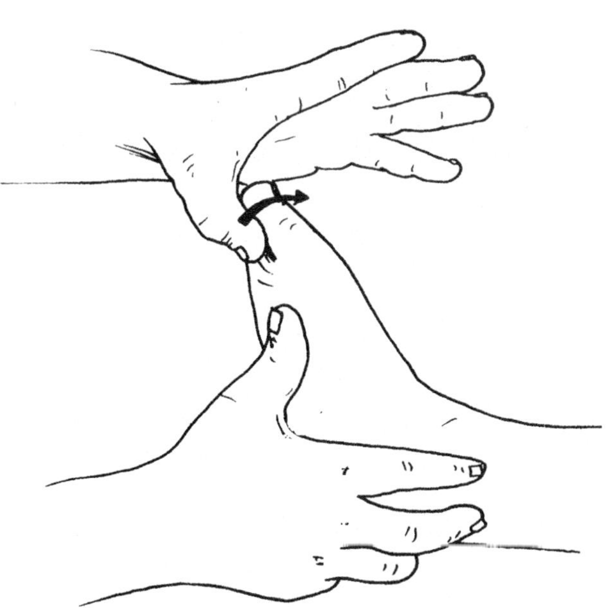

Fig. 3–9 Flexor hallucis longus test.

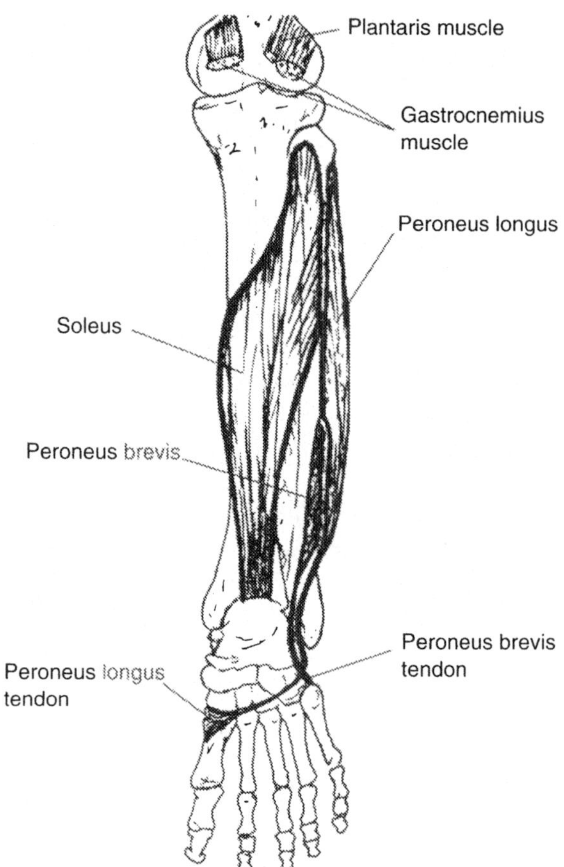

Fig. 3–10 Extensor muscles of the right leg and foot, posterior view.

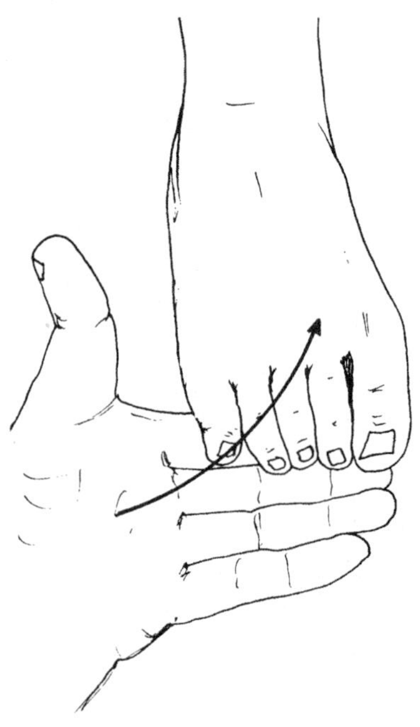

Fig. 3–11 Peroneus longus test.

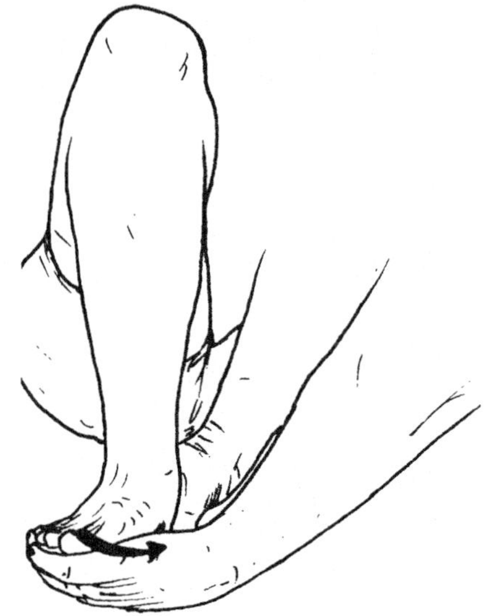

Fig. 3–12 Peroneus brevis test.

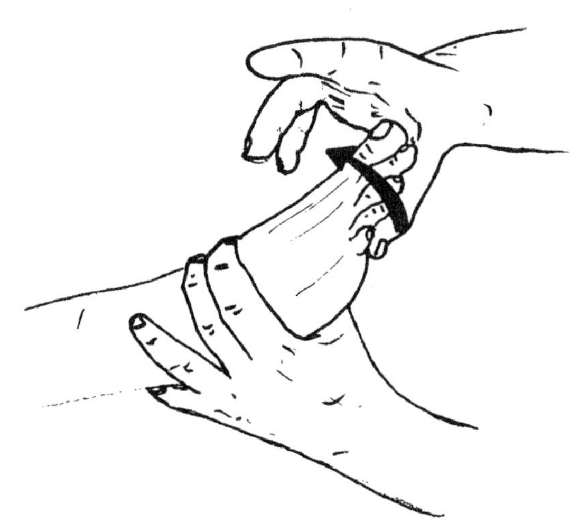

Fig. 3–13 Flexor digitorum longus test.

Another method of testing the posterior tibialis includes testing of the popliteus muscle as well. Place the heel on the table surface with the foot adducted. The examiner's hand should be under the forefoot to prevent the patient from dorsiflexing or plantar flexing the foot during the test. Abduct the foot against resistance without any ankle flexion (Fig. 3–16). This tests the posterior tibialis and the popliteus muscles together.

The triceps surae, comprising the gastrocnemius, soleus, and plantaris muscles, are the strong plantar flexors of the ankle (Fig. 3–17). The plantaris cannot be isolated for testing. The soleus may be tested with limited gastrocnemius influ-

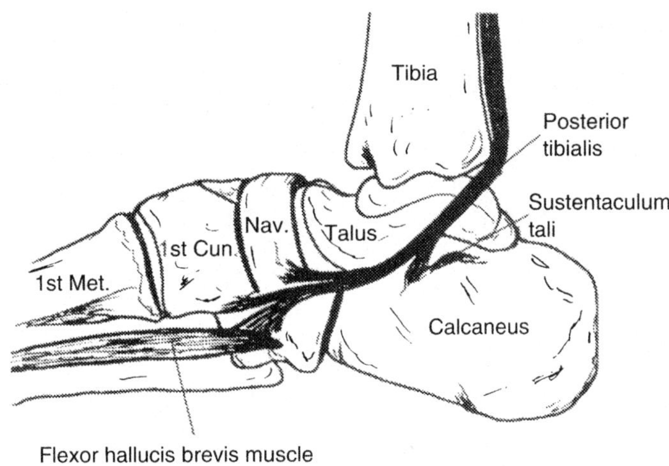

Fig. 3–14 Right ankle and foot, medial-plantar view.

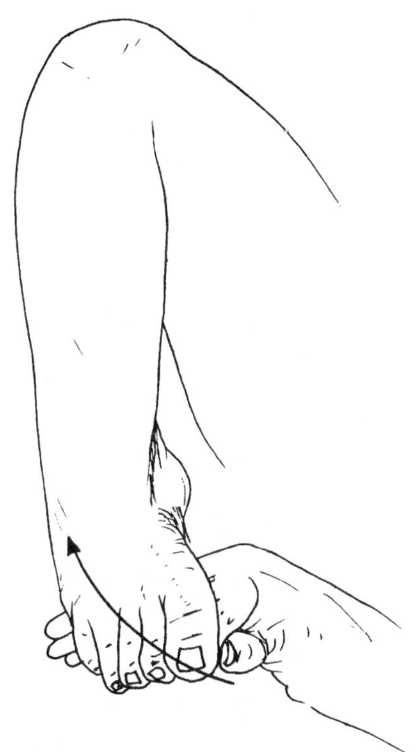

Fig. 3–15 Posterior tibialis test.

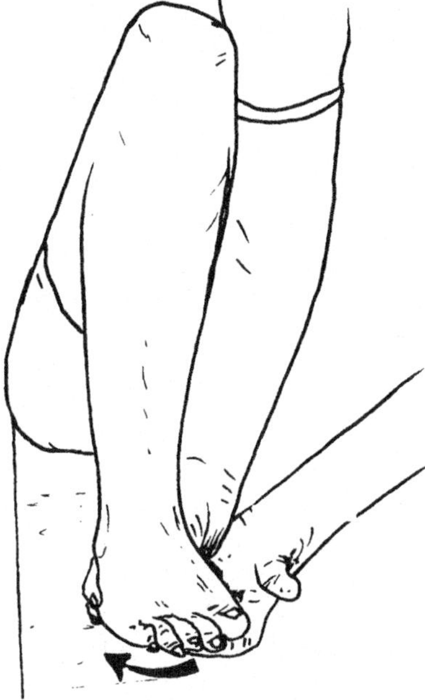

Fig. 3–16 Posterior tibialis test with adduction.

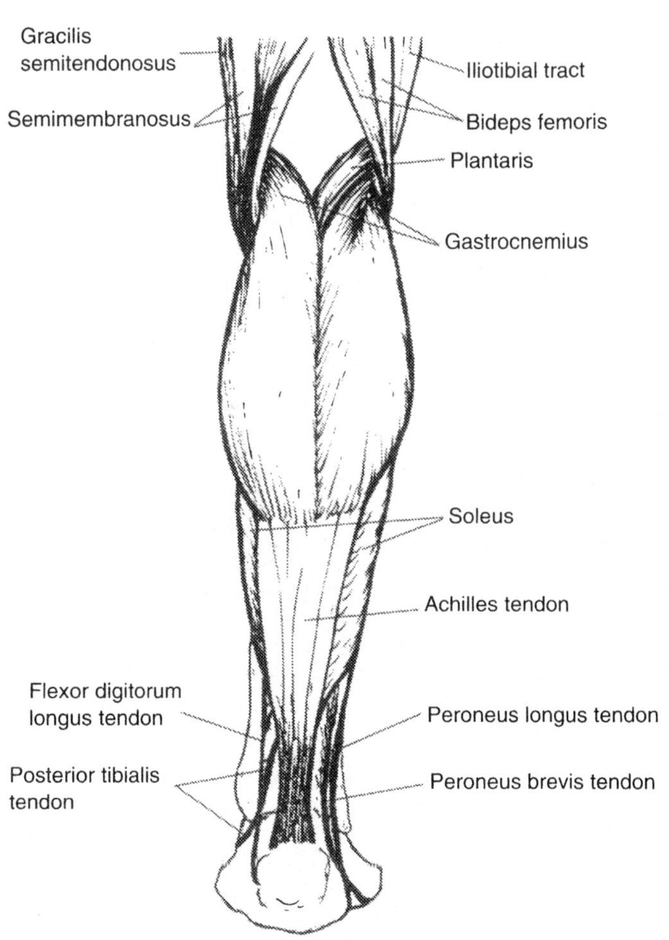

Fig. 3–17 Right leg, posterior view.

ence by flexing the knee past 100° (Fig. 3–18). Testing of the gastrocnemius (Fig. 3–19) is not possible without including the soleus and represents a test of the triceps surae as a group. The gastrocnemius, because of its two origins on the femur, may be strained or stretched unilaterally, as in a valgus knee, which will elongate the medial head. During the test, it must be kept in mind that the Achilles tendon turns on itself. The

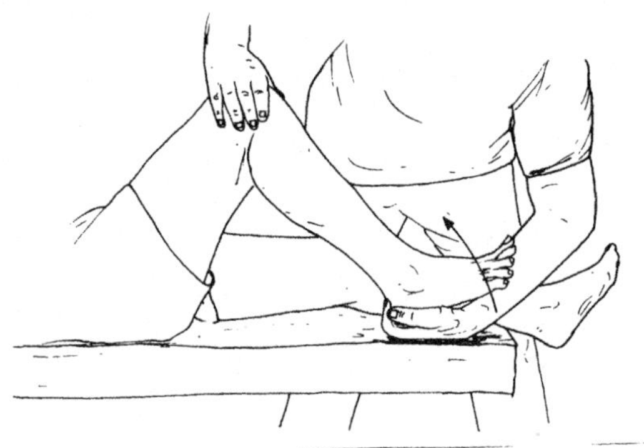

Fig. 3–18 Soleus test.

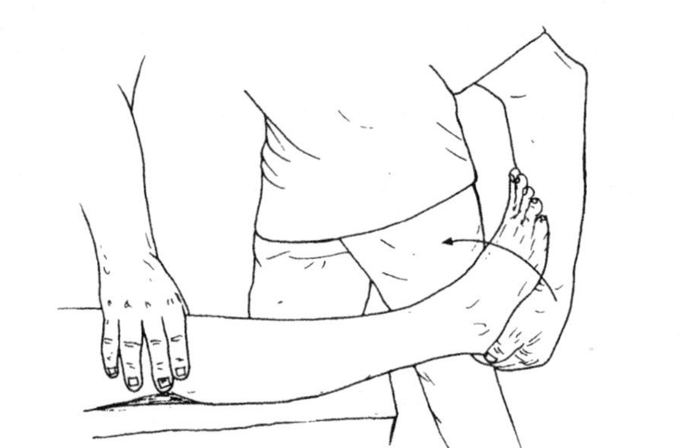

Fig. 3–19 Gastrocnemius test.

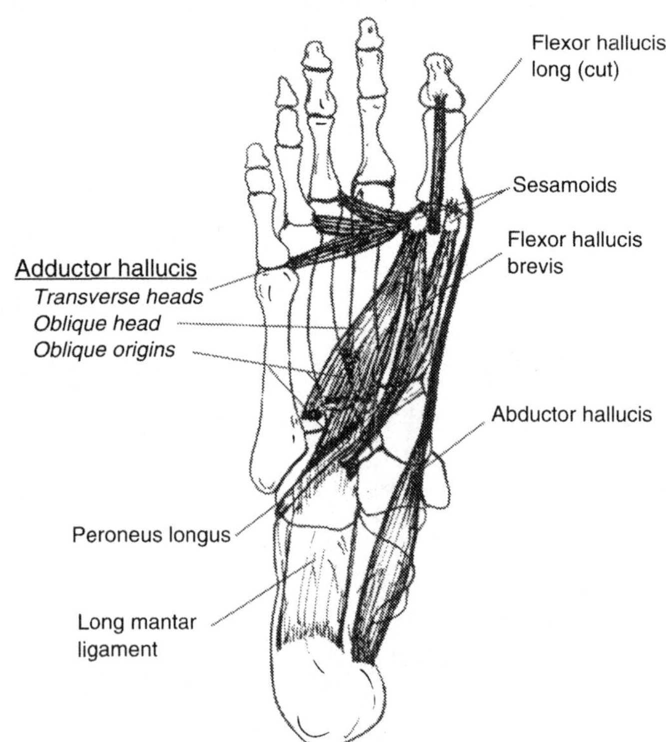

Fig. 3–20 Right foot showing deep muscles of the plantar surface.

tendons arising from the medial head are on the lateral side of the calcaneus insertion.

The strength of the adductor hallucis (Fig. 3–20) is much easier to test than that of the abductor. Test by placing a finger between the great toe and the second digit and asking the patient to squeeze and apply pressure medially (Fig. 3–21).

Test the abductor hallucis. With the foot resting on the table, secure the great toe and ask the patient to adduct the foot (Fig. 3–22). If the abductor hallucis is normal, the first digit will remain straight, without giving, during the test.

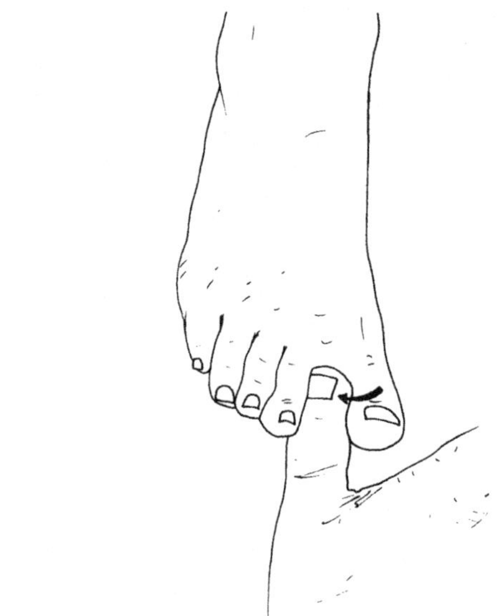

Fig. 3–21 Adductor hallucis test.

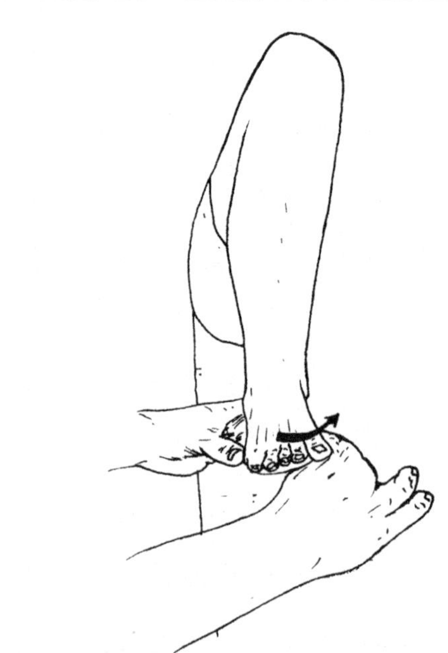

Fig. 3–22 Abductor hallucis test.

Muscle testing is an important part of the examination. Fixations and malfunction may be the direct result of muscle dysfunction. Foot problems are often the result of postural stress, as indicated in previous chapters. Testing and exercising procedures for muscles indirectly affecting the foot are discussed in Chapters 7 and 8.

REFERENCE

1. Oberg B, Bergman T, Tropp H. Testing of isokinetic muscle strength in the ankle. *Med Sci Sports Exerc.* 1989;19:318–322.

Chapter 4

Imaging

Lindsay J. Rowe, MAppSc (Chiropractic),
MD, DACBR (USA), FCCR (Can),
FACCR (Aust), FICC

This chapter reviews imaging of the most common abnormalities of the foot and ankle. Available imaging modalities are numerous, and many are utilized in the detection of specific disorders.

IMAGING METHODS

Plain Film Radiography

Standard radiography of the foot and ankle requires a minimum of frontal and lateral projections. Supplemental examinations are important to evaluate more anatomically complex regions, such as the tarsal structures.

Technical Considerations

A high-definition imaging system is required for the foot and ankle because of the anatomic detail needed. Kilovoltage should be between 50 and 60 kVp with fine-detail or single-emulsion extremity screens and films.

Ankle

Routine evaluation of the ankle includes the anteroposterior (AP), lateral, and mortise (15° to 20° internal oblique) views.

Thanks to Pat Leyland at the Medical Communications Unit, University of Newcastle and Royal Newcastle Hospital for Orthopedic Disorders for the fine photographic reproductions. Thanks to Sue Smith for her typographic expertise, Villadsen Health Services, and Kath Danes and Belinda of the John Hunter Hospital, Newcastle, for assistance with the literature and use of computer facilities.

AP view. The patient is supine with the foot placed vertically and slight dorsiflexion of the ankle. The central beam is perpendicular to the cassette and centered over the tibiotalar joint 1 to 2 cm proximal to the malleoli.[1] This demonstrates the tibiotalar joint and the distal tibia and fibula (Fig. 4–1). The talar dome and joint space are clearly visualized. The inferior tibiofibular articulation is not well demonstrated, but this is overcome with the medial oblique view.

Medial oblique view. Alternative names for this view include internal oblique and mortise. From the AP projection, the ankle is internally rotated 15° to 20°.[1] Dorsiflexion of the foot should also be maintained. The central beam is perpendicular to the cassette and centered over the tibiotalar joint 1 to 2 cm proximal to the malleoli.[1] This view demonstrates the entire talar dome, the fibulotalar joint, the lateral margin of the distal tibia, and the posterior portion of the lateral talar facet (Fig. 4–2).

Lateral view. The ankle is placed flat on the cassette with the medial side upward and in slight dorsiflexion. To ensure a true lateral view, it is necessary to have support under the knee. The central beam is perpendicular to the cassette and centered 1 to 2 cm proximal to the tip of the medial malleolus.[1] The base of the fifth metatarsal should be included.

The lower third of the tibia and fibula, the talar dome, the posterior subtalar joint, and the posterior malleolus are readily identified (Fig. 4–3). The base of the fifth metatarsal should also be closely inspected if visible because this is a common site for fracture after ankle trauma (eg, Jones' fracture). The pre-Achilles fat pad is identified as a large, triangular, radiolucent region anterior to the tendon. Hemorrhage and

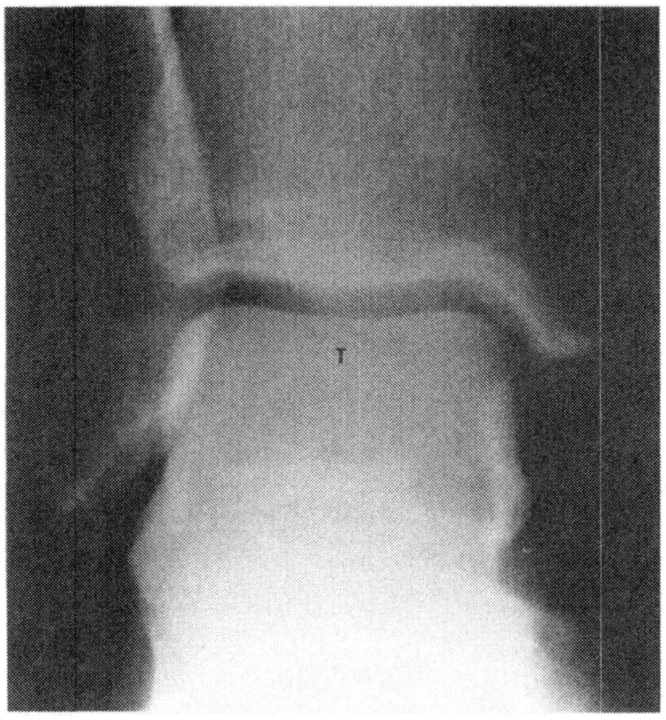

Fig. 4–1 Normal AP ankle. The distal tibia, fibula, and contained talar dome (T) are clearly demonstrated. Observe the congruous joint surfaces of the tibiotalar joint. The articular surface of the tibia is referred to as the plafond. *Comment:* The structures of the ankle are clearly demonstrated, although the tibiofibular joint and the lateral tibial margins are obscured, which requires inspection on the medial oblique view.

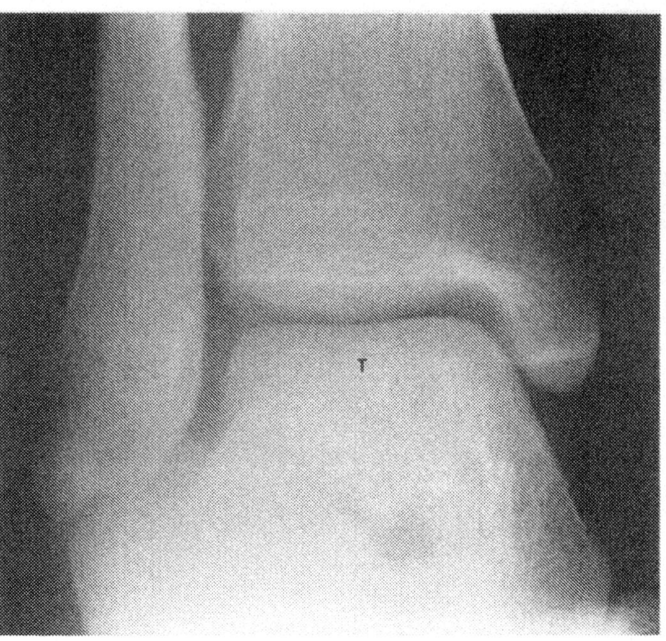

Fig. 4–2 Normal medial oblique ankle. With the foot rotated medially 15° to 20°, the entire ankle mortise can be identified. Note the depiction of the distal tibiofibular joint, the lateral tibia, both malleoli, and the talar dome (T). *Comment:* This is an extremely important view in cases of trauma to exclude a talar dome, distal fibular, or tibial fracture.

edema will infiltrate or distort this fat pad.[2] Ankle effusion is demonstrated as a teardrop-shaped soft tissue mass anterior to the tibiotalar joint.

Supplemental views. Ligamentous injury after trauma can be assessed with carefully obtained stress views. Varus–valgus stress views evaluate the medial and lateral stability of the ankle joint. In the AP position the ankle is placed into the varus and valgus positions, and the exposure is made in these positions. Comparison radiographs of the ankle are mandatory. A normal talar tilt up to 5° can be seen.[3] Criteria for instability include a 3-mm difference in the joint space[3–5] or a 10° difference in talar tilt between the injured and normal sides.[5, 6] AP (drawer) stress views are done in the lateral projection to indicate anterior talofibular ligament injury (positive drawer sign). A difference of 2 mm or more in comparison with the normal side suggests significant injury.[7]

Foot

Routine study of the foot includes AP (dorsiplantar), oblique, and lateral views.

AP view. The foot is place flat on the cassette. The central beam is positioned on the distal third metatarsal with the beam directed 15° cephaled.[1] A 1-mm aluminum filter can be utilized to prevent overexposure of the distal metatarsals and phalanges.[8] The osseous structures and articular relationships of the tarsometatarsal, metatarsophalangeal, and phalangeal joints are well demonstrated (Fig. 4–4).

Oblique view. With the knee flexed, the patient internally rotates the limb so that the lateral aspect of the foot is elevated 30° off the cassette.[1] A 30° wedge may be used for support. The central beam is perpendicular to the cassette and centered over the third metatarsal. This view separates the third to fifth tarsometatarsal joints, which are overlapping on the AP view (Fig. 4–5). The talonavicular and calcaneocuboid joints are also well seen. The sinus tarsi is also demonstrated.

Lateral view. The lateral aspect of the foot is placed against the cassette. The plantar surface of the foot should be perpendicular to the cassette. The central beam is directed through the tarsometatarsal junction. The tibiotalar joint, tarsal articulations, calcaneus, and forefoot are all well seen (Fig. 4–6).

Supplemental views. Phalanges, AP, oblique and lateral phalangeal views can be obtained with appropriate positioning and collimation for the axial calcaneal view.

In the supine position the foot is dorsiflexed as tolerated. This position may be supported with a strap beneath the forefoot held by the patient. The central beam is angled 40°

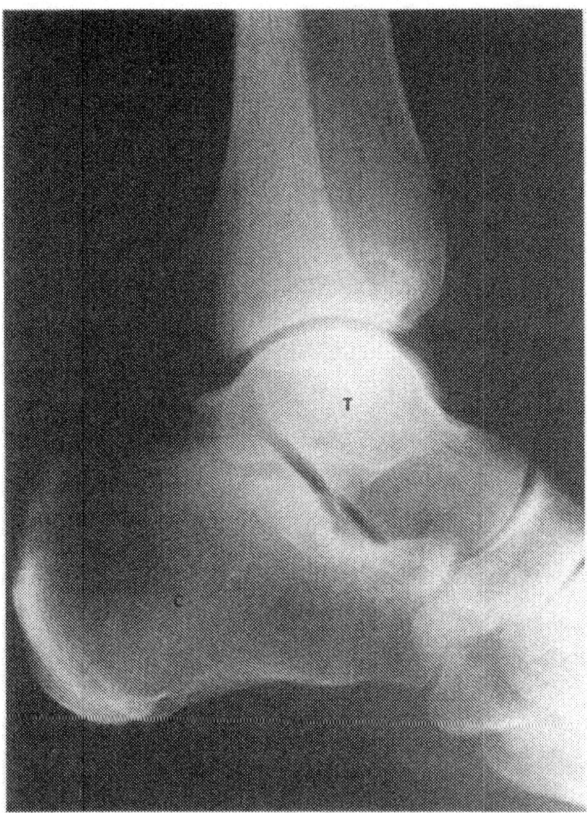

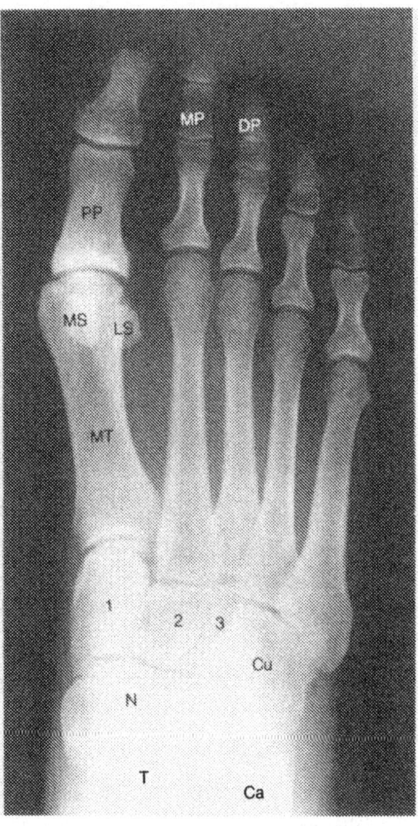

Fig. 4–3 Normal lateral ankle. The distal tibia, fibula, talar dome (T), calcaneus (C), and adjacent tarsal bones can all be identified. *Comment:* The soft tissues anterior and posterior to the ankle mortise should be observed with a bright light to identify evidence of effusion or edema.

Fig. 4–4 Normal AP foot. The bony and articular structures of the foot can be identified: head of talus (T), calcaneus (Ca), navicular (N), cuboid (Cu), cuneiforms (1, 2, 3), metatarsals (MT), medial (MS) and lateral (LS) sesamoids, and proximal, middle, and distal phalanges (PP, MP, DP). *Comment:* Note the overlapping structures at the tarsometatarsal junction, especially the third cuneiform and the second to fourth metatarsal bases. The medial oblique view shows these more clearly.

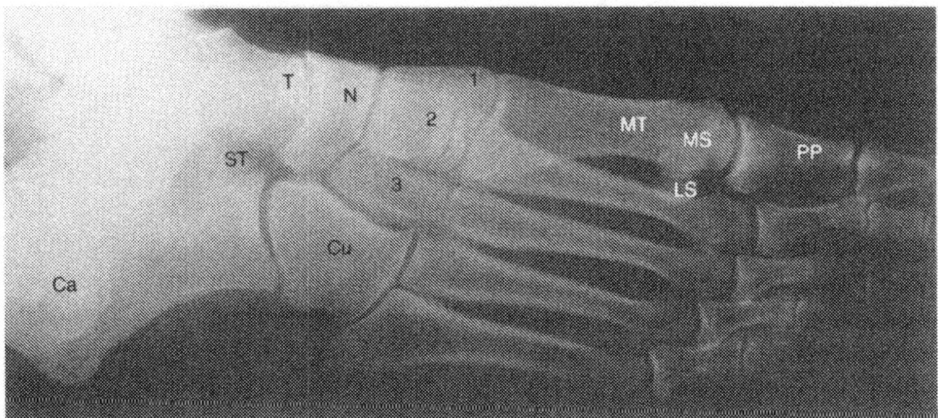

Fig. 4–5 Normal oblique foot. The osseous and joint components are depicted slightly differently. Observe the calcaneus (Ca), sinus tarsi (ST), head of talus (T), navicular (N), cuboid (Cu), cuneiforms (1, 2, 3), metatarsals (MT), medial (MS) and lateral (LS) sesamoids, and proximal phalanx (PP). *Comment:* Details of the tarsal bones, their joints, and their relationships are defined. Note the clarity of the tarsometatarsal junction, which is obscured on the AP view. The base of the fifth metatarsal is also effectively shown.

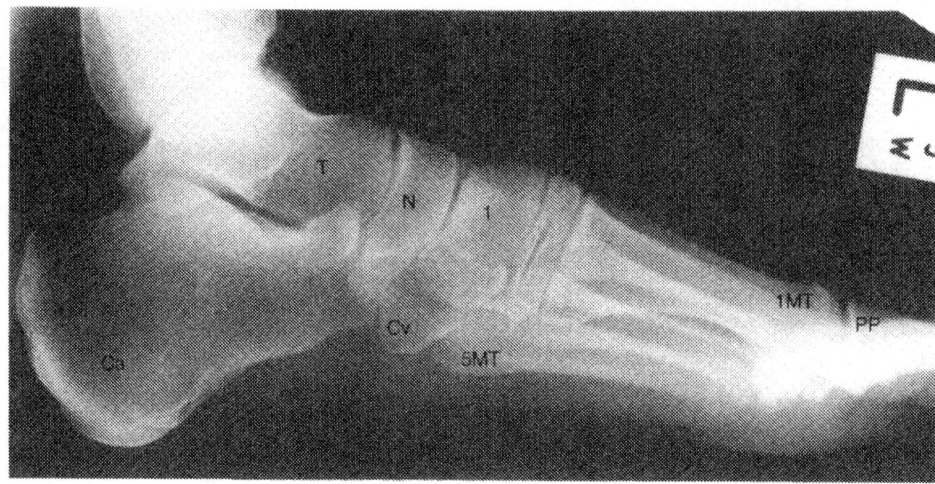

Fig. 4–6 Normal lateral foot. Note the calcaneus (Ca), head of talus (T), navicular (N), cuboid (Cu), first cuneiform (1), first metatarsal (1MT), fifth metatarsal (5MT), and proximal phalanx (PP). *Comment:* The bones and articulations of the hindfoot and midfoot can be seen, although considerable overlap of structures obscures some of them. This is most pronounced in the forefoot.

---

cephaled through the plantar surface of the fifth metatarsal base.[1,8] The calcaneus is portrayed in a PLAN projection; this is an especially useful view in identifying fractures (Fig. 4–7).

For the lateral calcaneal view, the central beam is centered on the calcaneus.

A wide variety of the techniques have been described for evaluation of the subtalar joint.[9–11] A tangential view of the hallux sesamoids is obtained with the foot dorsiflexed and the central beam directed through the plantar surface of the first metatarsal head.[12]

Anterior and weight-bearing views are obtained to evaluate structural changes that may not be detected on non–weight-bearing views. Modifications of the X-ray apparatus is often required for these views, especially to allow for the tube to be lowered significantly.

Arthrography

Technique

A joint is entered with a 22-gauge needle under local anesthetic anteriorly and medial to the dorsalis pedis artery.[3] Fluid is aspirated and is sent for laboratory examination. Between 6 and 8 mL of water-soluble medium is injected. If double-contrast technique is utilized, 1 mL of contrast medium is combined with 6 to 8 mL of air. After the injection, the ankle is exercised and observed fluoroscopically. Films are taken in the AP, lateral, and oblique projections. Stress views should also be taken during the procedure.[13]

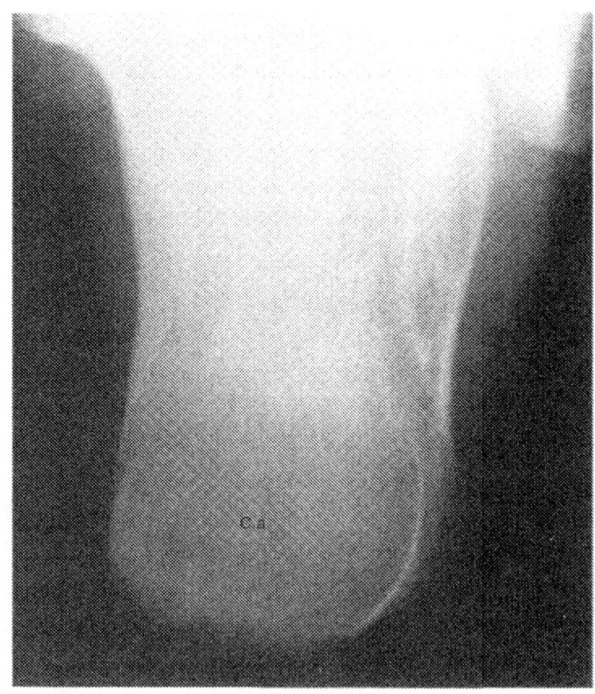

Fig. 4–7 Axial view of the calcaneus. The calcaneus (Ca) is depicted in a PLAN projection, which shows clearly its internal matrix and cortical margins. *Comment:* The axial view is especially useful in the detection of fractures because the cortices are seen in a tangential projection, so that their disruption or offset is more readily appreciated.

Applications

Ankle arthrograms are most frequently performed on patients with suspected ligamentous injury.[14] Arthrograms are useful for demonstrating other abnormalities, including articular cartilage lesions (talar dome fractures, osteochondritis dissecans), loose bodies, arthritis, and adhesive capsulitis.[3,7,15]

Computed Tomography

Technique

Computed tomography (CT) images of the foot and ankle are obtained with the feet perpendicular to the gantry table. The knees are extended, and the great toes are together.[16,17] For coronal images, the knees are flexed with the feet flat against the gantry table. Specific tarsal bones and joints may require a foot wedge, angling of the gantry, or both.

Typical examinations are performed using 5-mm thick slices, 120 kVp, and 20 to 50 mA with 3- to 5-second scan times. Thinner (1.5-mm) slices provide superior detail for reconstructions.

Applications

CT provides excellent bone detail and assessment of the complex articulations of the foot and ankle. It is the technique of choice for examination of the subtalar joint.[18,19] CT is also useful for imaging neoplasms of the foot and ankle. Magnetic resonance (MR), however, is the imaging method of choice for these lesions. Acute skeletal trauma and posttraumatic arthropathy, especially of the hindfoot (including the calcaneus), are well demonstrated with CT. CT is not helpful for soft tissue injury, such as ligamentous tears.[20]

MR Imaging

Technique

Images can be obtained in the coronal, sagittal, and oblique planes. A circumferential extremity coil is employed to achieve the maximum signal-to-noise ratio and the best spatial resolution.[21] Comparison with the opposite extremity should be included. In most situations, selection of T1- and T2-weighted sequences will provide the necessary diagnostic information.

Applications

Its superior soft tissue contrast, multiple image planes, excellent spatial resolution, and noninvasive nature give MR many advantages in foot and ankle imaging. MR is most commonly employed for evaluating neoplasms, trauma, infection, avascular necrosis, and chronic pain of unknown etiology.[22,23] It is particularly useful in the demonstration of ligament, tendon, cartilage, soft tissue, and even bone abnormalities.[24]

Nuclear Bone Scans

Technique

The two major radionuclides are *technetium* (^{99m}Tc) and *gallium* (^{67}Ga). ^{67}Ga scans are the method of choice in the evaluation of osteomyelitis. After intravenous injection of the isotope, the patient is placed under a scintillation camera, which detects gamma rays emitted from the body. A triphasic study is usually obtained with images immediately after injection (flow or perfusion study), within a couple of minutes (pool study), and a couple of hours later (delayed study). Special software can allow reformatting with tomography to provide improved image quality and multiplanar depiction (single-photon emission computed tomography or SPECT).

The isotope is absorbed onto the hydroxyapatite crystals within the bone matrix. For patients with suspected infection, a three-phase bone scan is of greatest value.[25] Areas of increased bone activity result in a concentration of the isotope. In a normal scan there is increased uptake within the metaphyses, particularly near joints. Similarly, the growth epiphyses will demonstrate increased uptake. Abnormalities such as fracture, infection, or tumor are depicted as focal areas of isotope concentration referred to as hot spots. In avascular necrosis a cold defect is demonstrated immediately on infarction and is followed by increased uptake during revascularization and repair.[26]

Applications

Nuclear medicine has high sensitivity and delivers a low radiation dose.[27] Bone scanning is utilized primarily for the diagnosis of trauma, particularly stress fractures, avascular necrosis, infection, tumors, compartmental evaluation of degenerative joint disease, and painful prosthesis or bone graft.[28] Tarsal coalition can be demonstrated with bone scan and confirmed with CT.[29] One of the major problems in the foot and ankle is the normal variations in isotope uptake of the developing growth centers.

MEASUREMENTS

Many lines and angles have been utilized for the assessment of foot and ankle disorders.[30] As in all body locations, measurements provide a guide only and cannot be the sole criterion for performing any specific treatment.[31] Length measurements on the AP film are influenced by the longitudinal arch, which foreshortens structures, although the lateral view is slightly more reliable.[31]

Ankle

Toygar's Angle

The Achilles tendon lies close to the overlying skin, such that the skin contour reflects the tension and integrity of the tendon. Normally the skin forms an obtuse angle (Toygar's angle) of at least 150° open posteriorly. When the Achilles tendon is disrupted, the skin contour becomes more concave, reducing the angle to less than 150°.[32]

Tibiotalar Joint Space

The gap between the tibial and talar joint surfaces is measured at the lateral and medial joint margins (Fig. 4–8). This should be done on varus–valgus stress studies, on which there should not be more than a 3-mm difference between the normal and injured sides.[7]

Talar Tilt

A line tangential to the talar dome and another along the adjacent tibial surface are drawn (Fig. 4–8). In the neutral position, greater than 6° indicates significant ligamentous injury. On valgus–varus stress views the normal range is 5° to 23°. If there is more than 10° difference when the right is compared with the left, this also indicates significant ligamentous damage.[33,34] An anterior drawer of 4 mm is also indicative of instability.[35]

Achilles Tendon Thickness

On a lateral view the thickness of the Achilles tendon is 4 to 8 mm at its attachment and 1 to 2 cm above.[36] Edema from inflammatory arthritis can thicken the ligament.

Fowler-Philip Angle

On a lateral view of the calcaneus, two lines are drawn. One line connects the posterosuperior margin with the tuberosity for the Achilles insertion; the other is drawn from the inferoposterior surface to the inferoanterior surface of the calcaneus (Fig. 4–9). The normal angle subtended is between 44° and 69°. Angles greater than this predispose to retrocalcaneal bursitis.[7]

Boehler's Angle

On a lateral view of the calcaneus, two tangential lines are drawn connecting the anterior, middle, and posterior tuberosities on the superior surface of the calcaneus (Fig. 4–9). The angle posteriorly is normally between 28° and 40°. A value less than 28° denotes a significant fracture deformity.[7,37]

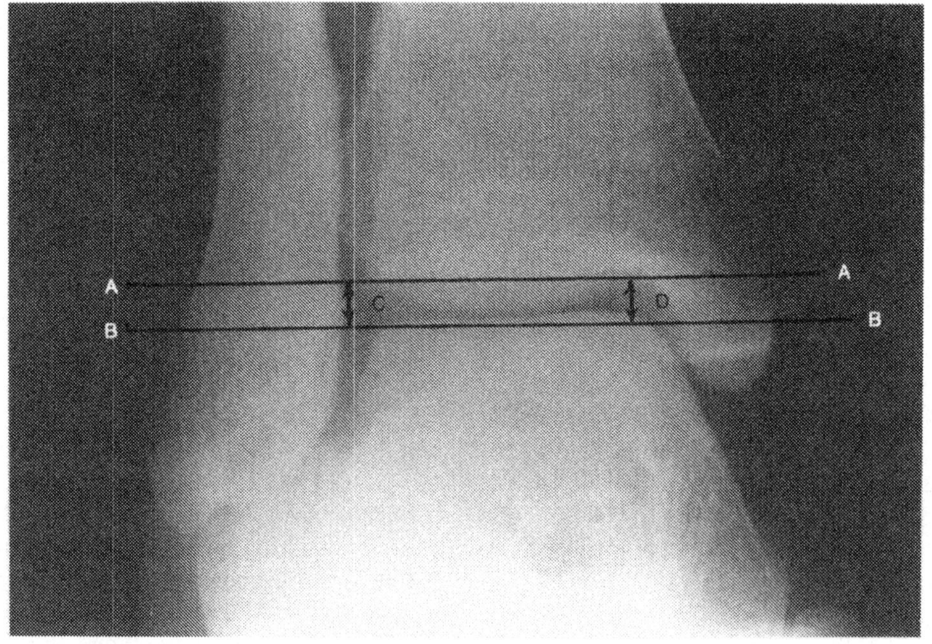

Fig. 4–8 AP measurements of the ankle: talar tilt. A line tangential to the tibial surface (*A–A*) and another along the adjacent talar dome surface (*B–B*) are drawn. These define the tibiotalar joint space. The gap between the tibial and talar joint surfaces is measured at the lateral (*C*) and medial (*D*) joint margins. *Comment:* Talar tilt can normally range up to 6° in the neutral position, and on valgus–varus stress views the normal range is 5° to 23°. If there is more than a 10° difference when the right is compared with the left, this also indicates significant ligamentous damage. The joint space should also be measured on varus–valgus stress studies, on which there should not be more than a 3-mm difference between the normal and injured sides.

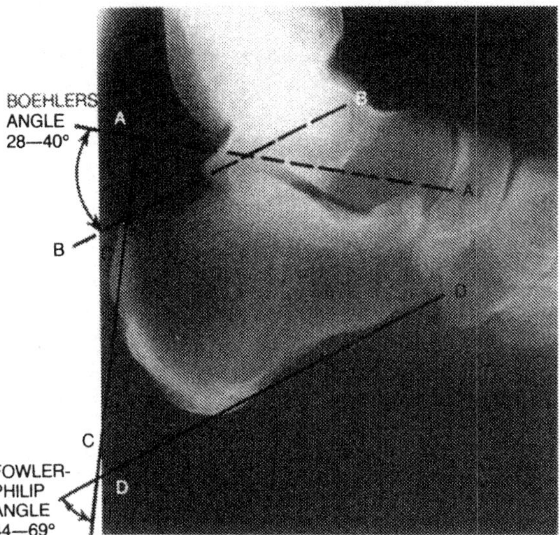

Fig. 4–9 Lateral calcaneal measurements. (1) *Boehler's angle.* Two tangential lines (*A–A* and *B–B*) are drawn connecting the anterior, middle, and posterior tuberosities on the superior surface of the calcaneus. The angle posteriorly is normally between 28° and 40°. (2) *Fowler-Philip angle.* Another line connects the posterosuperior margin with the tuberosity for the Achilles insertion (*C–C*), and a fourth is drawn from the inferoposterior surface of the calcaneus to the inferoanterior surface (*D–D*). The normal angle subtended is between 40° and 69°. *Comment:* A Boehler angle less than 28° denotes a significant fracture deformity. A Fowler-Philip angle greater than 69° predisposes to retrocalcaneal bursitis.

Tibial Slant

A line is drawn through the midshaft of the tibia and is intersected by another line made tangential to the articular surface of the tibia. These should be close to 90°.

Heel Pad Thickness

The measurement from the inferior surface of the calcaneus of the skin line is made at the narrowest dimension. If it exceeds 25 mm, this may indicate the presence of acromegaly.[7,37]

Axial Angles

The angle formed by the intersection of a line tangential to the surface of the talar dome with the articular surfaces of the tibia and fibula indicates the stability of the joint. The talofibular angle range is 43° to 63°, and the talotibial angle is 45° to 65°.[7,37]

Foot

On the AP view of the foot, a number of measurements can be obtained (Fig. 4–10).

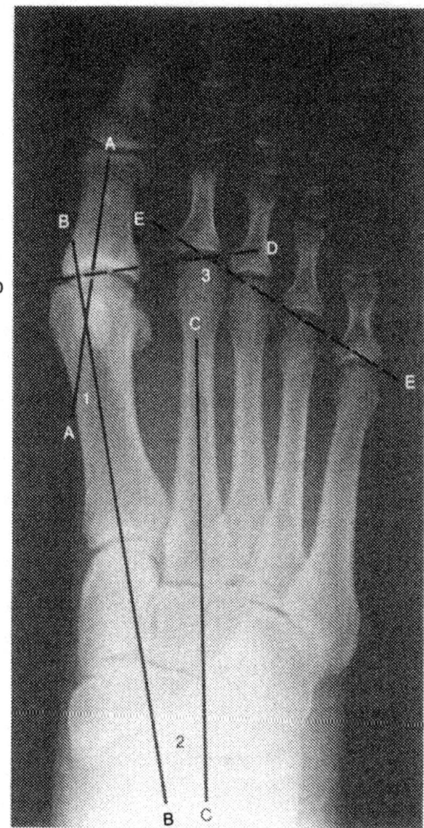

Fig. 4–10 AP foot measurements. (1) *Hallux abductus angle.* Two lines are drawn, with each line bisecting the shaft of the proximal phalanx (*A–A*) and the first metatarsal (*B–B*). The angle formed by their intersection is normal when it is 0° to 15°. (2) *Intermetatarsal angle.* Two lines drawn through the center of the first (*B–B*) and second (*C–C*) metatarsal shafts should diverge at 14°. (3) *Metatarsal angle.* A line is drawn intersecting the metatarsal head articular surfaces from the first to second (*D–D*) and fifth to second (*E–E*) rays. The angle subtended should be around 140°. *Comment:* A hallux abductus angle greater than 15° signifies hallux valgus. An intermetatarsal angle greater than 14° is usually associated with hallux valgus. A metatarsal angle of 140° demonstrates an even weight distribution in the forefoot.

Hallux Abductus Angle

Two lines are drawn, with each line bisecting the shaft of the proximal phalanx and the first metatarsal. The angle formed by their intersection is normal when it is 0° to 15°. An angle greater than 15° signifies hallux valgus.[7]

Intermetatarsal Angle (Metatarsus Primus Adductus Angle)

Two lines are drawn through the center of the first and second metatarsal shafts. These lines should diverge at 14°.[7]

Metatarsal Angle (Parabola)

A line is drawn intersecting the metatarsal head articular surfaces from the first to second and fifth to second rays. The angle subtended should be around 140°, demonstrating an even weight distribution in the forefoot.[7,8]

CONGENITAL ANOMALIES AND VARIANTS

Accessory Bones

Accessory bones are parts of prominences of the tarsal bones that are separated from the normal bone (Fig. 4–11). Accessory bones are secondary centers of ossification or result from nonunion of a fracture. They are usually asymptomatic and must be distinguished from fractures. Occasionally acute or repetitive trauma may initiate a fracture of the ossicle, separate it from its anchoring mechanism, or irritate adjacent tendons to cause a painful clinical syndrome.[38] The most common sites for this to occur are the hallux sesamoids, the os tibiale externum, the os peroneum, and the os trigonum.

Os Trigonum (Secondary Talus, Accessory Talus, or Os Intermedium Tarsi)

This bone is located at the posterior aspect of the talus (Fig. 4–12). It is called the os trigonum because it frequently appears triangular in shape. The flexor hallucis longus tendon passes in the groove of the os trigonum. The posterior tibio-talar and talofibular ligaments as well as the posterior capsule of the ankle and subtalar joints are attached to this ossicle. The bone is present in approximately 10% of the population, is usually bilateral, is variable in size, and is occasionally bipartite.

Os Sustentaculum

This is a small pyramidal ossicle located at the posterior and medial side of the sustentaculum tali.

Os Tibiale Externum (Accessory Scaphoid, Secondary Scaphoid, Accessory Navicular, or Secondary Navicular)

The ossicle lies at the medial aspect of the navicular and is usually bilateral. It is seen in 10% of children and fuses in all but 2% of adults. The area between the ossicle and the navicular is filled with connective tissue or fibrocartilage and at times may be a true joint space. The tibialis posterior tendon inserts into the ossicle rather than into the normal navicular site. As such this ossicle may be associated with pain if there is disruption, and with loss of the muscle action a pes planus may develop.

Os Supranaviculare (Dorsal Talonavicular Ossicle or Pirie's Ossicle)

This ossicle is usually triangular, lying within the joint space of the dorsal margin of the talonavicular joint.

A

B

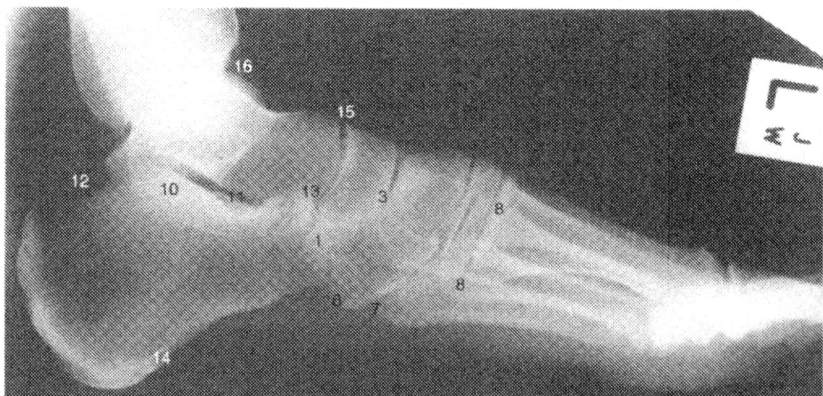

Fig. 4–11 Accessory bones of the foot. 1, os tibiale externum; 2, processus uncinatum; 3, os intercuneiforme; 4, pars peronea metatarsalia; 5, cuboides secundarium; 6, os peroneum; 7, os vesalianum; 8, os intermetatarseum; 9, supratalare; 10, talus accessories; 11, os sustenaculum; 12, os trigonum; 13, calcaneus secundarium; 14, os subcalcis; 15, os supranaviculare; 16, os talotibiale. *Comment:* Recognition of these ossicles is important to avoid confusion with fractures. Additionally, these accessory structures can develop painful clinical syndromes, which require close inspection of their appearance and location.

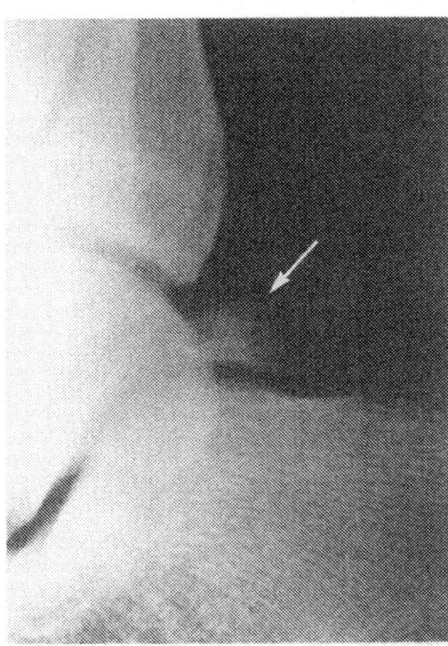

Fig. 4–12 Os trigonum. Note that the triangular bone is located at the posterior aspect of the talus (arrow). The posterior tibiotalar and talofibular ligaments as well as the posterior capsule of the ankle and subtalar joints are attached to this ossicle. *Comment:* An os trigonum is present in approximately 10% of the population, is usually bilateral, is variable in size, and is occasionally bipartite. It should not be confused with an intraarticular loose body.

Os Intermetatarseum (Os Intermetarsali)

This is usually an elongated ossicle located between the proximal ends of the first and second metatarsals.

Calcaneus Secondarium

At the dorsal and distal end of the calcaneus, an ossicle is placed to articulate with the cuboid and navicular bones.

Os Peroneum

This ossicle can be oval in shape and lies close to the cuboid within the tendon of the peroneus longus.

Os Vesalianum

This ossicle lies at the base of the fifth metatarsal. In children a secondary epiphysis forms close by, and in adults a fracture (Jones' fracture) through the base of the fifth metatarsal may simulate this bone.

Os Fibulare

At the distal tip of the fibula a solitary ossicle or multiple accessory ossicles can occur.

Os Tibiale

At the distal tip of the tibia a solitary ossicle or multiple accessory ossicles can occur.

Calcaneal Apophysis

The ossification of this secondary growth center begins in girls between 4 and 7 years of age and in boys between 7 and 10. Before its appearance, the opposing surface of the calcaneus is irregular and saw-toothed in appearance. The apophyses develop from multiple centers that subsequently coalesce to form one irregular apophysis, which may be traversed by fissures (Fig. 4–13). Before fusion of the apophysis to the calcaneus, the former is considerably more dense than the body of the latter. This appearance must not be confused with Sever's disease, an overuse syndrome that, contrary to some earlier reports, is not an osteochondrosis and has no radiographic findings.[39]

Pseudocyst of Calcaneus

A well-demarcated triangular area of lucency that may be delineated by a sclerotic line is often seen in the midportion of the calcaneus[40,41] (Fig. 4–14). A well-pronounced radiolucency may be seen in 7% of calcanei, a moderate one in 22%, and a faint one in up to 70%.[41] If this process is not too prominent, the differentiation between this variation and a simple bone cyst can be made.[40,42] A contained, circular, vascular foramen seen on a lateral projection is often found in the pseudocyst but not in other calcaneal lesions.[40] Further differentiation of the pseudocyst from a pathologic process is usually possible because the lesion is without symptoms referable to this location.

Irregularity of the Navicular

The navicular is the last of the tarsal bones to ossify and often possesses multiple ossification centers (Fig. 4–15). It commonly does not develop symmetrically bilaterally. Differentiation from avascular necrosis (Köhler's disease) is difficult and must be based on the presence of pain and residual bone deformity of the navicular.[43]

Fifth Metatarsal Apophysis

The secondary growth center at the base of the fifth metatarsal lies parallel to the long axis of the shaft. Between the ages of 5 and 12 years, this may simulate a fracture. Fractures in this region are transverse in orientation, however, allowing easy differentiation.

Bone Islands

Numerous terms have been used to describe these focal sclerotic bone lesions, including *enostosis*. These are asymptomatic, have no sex predilection, and can be found at any age. Approximately 10% of bone islands are found in the feet.[44] Approximately 30% change size when they are followed over a period of time. The majority range in size from

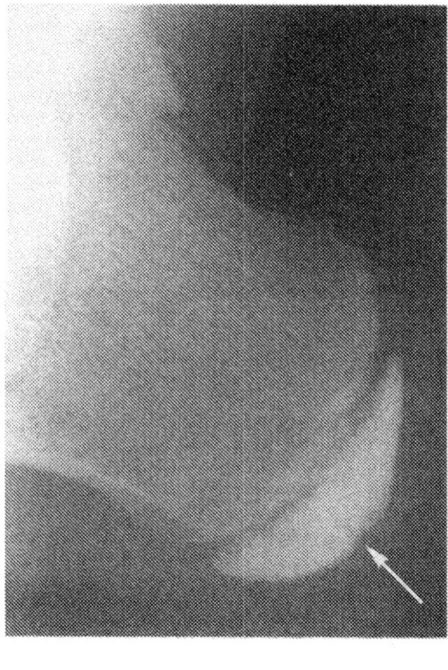

A

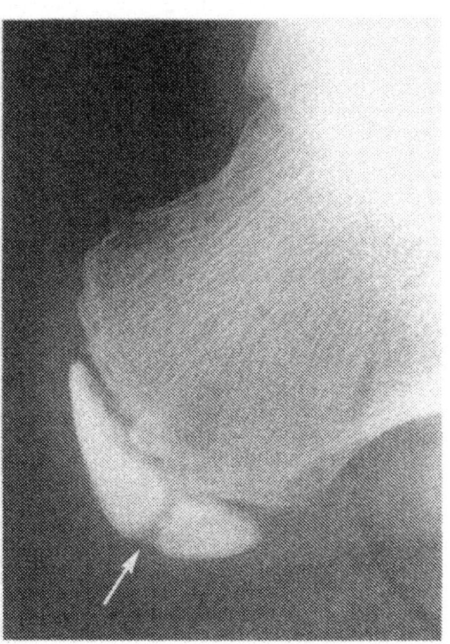

B

Fig. 4–13 Normal variant, calcaneal apophysis. In this 10-year-old boy the calcaneal apophyses bilaterally are densely sclerotic. (A) The apophysis is a single bony mass (arrow). Note the irregularity of the junction zone with the body of the calcaneus. (B) On the other side there is a cleft through the apophysis, which is a common variation (arrow). *Comment:* The apophyses develop from multiple centers that subsequently coalesce to form one irregular apophysis, which may be traversed by fissures. The ossification of this secondary growth center begins in girls between 4 and 7 years of age and in boys between 7 and 10 years.

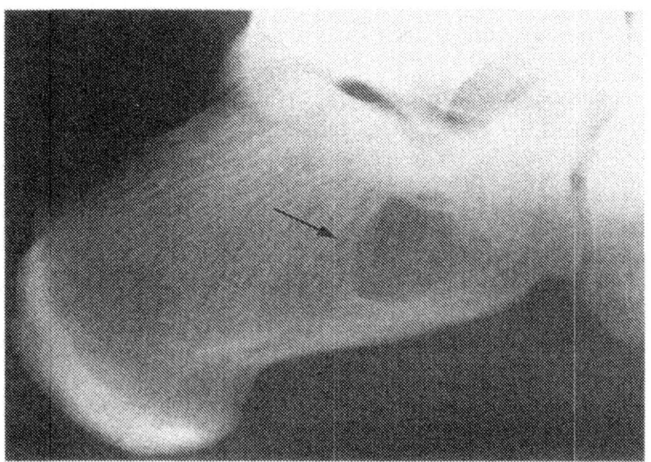

Fig. 4–14 Pseudocyst of the calcaneus. A well-demarcated triangular area of lucency is seen in the midportion of the calcaneus (arrow). *Comment:* A well-pronounced radiolucency may be seen in 7% of calcanei, a moderate one in 22%, and a faint one in up to 70%. Differentiation between this variation and a simple bone cyst can be difficult.

0.5 to 1.5 cm and are densely sclerotic. The margins are often spiculated (brush border; Fig. 4–16). They occasionally may be active on bone scans.[45]

Polydactyly

There is wide variation in forms of polydactyly. They may occur as an isolated finding or be associated with congenital dysplasias, such as Down and Ellis–van Creveld syndromes. Bilateral involvement is present in 50% of cases.[46] Polydactyly is termed preaxial if it is on the tibial or great toe side and postaxial if it is on the fibular or little toe side. Postaxial types account for 80%, preaxial for 15%, and central ray for 5%.[47]

Tarsal Coalition

The term *tarsal coalition* is applied to the condition where there is a bony, cartilaginous, or fibrous fusion between two or more tarsal bones with loss of motion between them.[48] It is a failure of segmentation of the primitive embryologic mesenchyme. It afflicts at least 1% of the population.[48] Approximately 40% of patients will have a first-degree relative with a similar condition, and it is bilateral in up to 80% of cases.[49]

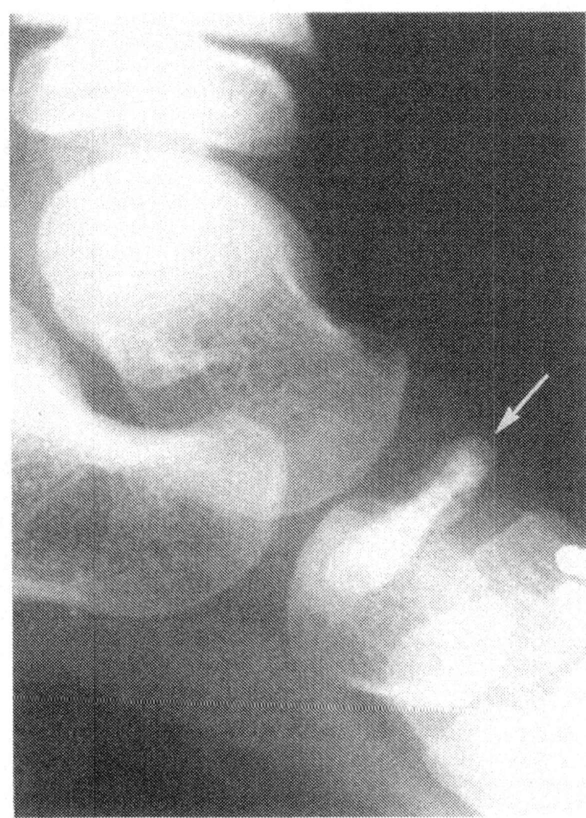

Fig. 4–15 Irregularity of the navicular. The navicular in this 5-year-old child is irregular, sclerotic, and fragmented (arrow). This is a normal growth variation. *Comment:* Differentiation from avascular necrosis (Köhler's disease) is difficult and must be based on the presence of pain and residual bone deformity of the navicular.

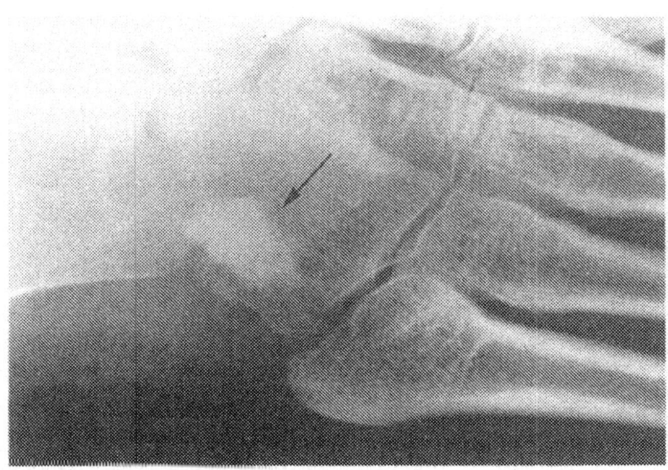

Fig. 4–16 Bone island in the cuboid. A distinct sclerotic focus is visible within the cuboid (arrow). Scrutiny of its margins shows its spiculated nature (brush border). *Comment:* Approximately 10% of bone islands are found in the feet. They need to be distinguished from osteoid osteoma.

They may be asymptomatic or cause vague foot pain, especially after standing or exercise. Muscle spasm, restricted subtalar mobility, and pes planus or cavus can all be associated.

The most common type of coalition is the calcaneonavicular fusion.[48] Less common fusions occur at the talocalcaneal, talonavicular, and calcaneocuboid joints. Rare sites include the cuboidonavicular, naviculocuneiform, talocuboid, and cuboidocuneiform articulations. CT and bone scans are usually required to determine accurately the site of coalition.[48] At the site of coalition a bony bridge can be seen. In the presence of cartilaginous or fibrous union, the cortical margins are irregular and lack cortical definition. The method of choice for tarsal coalition is CT scan. A coronal scan with 2- to 4-mm contiguous slices will usually demonstrate the site of union.

Calcaneonavicular Coalition

The medial oblique view of the foot is required for diagnosis; the bony bridge extending between the calcaneus and navicular can be seen.[48] Secondary signs include hypoplasia of the talar head.

Talocalcaneal Coalition

The most common sites for fusion are at the middle facets. On conventional radiographs the coalition is usually obscured. A lateral projection and specific subtalar views, although useful, may not show the abnormality. CT is usually necessary for diagnosis.

Associated radiographic features of talocalcaneal coalition have been described.[48,50] These include a talar beak, narrowing of the posterior talocalcaneal space, rounding of the lateral process of the talus, failure to see the middle facet of the subtalar joint on the lateral view, asymmetry of the anterior part of the subtalar joint, and ball-and-socket tibiotalar articulation. The talar beak is a bony projection extending ventrally that bridges the talonavicular articulation; it is a reliable sign of tarsal coalition (Fig. 4–17).

TRAUMATIC DISORDERS

Soft Tissue Trauma

Soft tissue injuries of the foot and ankle are common. The most frequent injury is disruption of the lateral ligaments of the ankle. Routine imaging is not effective in determining ligamentous injury.[51] Stress views in both AP and lateral positions are useful examinations.[13,52] Up to 25% of ankles with verified ligament disruption will have normal stress radiographs.[5]

In valgus and varus positions, normal talar tilt ranges from 5° to 23°.[7,33] Comparison with the normal side is essential, with more than 10° greater tilt being significant of ligamentous dis-

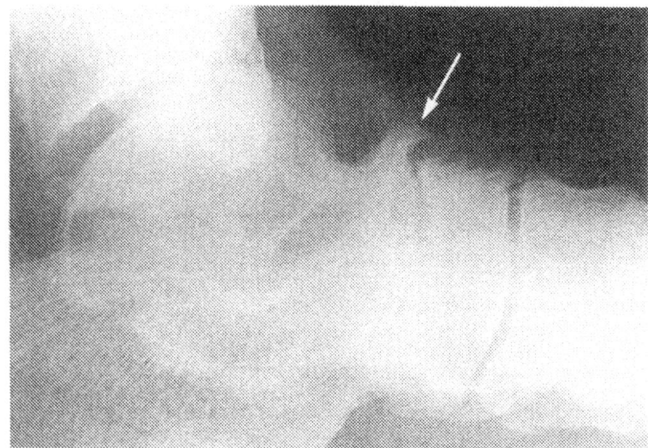

Fig. 4–17 Tarsal coalition, talar beak. This can be seen as a bony projection extending ventrally and bridging the talonavicular articulation (arrow). Also note the lack of visualization of the subtalar joint space. *Comment:* The talar beak is a reliable sign of tarsal coalition.

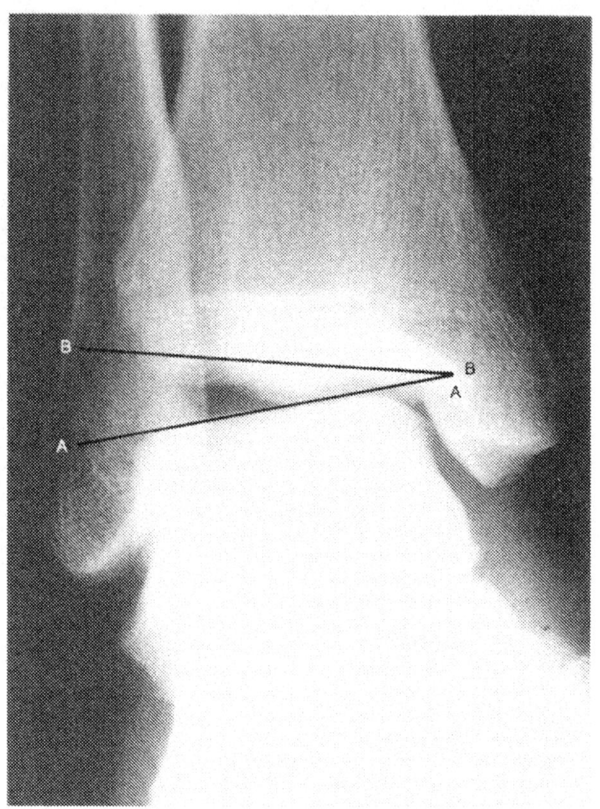

Fig. 4–18 Abnormal talotibial tilt. The ankle is in neutral position. Observe the tilt of the talar surface (*A–A*) in relation to the tibia (*B–B*). *Comment:* This magnitude of talar tilt in the neutral position signifies significant instability. On valgus and varus positions, normal talar tilt ranges from 5° to 23°. Comparison with the normal side is essential, with more than 10° greater tilt on the injured side being significant of ligamentous disruption.

ruption.[33] If there is greater than 6° tilt in the neutral position or more than a 3-mm difference in joint space, this is also indicative of probable ligament damage[53] (Fig. 4–18).

Signs of soft tissue swelling consist of displacement of the skin line, blurring of the fascial plane lines, infiltration of the pre-Achilles fat, and the presence of a teardrop-shaped soft tissue density anterior to the ankle mortise on the lateral view[2] (Fig. 4–19). Myositis ossificans is unusual in the foot and ankle but can be observed in the Achilles tendon, interosseous membrane, and intermetatarsals (Fig. 4–20).

Arthrography can produce diagnostic accuracy in close to 95% of all ligament tears.[7] CT and MR imaging are useful in evaluating tendons around the ankle but are less effective in visualizing the capsule and ligaments.[24]

Fractures

Pediatric Ankle Fractures

In children the growth plates are two to five times weaker than the ligaments, so that fractures of the growth plate occur more commonly than ligament injuries.[54] Fusion of the distal tibial epiphysis begins at age 12 in girls and age 13 in boys. Fusion does not occur symmetrically; it begins centrally and progresses peripherally over a period of 18 months.

Salter-Harris fractures. Fractures are classified by the Salter-Harris system, which describes their relationship to the adjacent growth plate.[55] Type I is a separation of the growth plate (slipped epiphysis), usually in children younger than 5 years, and has an excellent prognosis. Type II is the most com-

mon fracture, extending through the metaphysis and disrupting the growth plate; it usually occurs in patients older than 10 years of age. The Type III fracture extends through the epiphyses and enters the growth plate. Type IV involves a fracture extending through the metaphysis, growth plate, and epiphysis. Type V fractures are compression injuries of the growth plate.

Greenstick fractures. These are readily recognized by a buckling of trabecular patterns and a bulging of the cortex (torus fracture). These may involve the tibia or fibula.

Toddler's fracture. This is a combined fracture of the tibia and fibula up to 10 cm above the ankle joint. It usually occurs between 9 months and 3 years of age.

Juvenile Tillaux' Fracture. This is a Salter-Harris Type III fracture of the lateral tibial epiphysis.

Triplane Fracture. This is a three-fragment fracture involving the tibial shaft and the anterolateral tibial epiphysis, with the remaining tibial epiphyseal fragment attached to the fibula.

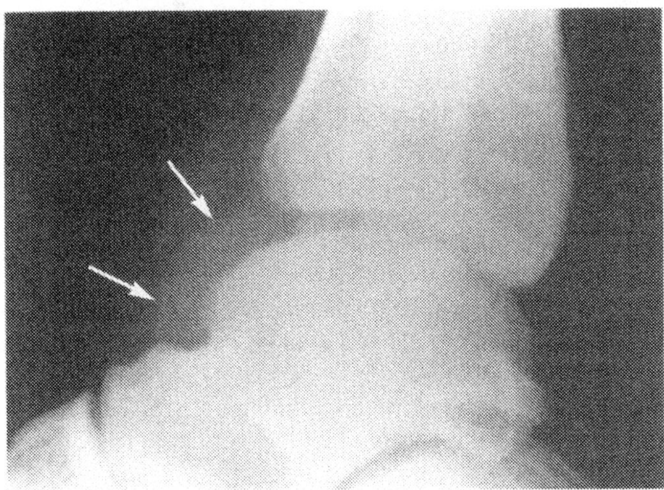

Fig. 4–19 Ankle joint effusion (teardrop sign). On the lateral projection, evidence for the presence of a joint effusion can be identified by this piriform soft tissue density at the anterior joint margin (arrows). *Comment:* The teardrop is a reliable sign of joint effusion, and a search for fracture close to the joint surface should be instigated. Ligamentous injuries also precipitate this sign.

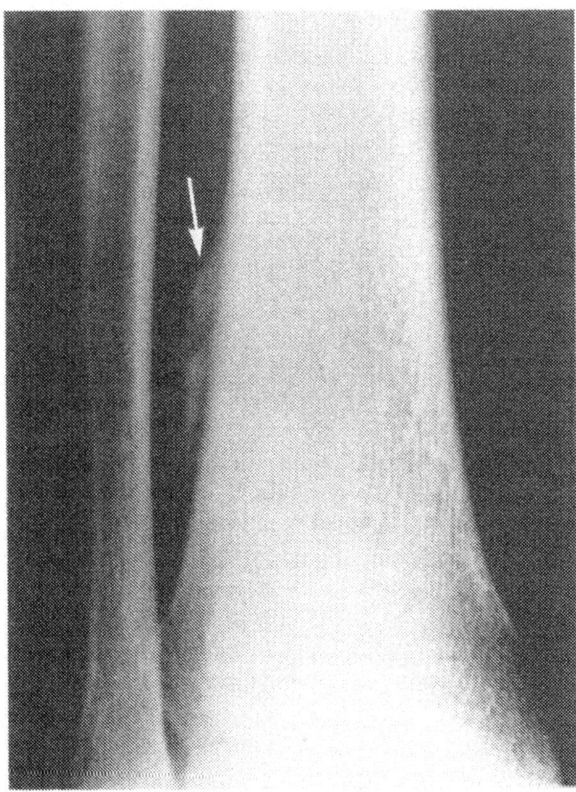

Fig 4–20 Myositis ossificans, interosseous membrane. A curvilinear area of ossification extends from the tibia (arrow). *Comment:* Myositis ossificans is unusual around the foot and ankle. In this case the inversion injury some 6 months earlier caused significant diastasis and hemorrhage of the distal tibiofibular joint.

Adult Ankle Fractures

The Weber classification is commonly used to describe fractures in the adult ankle. It uses the level of fibular fracture in predicting the degree of tibiofibular syndesmosis injury and mortise displacement and is divided into three types: A, B, and C.[56]

Type A are fractures of the fibula below the tibiotalar joint and do not involve the syndesmosis. Type B occur at the joint level, producing an oblique fibular fracture (Fig. 4–21). Two categories of Type C fractures are described. Type C1 are oblique fibular fractures above the level of the distal tibiofibular

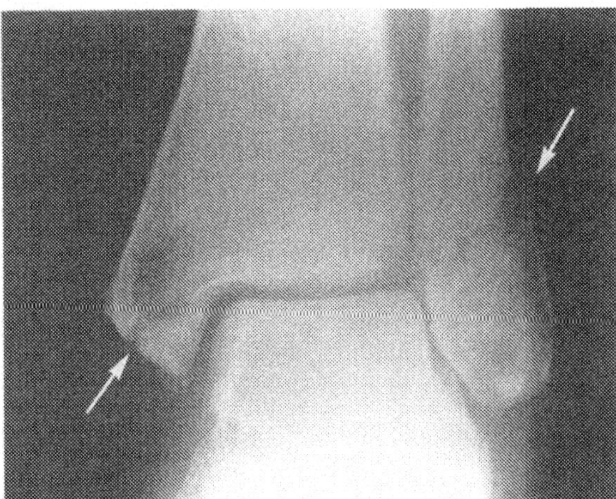

A

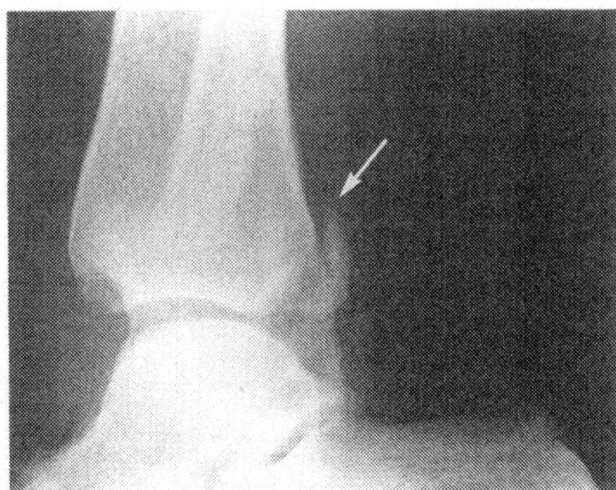

B

Fig. 4–21 Weber Type B fracture. (**A**) The fracture of the fibula is at the level of the ankle mortise (arrow). An additional fracture is evident at the tip of the medial malleolus. (**B**) On the lateral film there is also fracture of the posterior malleolus (arrow). *Comment:* The presence of the fibular fracture at the level of the joint makes this an unstable fracture, which usually requires internal fixation. With the presence of a trio of malleolar fractures, this could also be described as a trimalleolar fracture.

ligaments (Fig. 4–22). Type C2 lesions present with higher fibular fractures and therefore coexist with more extensive rupture of the syndesmosis. Type A injuries can be treated by closed methods; Types B and C usually require internal fixation.

Fractures are often described according to whether the medial, lateral, or posterior malleolus is involved. When two malleoli are affected, it is designated as a bimalleolar fracture; three malleolli are a trimalleolar fracture. Inversion injuries of the ankle not infrequently produce fracture of the proximal fibula (Maisonneuve's fracture).

The osteoligamentous complex of the three bones (tibia, fibula, and talus) and their ligaments maintain stability of the joint (Neer's ring analogy).[7] If the ring is broken in one place, the joint remains stable; a break in two places renders it unstable (eg, bimalleolar fracture or one malleolus fracture and one ligament injury). Unstable joints should be reduced and internally fixed.

Talus

Traumatic lesions of the talus in children are unusual. The most common fracture of the talus is a chip or avulsion fracture of the talar dome.

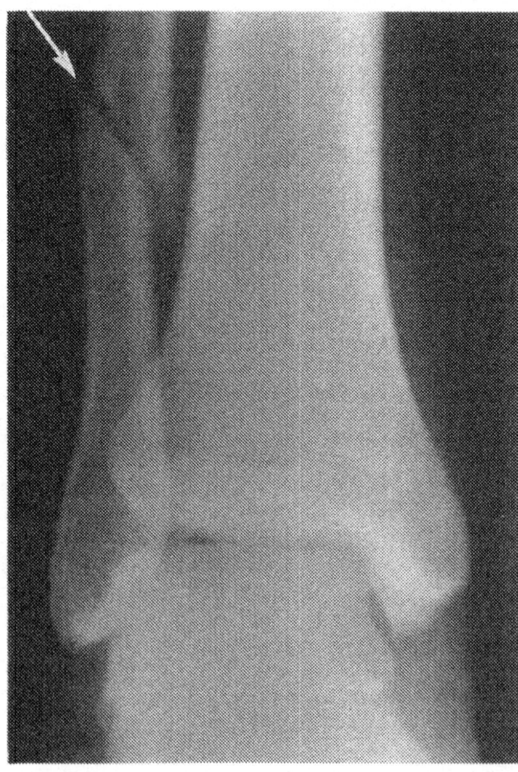

Fig. 4–22 Weber type C1 fracture. The fibular fracture is above the distal tibiofibular syndesmosis (arrow). *Comment:* This type of fracture may be unstable and may require internal fixation, depending on examination findings.

Talar dome fractures. These have been referred to as a form of osteochondritis dissecans. Less than 10% occur in children younger than 16 years.[57] Inversion injuries tend to precipitate fracture of the lateral talar dome. The best view for demonstration is the medial oblique projection (Fig. 4–23).

Talar neck fractures. The second most common fracture is through the neck of the talus (aviator's fracture). Up to 20% of patients have associated fracture of the medial malleolus.[58] The more severe the displacement at the fracture site, the greater the incidence of tibiotalar arthritis, subtalar arthritis, malunion, nonunion, and avascular necrosis. Follow-up radiographs 2 years after injury in adults should be obtained to assess for avascular necrosis; in children this should be at 6-month intervals.[7]

Calcaneus

The calcaneus is the most commonly fractured tarsal bone.[7] Fractures usually result from falls or motor vehicle accidents causing compression injuries. On the lateral projection, assessment of Boehler's angle will reveal the injury if an angle of less than 28° is found (Fig. 4–24). Not all calcaneal compression fractures reduce Boehler's angle, so that a careful search on all available views is required to identify a fracture line. CT of comminuted fractures is essential to identify whether any tendons, especially the peroneal tendons, are trapped.

Up to 75% of these fractures are intraarticular into the subtalar joint and involve the body of the calcaneus. The remaining 25% involve the calcaneal processes and spare the subtalar joint. Additional fractures occur in up to 50% of cases; notably, 10% of patients have a compression fracture or a posterior element fracture in the thoracolumbar spine.[59]

Fractures of the calcaneal processes are often avulsions. The anterior process is the one most commonly avulsed. Avulsion of the posterior calcaneal tuberosity is called a beak fracture.

Fifth Metatarsal

Depiction of fractures in the proximal fifth metatarsal often requires AP, medial oblique, and lateral views. The proximal portion of the fifth metatarsal is a common site for fracture; two types are described. An avulsion fracture involves the most proximal bulbous tip of the metatarsal; it is due to an inversion injury exerting traction via the insertion of the peroneus brevis tendon and the lateral cord of the plantar aponeurosis. These usually heal well without complication. A transverse fracture through the base of the fifth metatarsal is referred to as a Jones' or dancer's fracture. Unlike the more proximal avulsion, these are notorious for slow healing and nonunion as a result of reduced blood supply to the region.[60]

Phalanges

Direct trauma is the most common cause of fracture. Dropping a heavy object on the foot and kicking a piece of furni-

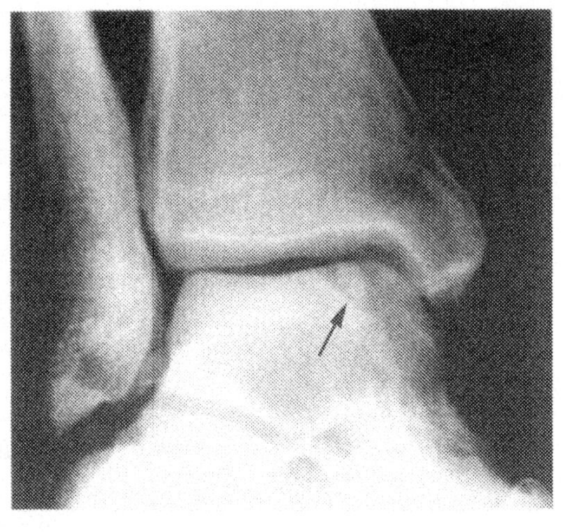

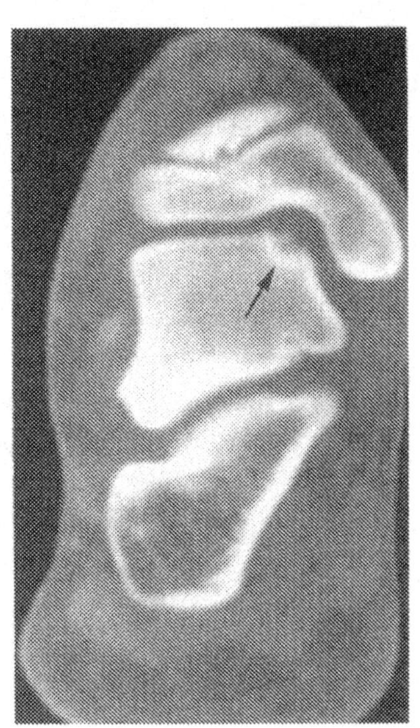

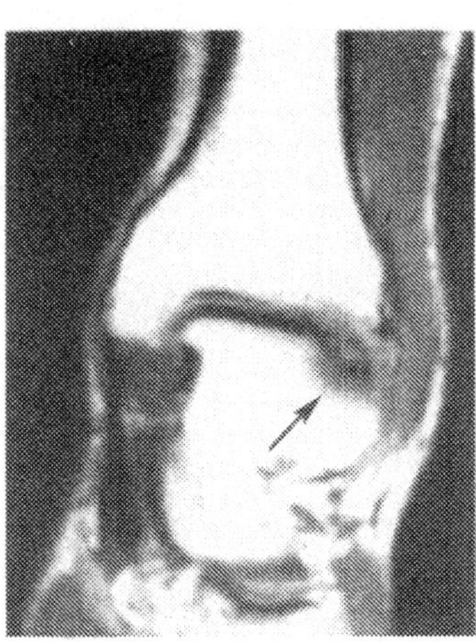

A   B   C

Fig. 4–23 Talar dome fracture. (**A**) An isolated bony fragment is visible at the medial margin of the talar dome (arrow). (**B**) CT and (**C**) MR examination in a different patient of the lateral talar dome (arrows) clearly delineate the defect. *Comment:* These talar dome lesions are often overlooked and can lead to chronic ankle disability. Adequate plain film study is pivotal in its detection.

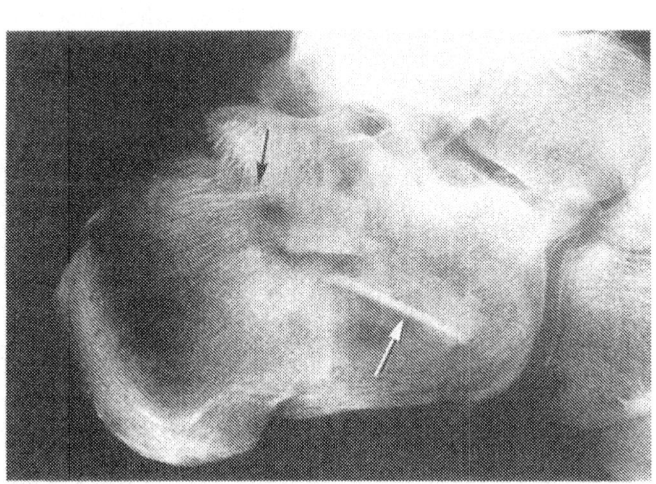

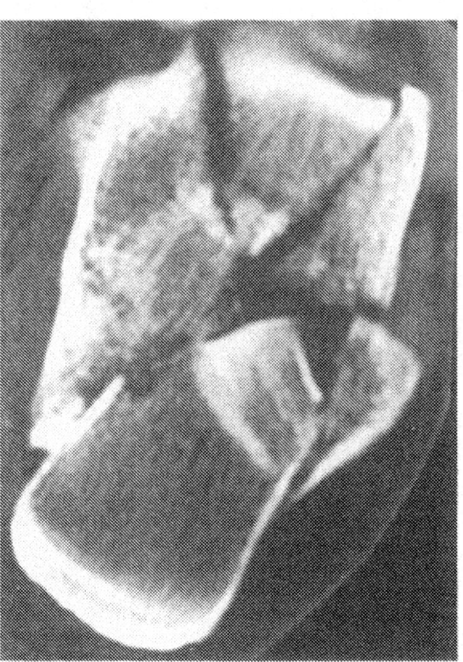

A   B

Fig. 4–24 Comminuted calcaneal fracture. (**A**) On the lateral view, observe the multiple fracture lines (arrows) and the diminished Boehler's angle. (**B**) On CT examination, the degree of fragmentation can be fully appreciated. *Comment:* The calcaneus is the most common bone of the tarsals to fracture. Such fractures often cannot be fully appreciated on lateral views and require the application of Boehler's angle, the axial calcaneal view, and, where indicated, CT.

ture, especially at night (bedroom fracture), are frequent mechanisms of injury (Fig. 4–25). Kicking the ground during sport, especially on artificial turf, commonly traumatizes the first metatarsophalangeal joint (turf toe), precipitating anything from a joint sprain to a fracture of the phalanx or even a dislocation.

Stress Fractures

All bones except the phalanges have been documented to develop stress fractures. In athletes, the distal tibia is the most common site, being involved in 50% of cases; 25% occur in the tarsals and 10% in the metatarsals.[61] Almost 20% are bilateral. Military recruits most commonly develop fractures of the metatarsal shafts and calcaneus. Of metatarsal stress fractures, the second and third metatarsals account for at least 90%, the first for 7%, and the fourth and fifth for 3%.[62]

Plain film changes occur, at the earliest, 2 weeks after the onset of pain; bone scans detect changes within 24 hours.[7] The major features consist of fluffy periosteal new bone, a subtle (often absent) fracture line, or a band of sclerosis[63] (Fig. 4–26). The extensiveness of the periosteal reaction may simulate an aggressive neoplasm.

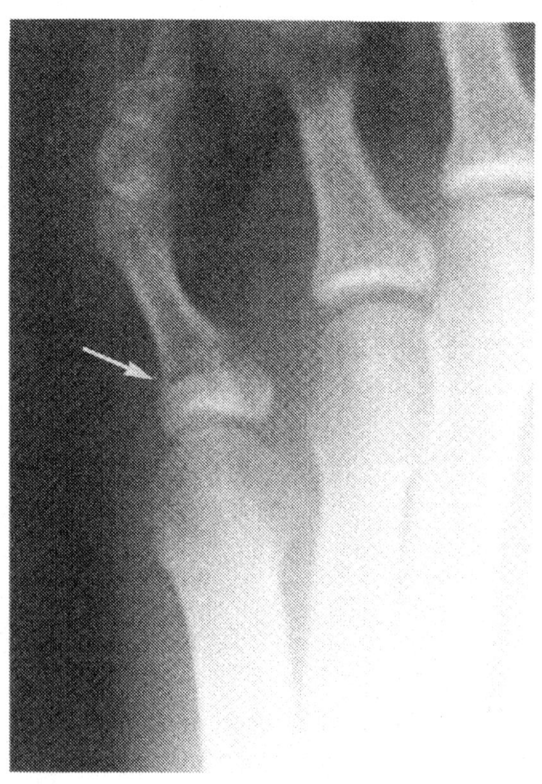

Fig. 4–25 Fracture of the proximal phalanx (bedroom fracture). At the base of the fifth proximal phalanx, a fracture can be seen (arrow). *Comment:* Such fractures of the toes are extremely common and occur when an object is kicked inadvertently.

Dislocations

Dislocations are encountered through any joint, in particular the tibiotalar, subtalar, talonavicular (swivel dislocation), midtarsal (Chopart's dislocation), tarsometatarsal (Lisfranc's dislocation), metatarsophalangeal, and interphalangeal joints (Fig. 4–27).

VASCULAR DISORDERS

Freiberg's Infraction

The underlying pathologic disorder in Freiberg's infraction is avascular necrosis. It affects females more than males in a ratio of approximately 4:1, which may be partially due to high-heeled shoes.[64] The majority first manifest in adolescence (13 to 18 years), although the condition has been reported in adults. The second metatarsal head is the most common site; occasionally the third metatarsal head is involved, with the remaining heads being rare sites. It may occur bilaterally. Precipitating events include dancing, gymnastics, marching, and direct trauma.

The radiographic signs include flattening of the metatarsal head, a subchondral fracture (crescent sign), fragmentation, loose bodies, widening of the adjacent joint space, and thickening of the metatarsal cortex (Fig. 4–28).

Sesamoid Avascular Necrosis

The medial hallux sesamoid frequently undergoes avascular necrosis as a sequela to repetitive trauma. This may include running, dancing, playing sports on hard surfaces, and wearing poorly supportive footwear. Females are affected more commonly.

A specific axial view beneath the plantar surface of the toes is required to demonstrate the changes within the sesamoid bones (Fig. 4–29). This consists of subchondral fracture (crescent sign), sclerosis, and fragmentation. These signs usually are best demonstrated in the medial sesamoid.

Sever's Disease

Initially Sever's disease was considered osteonecrosis of the calcaneal apophysis. The normal variation in ossification of the calcaneal apophysis renders it sclerotic and fragmented, which accounts for the confusion (see Fig. 4–13).

Köhler's Disease

True Köhler's disease is considered avascular necrosis of the tarsal navicular. In young children the navicular can appear sclerotic, irregular, and fragmented. When associated with pain and flatfoot and when the condition is not bilateral,

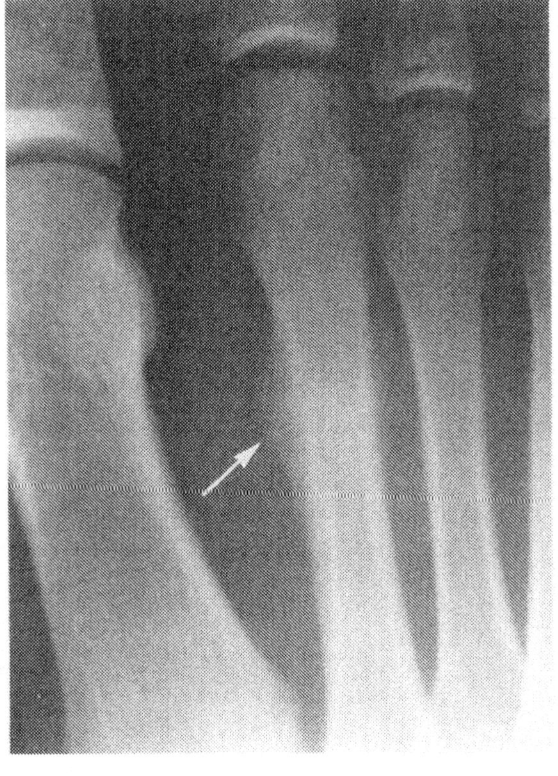

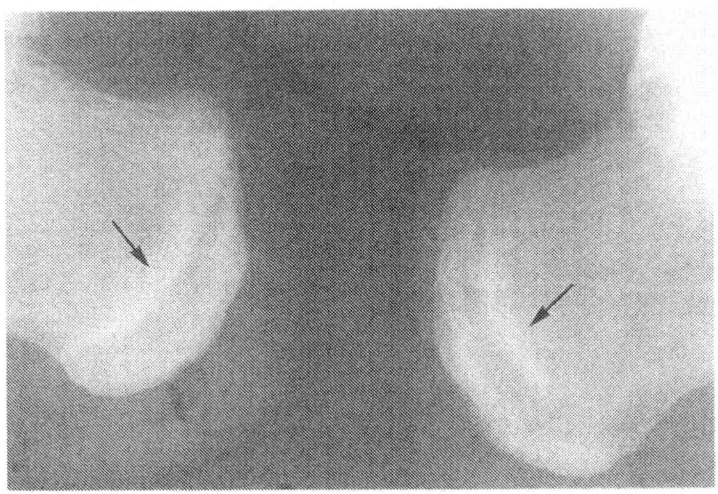

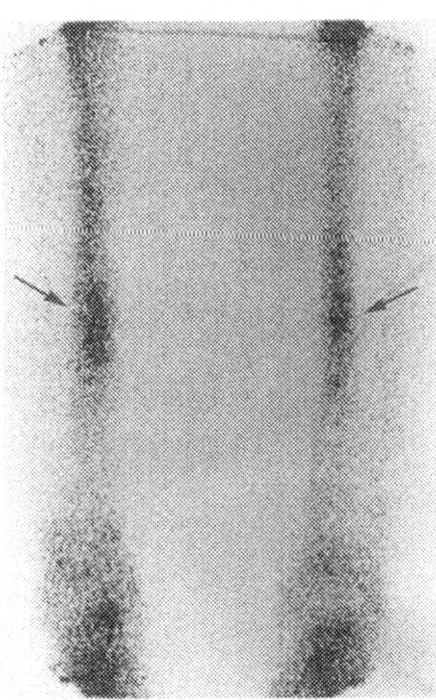

Fig. 4–26 Stress fractures. (**A**) Metatarsal. The only feature on this film 3 weeks after the onset of pain is the fluffy periosteal reaction (arrow). No fracture line is visible. (**B**) Calcaneus. A curvilinear band of sclerosis is evident bilaterally (arrows). (**C**) Tibias, nuclear bone scan. There is focal uptake of isotope in both tibias (arrows). *Comment:* The most common sites for stress fractures are the second metatarsal, the calcaneus, and the tibia. The spectrum of manifestations demonstrated is typical of these injuries.

then the diagnosis is certain. If bilateral and asymptomatic, then it is considered a normal variation in ossification (see Fig. 4–15).

Avascular Necrosis of the Talus

This may occur as a posttraumatic or idiopathic phenomenon. The blood supply renders the talar body susceptible to avascular necrosis, particularly after fractures of the neck of the talus. Up to 50% or more of talar neck fractures can precipitate avascular necrosis of the talar body.[65] The radiographic appearance is a sclerotic and collapsed talar dome and body. The head of the talus usually remains remarkably normal in appearance; this is a good differential feature from Paget's disease, which it may simulate (Fig. 4–30). A good prognostic sign for the preservation of blood supply to the talar body after fracture is the appearance of a linear radiolucency within a few days paralleling the articular surface of the talar dome (Hawkins' sign; Fig. 4–31).

Venous Insufficiency

Chronic venous stasis of the lower limb characteristically produces wavy periostitis involving the distal tibia[66] (Fig.

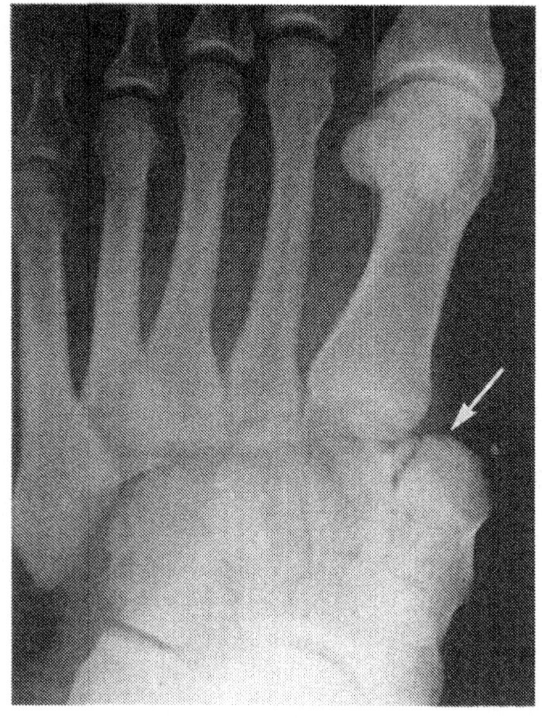

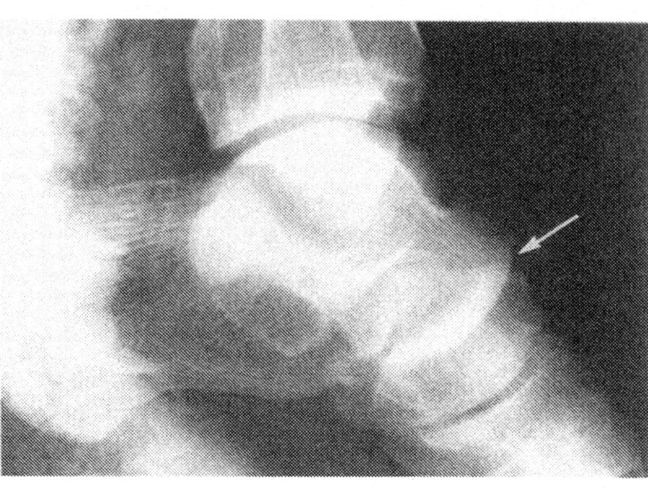

A   B

Fig. 4–27 Dislocations of the foot. (**A**) Lisfranc's dislocation. Note that the dislocation has occurred through the tarsometatarsal junction (arrow). (**B**) Chopart's dislocation. The separation has occurred through the intertarsal joints of the talonavicular (arrow) and calcaneocuboid joints. *Comment:* These types of injuries most commonly follow falls from a height or down stairs, stepping off a curb, or motor vehicle accidents. They also may accompany neuropathic arthropathy.

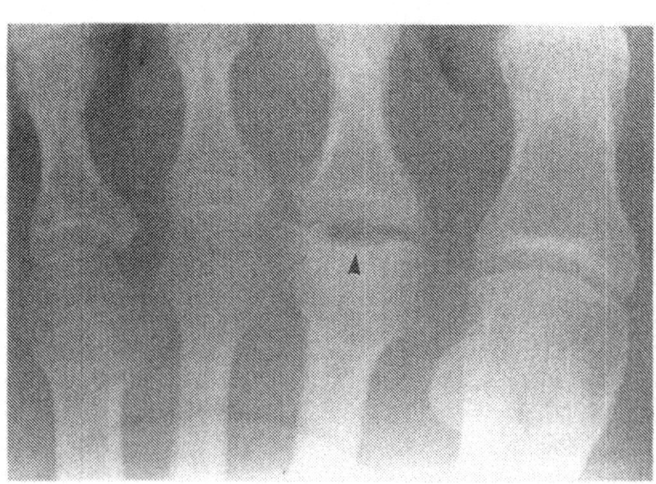

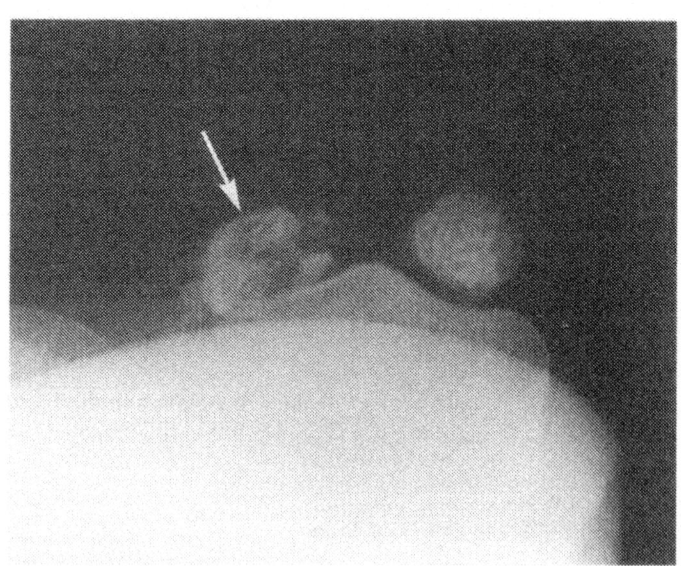

Fig. 4–28 Freiberg's infarction. Note the flattening of the metatarsal head, the widening of the adjacent joint space, and the thickening of the metatarsal cortex (arrow). *Comment:* The underlying pathologic disorder is avascular necrosis. It affects girls more often than boys in a ratio of approximately 4:1, first manifesting in adolescence and usually involving the second metatarsal head.

Fig. 4–29 Avascular necrosis of the medial sesamoid bone. There is sclerosis and fragmentation of the medial sesamoid bone (arrow). *Comment:* The medial hallux sesamoid frequently undergoes avascular necrosis as a sequela to repetitive trauma, including running, dancing, playing sports on hard surfaces, and wearing poorly supportive footwear.

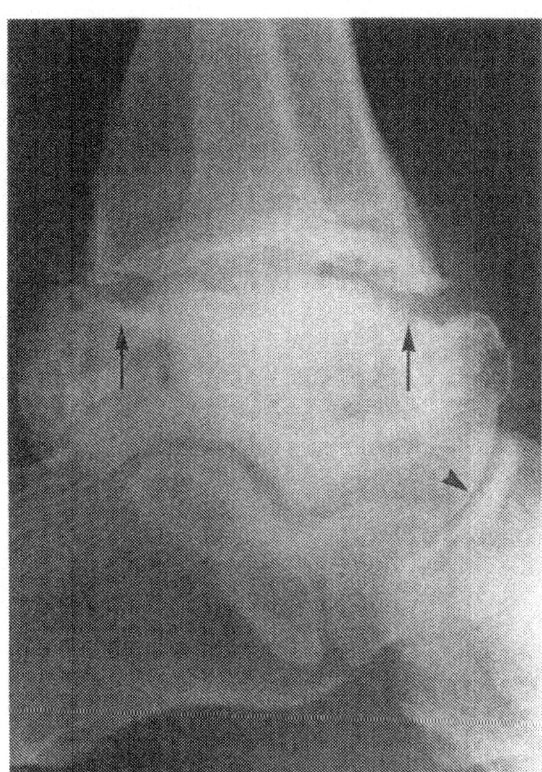

Fig. 4-30 Avascular necrosis of the talus. The talar dome and body are sclerotic and collapsed (arrows). The head of the talus is relatively normal in appearance (arrowhead), which is a good differential feature from Paget's disease (which it may simulate). *Comment:* This may occur as a posttraumatic, corticosteroid-induced, or idiopathic phenomenon. The blood supply renders the talar body susceptible to avascular necrosis, particularly after fractures of the neck of the talus.

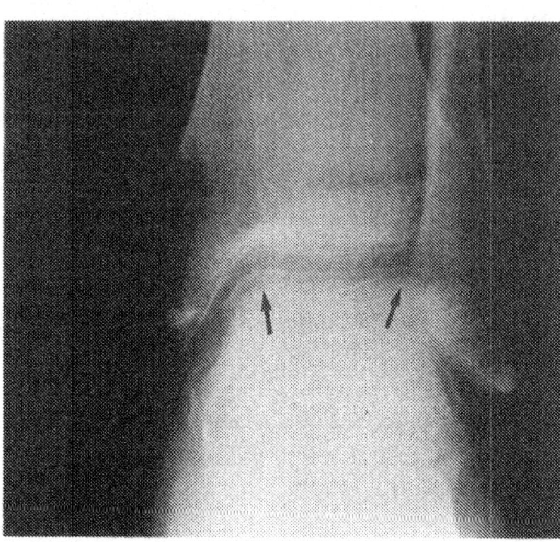

Fig. 4–31 Hawkin's sign. A distinctive linear radiolucency is seen immediately below the articular surface of the talus (arrows). *Comment:* This is a good prognostic sign for the preservation of blood supply to the talar body after fracture.

4–32). The mechanism is thought to relate to hypoxia. Additional features include phleboliths, soft tissue calcification, edema, and skin ulcers.

INFECTIONS

The term *osteomyelitis* is reserved for infections involving bone. Osteomyelitis may be acute or chronic. A localized chronic form of osteomyelitis is referred to as Brodie's abscess; a generalized chronic form is termed Garre's sclerosing osteomyelitis. Infection of a joint cavity is designated as septic arthritis. Osteomyelitis and septic arthritis may coexist. The causative organism most commonly is *Staphylococcus aureus*, although any organism can infect.

Osteomyelitis

Infection of bone can follow penetrating wounds, fractures, surgery, and hematogenous spread. A common predisposing condition is diabetes mellitus, which can account for up to 30% of foot osteomyelitis.[67] Diabetic infections commonly occur at pressure points (eg, the metatarsal heads and the heel), where ischemic changes tend to localize. In the foot the most common bone for osteomyelitis is the calcaneus.[68]

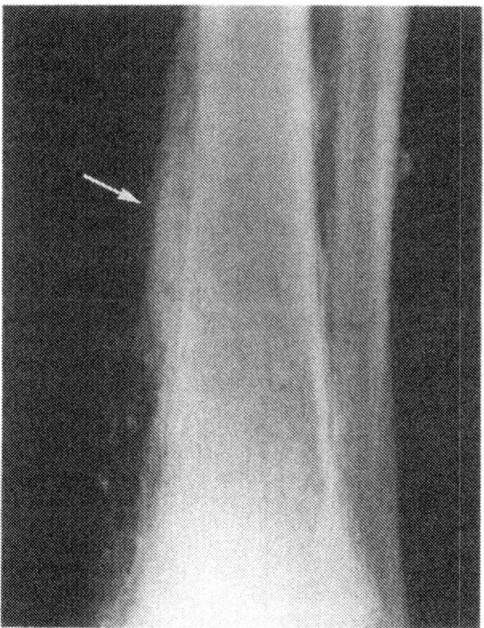

Fig. 4–32 Venous insufficiency with periostitis. Prominent wavy periostitis is visible throughout the distal tibia (arrow). *Comment:* Chronic venous stasis of the lower limb characteristically produces wavy periostitis involving the distal tibia, thought to relate to hypoxia. Additional features include phleboliths, soft tissue calcification, edema, and skin ulcers.

The earliest radiographic feature (within 2 to 3 days) is overlying soft tissue swelling. There is a radiographic latent period of 10 to 14 days before bony changes can be seen.[69] In the tubular bones, marked periosteal new bone (involucrum) can be seen.[70] A moth-eaten pattern of bone destruction is also observed. Joints are frequently involved early, as manifested by destruction of the articular cortex (Fig. 4–33). Within the tarsal bones, particularly the calcaneus, sequestra are common. At the site of surgical pin insertion, a ring sequestrum can be seen.[71] Isotopic bone scans are the procedure of choice in detection of early osteomyelitis within days of onset of clinical symptoms. Areas of osteomyelitis always show increased uptake (hot spots).

Brodie's Abscess

A localized infection less than 2 cm in diameter and surrounded by a bony response is characteristic of a bony abscess (Fig. 4–34). The distal tibia is the most common site of in-

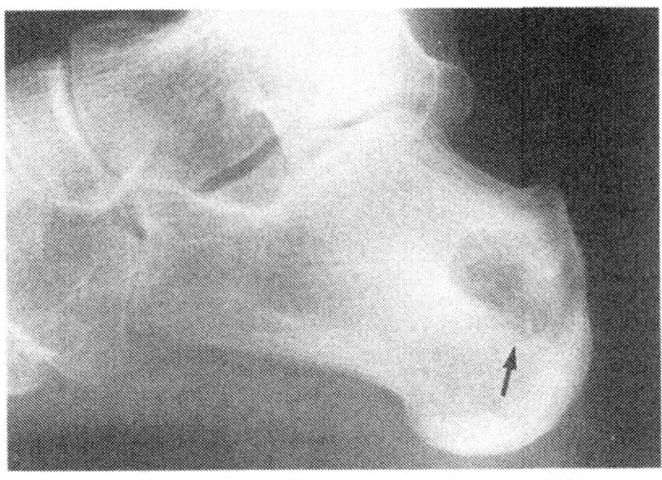

Fig. 4–34 Brodie's abscess, calcaneus. A localized, radiolucent, geographic lesion is evident at the posterior aspect of the calcaneus (arrow). Observe the surrounding zone of sclerosis. *Comment:* The distal tibia is the most common site of involvement followed by the calcaneus, where up to 20% demonstrate a central bony sequestrum.

volvement. The second most common site is the calcaneus, where up to 20% of lesions demonstrate a central bony sequestrum.[72]

Septic Arthritis

Joint infection can occur in penetrating injuries, immunocompromised patients (including diabetics, those on corticosteroid therapy, and those with acquired immunodeficiency syndrome), and osteomyelitis. The earliest signs occur in the soft tissues with swelling and joint effusions. Local hyperemia precipitates juxtaarticular osteopenia early in the process with erosive destruction of the articular cortex and loss of the joint space (Fig. 4–35). Diminution of the joint space may begin as early as 2 to 3 days after the onset of infection, especially in the ankle. Infection in an articulation of the foot or ankle can rapidly spread to involve multiple bones and joints. [67]Ga scans are particularly useful in demonstrating septic arthritis.

ARTHRITIC DISORDERS

Degenerative Joint Disease

Degenerative joint disease (DJD, osteoarthritis) is the most common arthropathy of the skeleton. In its primary form, usual sites include the spine, hips, knees, acromioclavicular joint, first metacarpal–trapezium joint, first metatarsophalangeal joint, and interphalangeal joints of the hand.[73]

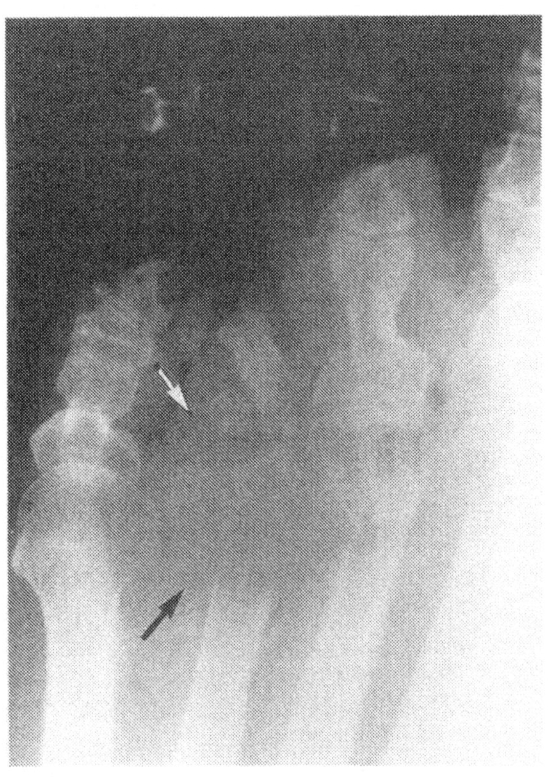

Fig. 4–33 Osteomyelitis, metatarsal heads. There is destruction of the fourth and third distal metatarsals as well as the proximal phalanx of the fourth digit (arrows). *Comment:* A common predisposing condition is diabetes mellitus, which can account for up to 30% of foot osteomyelitis. Many cases occur at pressure points (eg, the metatarsal heads and the heel), where ischemic changes tend to localize.

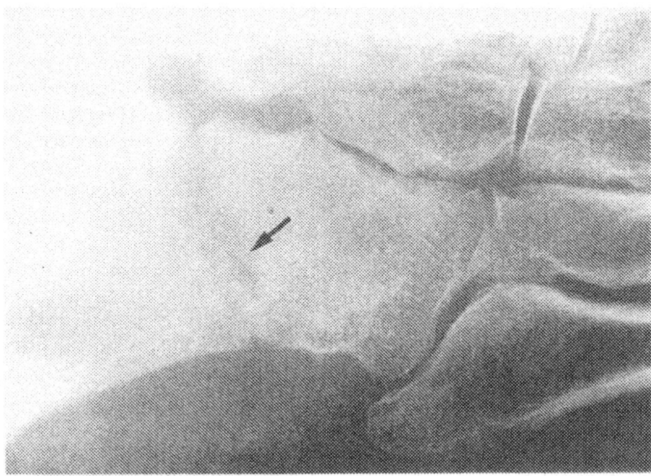

Fig. 4–35 Septic arthritis of the calcaneocuboid joint. This adult man developed a sudden onset of localized pain and swelling over the lateral foot; this radiograph was taken 5 days later. There is loss of the articular cortex on both sides of the joint with obliteration of the joint cavity (arrow). *Comment:* Joint infection can occur in penetrating injuries, immunocompromised patients (including diabetics, those on corticosteroid therapy, and those with acquired immunodeficiency syndrome), and osteomyelitis.

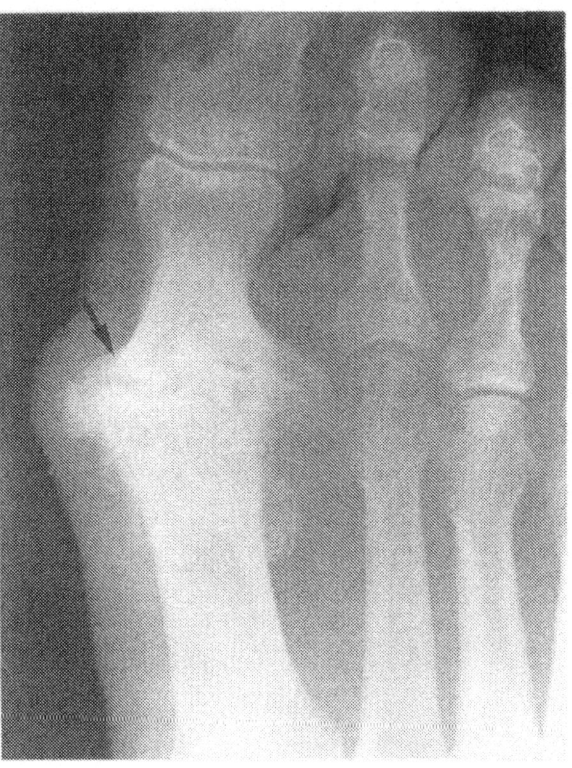

Fig. 4–36 DJD, first metatarsophalangeal joint. The radiologic hallmarks include osteophytes, subchondral sclerosis, asymmetric joint space narrowing, and subchondral cysts (arrow). *Comment:* At this joint the combination of DJD, stiffness, and painful dorsiflexion is referred to as hallux rigidus.

In the foot and ankle, DJD is common only at the metatarsophalangeal joint of the great toe[74] (Fig. 4–36). At this joint, the combination of DJD, stiffness, and painful dorsiflexion is referred to as hallux rigidus.[75] If DJD is found at any other joint, including the ankle mortise, then an underlying cause should be sought. Examples include DJD at the subtalar or tarsometatarsal joints due to neuropathic arthropathy, DJD at the talonavicular joint with a talar beak due to tarsal coalition, and DJD at the ankle due to trauma, inflammatory arthritis, pseudogout, or avascular necrosis of the talus. The radiologic hallmarks include osteophytes, subchondral sclerosis, a symmetric joint space narrowing, subchondral cysts, and loose bodies.

First Metatarsophalangeal Joint

At the metatarsophalangeal joint, there frequently coexists a hallux valgus deformity and a broad-based, often cystic bony exostosis (bunion; Fig. 4–37). Associated features of hallux valgus include a rounded first metatarsal head, a hallux abductus angle of more than 15°, and an intermetatarsus angle of greater than 14°.[7] Involvement of the hallux sesamoids is common.[76]

Plantar Spur

The pathogenesis of the plantar spur remains speculative, although it seems likely that it is the result of a traction periostitis at the insertion of the plantar fascia.[7] The incidence of plantar spurs increases with age, being rare in patients younger than 30 years and uncommon in those younger than 40 and thereafter rapidly increasing in incidence to age 65.[77] Almost 50% of patients will be overweight by 25 lb or more. At least 25% of spurs are bilateral.[78]

On a lateral view the spur is visible as a triangular, tapered excrescence extending forward from the plantar surface of the calcaneus (Fig. 4–38). It exhibits a smooth, often corticated margin, in contrast to inflammatory plantar enthesopathies such as in psoriasis, Reiter's syndrome, and even ankylosing spondylitis. Increased uptake on blood pool nuclear scans may be an indicator for injection therapy.[7]

Diffuse Idiopathic Skeletal Hyperostosis

Exuberant ossification at both the plantar surface and the Achilles tendon insertion frequently accompanies diffuse idiopathic skeletal hyperostosis. Radiographs of the spine and pelvis will confirm its presence.

Neuropathic Arthropathy

Central or peripheral loss of sensation and joint proprioception can precipitate rapidly advancing destructive DJD. The

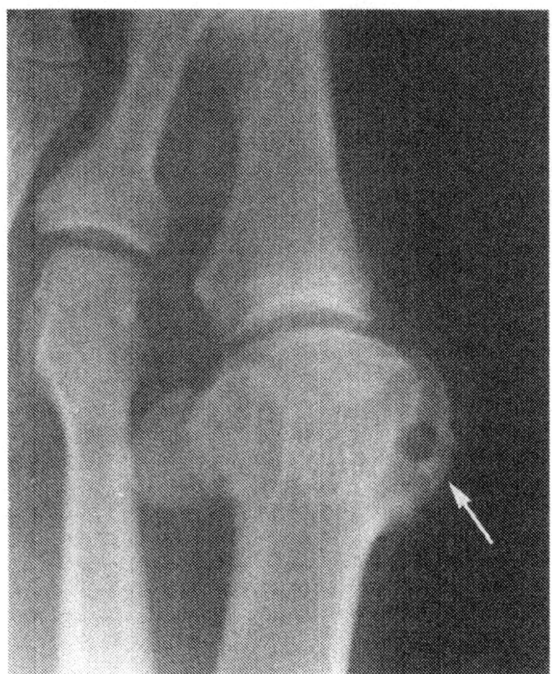

Fig. 4–37 Bunion, first metatarsophalangeal joint. At the metatarsophalangeal joint there frequently coexist a hallux valgus deformity and a broad-based, often cystic bony exostosis (bunion, arrow). *Comment:* This cystic appearance can be confused with early gout.

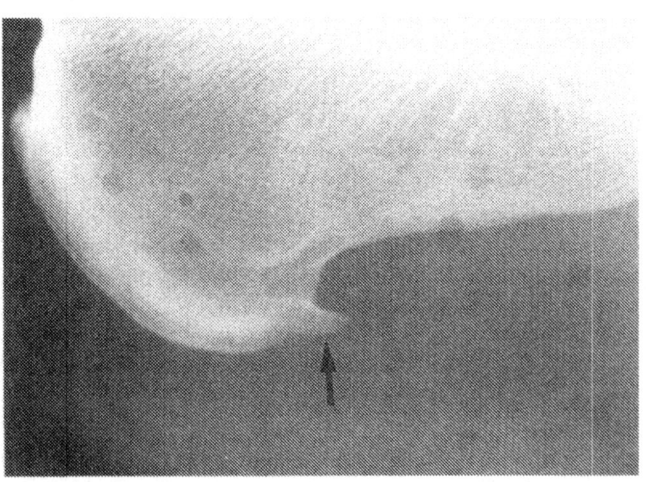

Fig. 4–38 Plantar spur. The spur is visible as a triangular, tapered excrescence extending forward from the plantar surface of the calcaneus (arrow). It exhibits a smooth, corticated margin. *Comment:* The pathogenesis remains speculative, although it seems likely that the spur is the result of a traction periostitis at the insertion of the plantar fascia. The definite smooth margin contrasts with the fluffy, irregular border of an inflammatory spur, such as that in psoriasis and Reiter's syndrome. (See also Fig. 4–44.)

most common cause of neuropathic arthropathy of the foot and ankle in adults is diabetes mellitus; in children it is spina bifida. Other less common causes include tabes dorsalis, alcoholism, Charcot-Marie-Tooth disease, amyloid neuropathy, and congenital indifference to pain.[79] Two morphologic types are recognized: hypertrophic and atrophic.

Hypertrophic Neuropathic Arthropathy

The radiologic hallmarks of hypertrophic neuropathic arthropathy are distension, debris, disorganization, dislocation, density, and destruction (the "six Ds"; Fig. 4–39). This is the most common type, and it typically occurs in the intertarsal, subtalar, and metatarsophalangeal joints. The medial side of the foot exhibits more pronounced changes than the lateral side.

Atrophic Neuropathic Arthropathy

This form if characterized by bone resorption adjacent to the joints, usually in the metatarsophalangeal region. The articular ends of the bones are tapered (licked candy stick appearance) or appear surgically amputated. The joint spaces are widened, and there is normal to decreased bone density with little debris.

Synoviochondrometaplasia

Synoviochondrometaplasia is a benign articular disorder characterized by the transformation of the synovium to produce cartilaginous intraarticular loose bodies. It is of unknown etiology, although it frequently coexists with DJD. Males are affected more commonly than females (male:female ratio, 3:1), typically through the third to fifth decades of life. The ankle is the fourth most common site of involvement after the knee, elbow, and hip.[73]

Radiographically, the appearance is characteristic with a single or, more often, multiple circular to ovoid radiopacities that exhibit smooth margins (Fig. 4–40). Internally they may be laminated into concentric rings or exhibit foci of radiolucency. Rarely, there may be some intraarticular bone erosion.

The condition should be differentiated from the variant os trigonum and from the malignancies of chondrosarcoma and synovioma.

Gout

Hyperuricemia results in crystal deposition within joint cartilage, synovium, and capsule and in subchondral bone. At least 85% of patients with gout develop foot and ankle involvement, with the majority of cases occurring in the metatarsophalangeal joint of the great toe.[74]

Acute gout (podagra) rarely exhibits radiographic changes. With the common usage of hyperuricemic agents, the findings

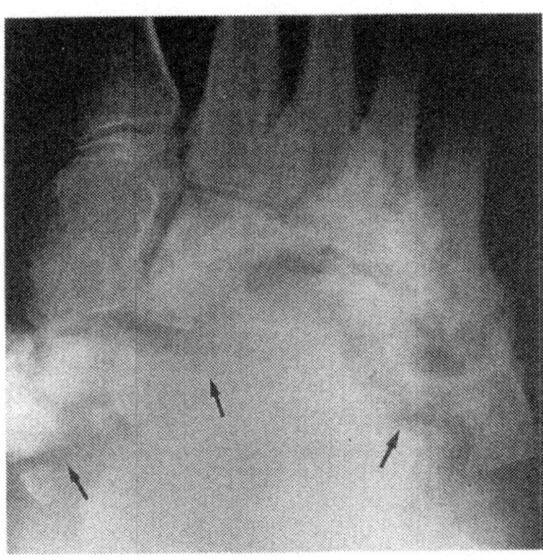

A

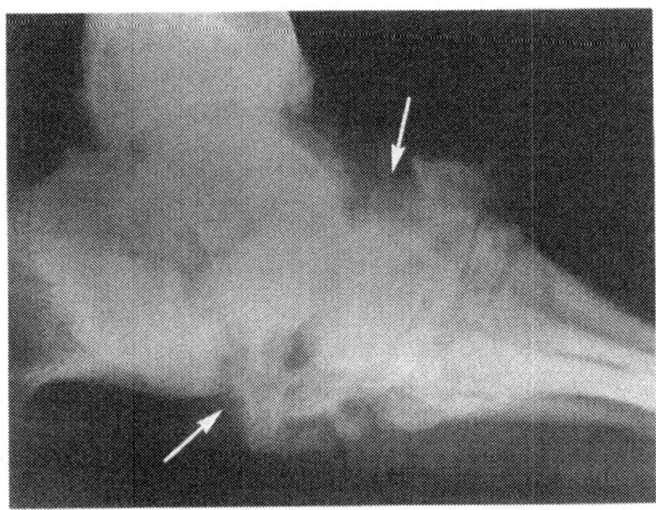

B

Fig. 4–39 Neuropathic arthropathy. (**A**) On the AP view, observe the extreme fragmentation and sclerosis at the tarsometatarsal junction (arrows). (**B**) The lateral view reveals destruction and collapse of the subtalar and intertarsal joints (arrows). *Comment:* The radiologic hallmarks of hypertrophic neuropathic arthropathy are distension, debris, disorganization, dislocation, density, and destruction (the "six Ds").

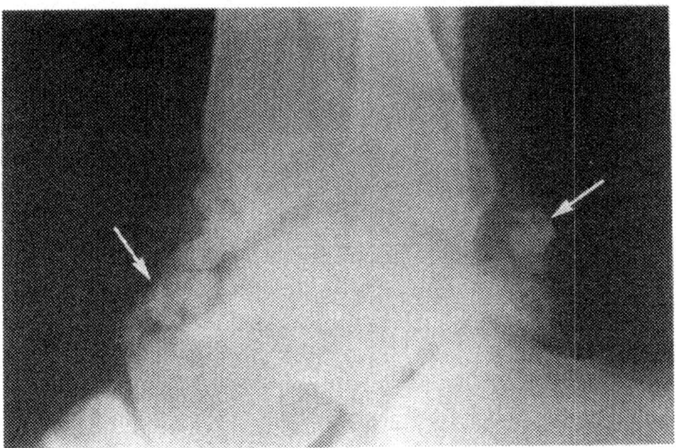

Fig. 4-40 Synoviochondrometaplasia, ankle joint. Multiple circular and ovoid radiopacities with smooth margins are present at the anterior and posterior joint margins (arrows). *Comment:* Synoviochondrometaplasia is a benign articular disorder characterized by the transformation of the synovium to produce cartilaginous, intra-articular loose bodies. The ankle is the fourth most common site of involvement after the knee, elbow, and hip.

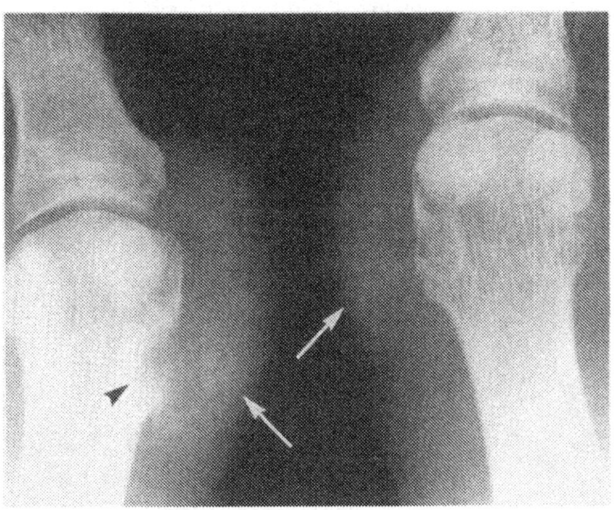

Fig. 4–41 Gout, first metatarsophalangeal joint. Soft tissue densities are visible medially (arrows). There is an extrinsic bone erosion from the adjacent tophus (arrowhead) with a characteristic overhanging edge. *Comment:* These features are of chronic tophaceous gout; acute gout (podagra) rarely exhibits any radiographic changes.

---

of chronic tophaceous gout are unusual. Hallmarks of gout at the great toe include preservation of the joint space until late in the disease, extrinsic periarticular bony erosions with a distinctive lip of bone at the edge (overhanging edge), intraosseous cystic lesions, and generally normal bone density[73,74] (Fig. 4–41).

Rheumatoid Arthritis

Rheumatoid arthritis is a common inflammatory joint and connective tissue disorder. Onset is usually between the ages of 20 and 60 years with a peak incidence between 40 and 50 years. Under 40 years of age, women are affected three times more commonly than men; after 40 the gender incidence equalizes.

The foot may be the initial site of occurrence in at least 10% to 20% of cases.[7,73,74] Involvement of the feet and hands may be a reflection of coexisting cervical spine involvement.[73,74] The metatarsophalangeal joints are the most frequent site of involvement, especially the fifth.[7,73,74] The interphalangeal joint of the great toe and the intertarsal joints later are also favored sites.

On plain film examination in the early stages, high-quality images and adequate views are necessary. Signs of involvement include initial juxtaarticular osteoporosis that progresses to be generalized, marginal erosions, uniform loss of joint space, and deformity.

In the foot the predominant sites of involvement are the metatarsophalangeal joints. Marginal erosions are due to bony erosion from invading pannus and are best seen on the medial margins of the metatarsal heads except the fifth, where they are on the lateral side (Fig. 4–42A). Involvement of the hallux sesamoid bones is common.[76] Intraosseous cysts can be prominent and are linked to pannus extension beyond the joint confines. Deformities develop later, including a splayed foot and flexion and fibular deviation of the digits. Ankylosis is seen later in the disease, typically at the intertarsal joints. Fusion of the interphalangeal and metatarsophalangeal joints is rare.

At the ankle the major feature late in the disease is the uniform loss of joint space and osteoporosis (Fig. 4–42B). Mar-

ginal erosions are infrequently seen, although erosion at the tibiofibular syndesmosis insertion does occur. At the calcaneus, erosion at the posterior surface near the insertion of the pre-Achilles bursa can be seen as well as edema into the adjacent fat. Rheumatoid nodules can be seen near the Achilles tendon. Insufficiency fractures can be seen throughout the foot, such as at the metatarsals or calcaneus, due to osteoporosis and corticosteroid effects.

Psoriatic Arthritis

Less than 10% of patients with psoriasis develop arthritis. Nail involvement characterized by discoloration, thickening, ridging, and pitting correlates with the development of arthritis in 90% of cases, usually of the small joints of the hands and feet (typically simultaneously).[73,80]

The interphalangeal joints are the favored sites of involvement, although no joint is necessarily spared. Erosion of the distal bone often coexists with cupping of the reciprocal joint surface (pencil-in-cup deformity, balancing pagoda appearance, pestle-and-mortar deformity; Fig. 4–43). Widening of the joint space is due to fibrous deposition, and a reliable sign of psoriasis is involvement of all joints on a single ray (ray sign). A homogeneously sclerotic phalanx (ivory phalanx) due to endosteal new bone occasionally is encountered. Osseous joint fusion is common at the interphalangeal joints. Fluffy

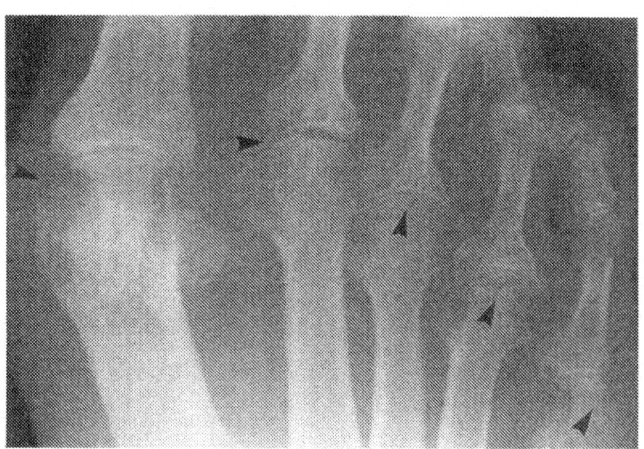

A

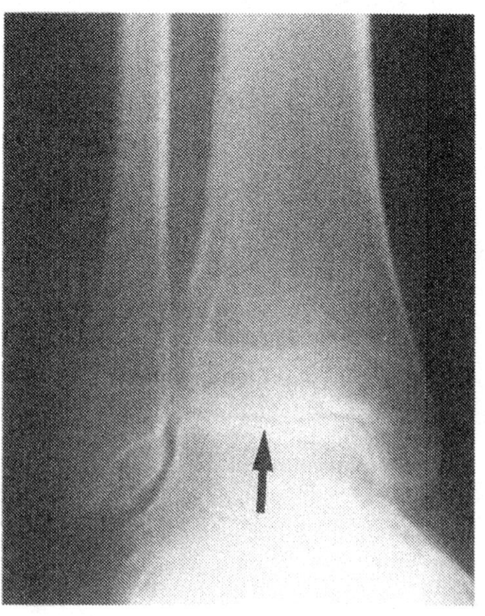

B

Fig. 4–42 Rheumatoid arthritis. **(A)** Prominent marginal erosions are evident at the metatarsophalangeal joints (arrowheads). **(B)** There is characteristic symmetric narrowing of the joint space (arrow). *Comment:* The foot may be the initial site of occurrence in at least 10% to 20% of cases. Marginal erosions are due to bony erosion from invading pannus and are best seen on the medial margins of the metatarsal heads except the fifth, where they are on the lateral side.

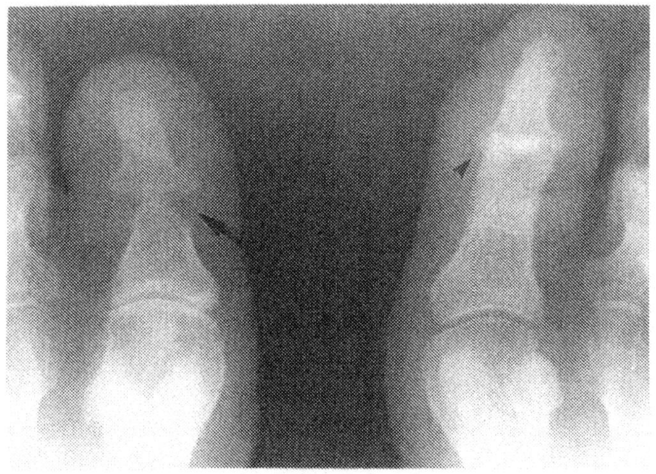
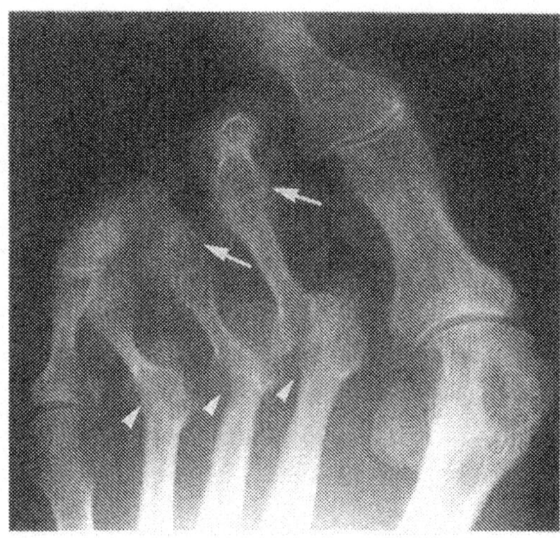

A

B

Fig. 4–43 Psoriatic arthritis. (**A**) Great toe involvement is common in psoriasis. Note the developing pencil-in-cup deformity (arrow) and ankylosis (arrowhead). (**B**) The metatarsophalangeal joints are dislocated (arrowheads). Note the normal bone density and the interphalangeal joint fusion (arrows). *Comment:* These features of bone erosion, joint fusion, and normal bone density in an asymmetric fashion are characteristic of psoriatic arthropathy.

periostitis, especially of the distal tufts and calcaneus, is readily recognizable. Bone density usually remains normal despite the severity of the disease.

Reiter's Syndrome

The vast majority of Reiter's syndrome patients are men between 20 and 40 years of age. The cause is unknown, although venereal transmission of a *Chlamydia* organism has been implicated. The syndrome can also be precipitated by severe diarrhea. The classic triad consists of conjunctivitis, urethritis, and arthritis that usually affects the lower extremity in an asymmetric fashion. There may or may not be a skin rash on the soles of the feet (keratodermia blennorrhagica).

At the calcaneus there are two target areas of involvement: the Achilles and plantar aponeurosis insertion areas. At both these sites there may be erosive and proliferative periostitis changes. A resultant plantar spur has irregular, fluffy margins, in contrast to the smoothly marginated degenerative spur (Figs. 4–38 and 4–44).

In the toes all joints can be affected, usually in a nonuniform manner. The great toe is a favored site. Diffuse soft tissue swelling, cortical erosions, and fluffy periostitis are the major features. At the ankle effusion, some uniform loss of joint space and even periostitis can be seen.

NEOPLASTIC DISORDERS

Tumors of the foot and ankle are uncommon and represent less than 3% of primary skeletal neoplasms.[81]

Malignant Tumors

The most common bone malignancy of the foot is osteosarcoma. Metastasis to the foot is rare but is most common from primary carcinoma of the lung.

Osteosarcoma

Osteosarcoma is slightly more common in males and tends to occur between the ages of 10 and 25 years. The major variation on this age predilection is the occurrence of secondary osteosarcoma arising in preexisting Paget's disease or previously irradiated bone. Usually this occurs in the sixth decade, giving a later age peak, and accounts for the bimodal age distribution of presentation. Unresolving pain and progressive swelling are the usual symptoms.

Less than 3% of osteosarcomas occur in the foot and ankle; in this area the most frequently involved bone is the tibia followed by the fibula, the tarsals (especially the calcaneus), and the metatarsals.[81] The appearance is variable, although the most frequently encountered form of moth-eaten destruction, spiculated periosteal response, and a dense soft tissue bone mass is highly characteristic (Fig. 4–45). This appearance in a metatarsal shaft mimics closely that of a stress fracture.

Ewing's Sarcoma

This is the second most common malignancy of the foot and ankle.[81] The highest incidence occurs in the first and second decades of life, with less than 9% of lesions involving the foot and ankle. The most common bones affected are the tibia and fibula followed by the tarsals, metatarsals, and phalanges.

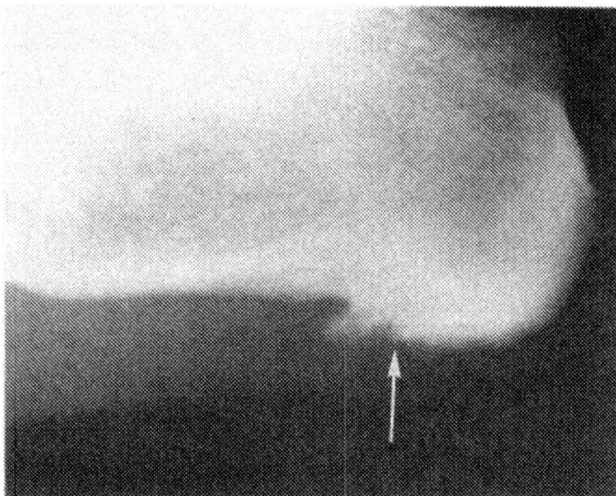

Fig. 4–44 Reiter's syndrome, calcaneal spur. Along the plantar surface of the calcaneus, there is an irregular proliferation of periosteal new bone (arrow). *Comment:* At the calcaneus there are two target areas of involvement: the Achilles and plantar aponeurosis insertion areas. At both these sites, there may be erosive and proliferative periostitis changes. A resultant plantar spur has irregular, fluffy margins, in contrast to the smoothly marginated degenerative spur.

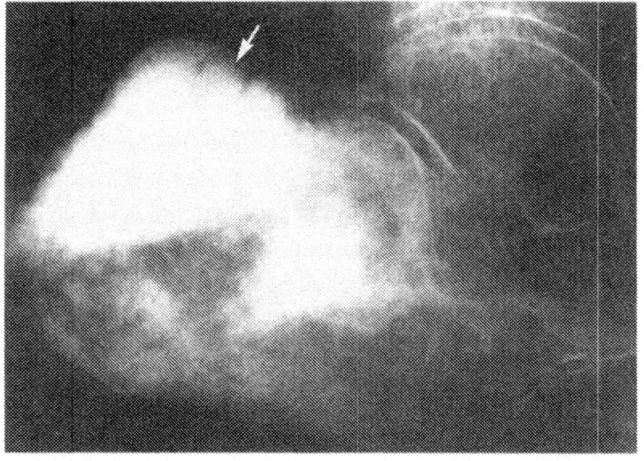

Fig. 4–45 Osteosarcoma of the calcaneus. The calcaneus is diffusely sclerotic. Most notable is the dense sarcomatous new bone extending off the superior aspect of the calcaneus (arrow). *Comment:* Less than 3% of osteosarcomas occur in the foot and ankle. The most frequently involved bone in this area is the tibia followed by the fibula, tarsals (especially the calcaneus), and metatarsals.

Generally these present as diaphyseal lesions with an admixture of moth-eaten destruction and patchy sclerosis. Overlying is a characteristic multilaminated periosteal response that may appear eroded from the outside, creating a saucerization effect (Fig. 4–46). An absence of matrix calcification aids in the differentiation from osteosarcoma.

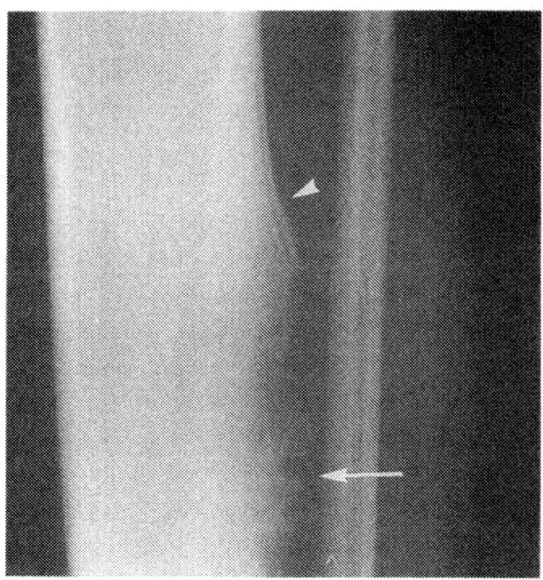

Fig. 4–46 Ewing's sarcoma, tibia. The diaphyseal lesion has an admixture of moth-eaten destruction and patchy sclerosis. Overlying is a characteristic multilaminated periosteal response (arrowhead), which may appear eroded from the outside, creating a saucerization effect (arrow). *Comment:* This is the second most common malignancy of the foot and ankle after osteosarcoma. The most common bones affected are the tibia and fibula followed by the tarsals, metatarsals, and phalanges.

Metastatic Carcinoma

Dissemination of carcinoma distal to the knee is distinctly uncommon. Involvement of the hands and feet (acral metastases) is usually from primary carcinoma of the lung, although any tumor potentially could manifest in this way. Imaging findings are variable but usually involve an osteolytic pattern of destruction with no soft tissue mass (Fig. 4–47).

Benign Tumors

Benign tumors of the foot and ankle are slightly more common than malignant tumors.[81] The two most common benign tumors of the foot and ankle, occurring with an almost equal frequency, are osteochondroma and nonossifying fibroma.

Osteochondroma

An osteochondroma is the most common benign skeletal neoplasm. It is most common around the knee. Less than 5% involve the foot and ankle.[81] Of these, lesions of the distal tibia and fibula make up the majority. An osteochondroma arising beneath a nail bed is called a subungual exostosis. More than 85% of these occur beneath the nail of the great toe.[81] An osteochondroma discovered at the foot or ankle should instigate a skeletal survey, including examination of family mem-

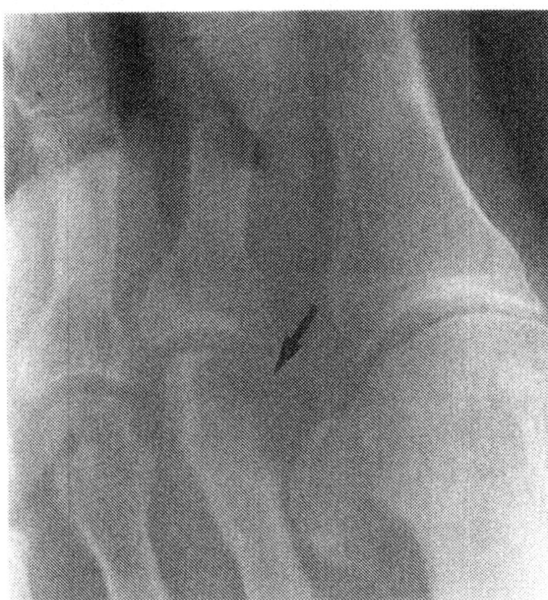

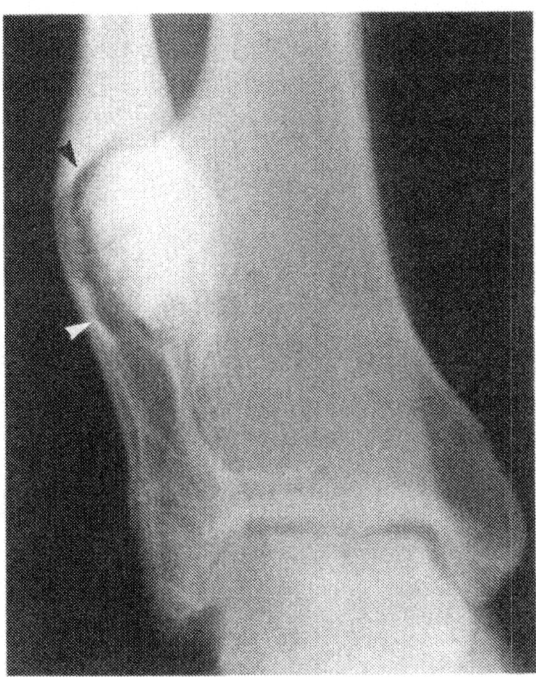

Fig. 4–47 Metastatic carcinoma, metatarsal. At the distal second metatarsal there is an osteolytic pattern of destruction with no soft tissue mass (arrow). *Comment:* Dissemination of carcinoma distal to the knee is distinctly uncommon. Involvement of the hands and feet (acral metastases) is usually from primary carcinoma of the lung, as in this case, although any tumor potentially could manifest in this way.

Fig. 4–48 Osteochondroma, distal tibia. A bony exostosis with calcification of the overlying cartilaginous cap has created an extrinsic bone erosion of the adjacent fibula (arrowheads). *Comment:* An osteochrondroma is the most frequent benign skeletal neoplasm. It is most common around the knee, with less than 5% involving the foot and ankle. An osteochondroma discovered at the foot or ankle should instigate a skeletal survey (including examination of family members) for the presence of hereditary multiple exostoses.

bers, for the presence of hereditary multiple exostoses. Less than 1% can become malignant. Other causes for the lesion becoming symptomatic include compression of neurovascular structures, bursa formation, altered joint mechanics, joint deformity, and fracture of the lesion.

The lesion is composed of an osseous base confluent with the underlying bone and an overlying cartilaginous cap. Two forms are seen: sessile and pedunculated. The sessile form appears as a broad-based protuberance, and the pedunculated variety exhibits a distinctive stalk. Located in the metaphysis, they tend to orient away from the nearest joint, have a thin or even absent overlying cortex, and often demonstrate foci of calcification. Tibial or fibular lesions can produce extrinsic pressure erosions on the adjacent bone and produce tilting of the ankle mortise (tibiotalar slant deformity; Fig. 4–48).

Nonossifying Fibroma

These fibrous lesions are almost exclusively found in the lower extremity, with two thirds arising at the knee and the other third at the ankle.[81] They are rare beyond the tibia and fibula. They are invariably encountered in the second decade of life either as an incidental radiographic finding or in association with a pathologic fracture. They continue growth in parallel with skeletal growth and at adulthood tend to heal

spontaneously. On their own without fracture complication, they are asymptomatic. Multiple nonossifying fibromas do occur and have been found in association with neurofibromatosis.

The most distinctive features consist of a metaphyseal geographic lesion that tends to be eccentrically placed and slightly expansile, has a marked scalloped and sclerotic border, and tapers away from the joint (flame-shaped appearance; Fig. 4–49). The long axis of the lesion parallels that of the bone of origin. Large lesions may occupy the entire circumference of the bone and have a greater chance for pathologic fracture.

Management is often a dilemma because most are asymptomatic and will undergo a natural involution once skeletal maturity is reached. Large lesions may be assessed as a high fracture risk and can be curetted and bone grafted. The majority require no intervention.

Osteoid Osteoma

This is a painful lesion, occurring in the 5- to 25-year age group and affecting males four times as often as females. About 10% of osteoid osteomas are found in the foot and

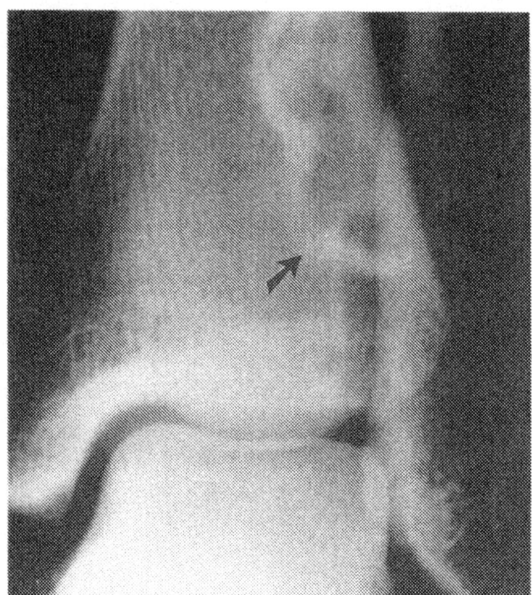

Fig. 4–49 Nonossifying fibroma, distal tibia. The most distinctive features consist of a metaphyseal geographic lesion that tends to be eccentrically placed and is slightly expansile, has a marked scalloped and sclerotic border, and tapers away from the joint (flame-shaped appearance; arrow). *Comment:* These fibrous lesions are almost exclusively found in the lower extremity, with two thirds arising at the knee and the other third at the ankle.

ankle.[81] More than half of these involve the distal tibia, a quarter the tarsals, and less than 10% the phalanges. A clinical hallmark is the rapid and dramatic relief provided by the ingestion of aspirin.

The lesion itself can be difficult to localize on plain films, and up to a quarter are not detectable.[82] On bone scan there is avid isotope uptake. The lesion is usually less than 1 cm in size and consists of a radiolucent center (nidus), often with a central focus of calcification, and surrounding sclerosis (Fig. 4–50). Its proximity to the cortex will dictate how much solid periosteal new bone will be found; subperiosteal and cortical lesions will produce a considerable amount, whereas cancellous and intraarticular lesions will produce little to none. The main differential considerations are Brodie's abscess and bone islands.

Giant Cell Tumor

This tumor is more common in women in the age range of 20 to 40 years. It is classified as a quasi-malignant tumor because up to 20% can become frankly malignant; this is more often the case in men. Only about 6% of giant cell tumors are found in the foot and ankle, with more than 90% of these occurring in the distal tibia.[81]

The radiographic appearance can be misleading, with benign-looking lesions being malignant. The tumor can readily

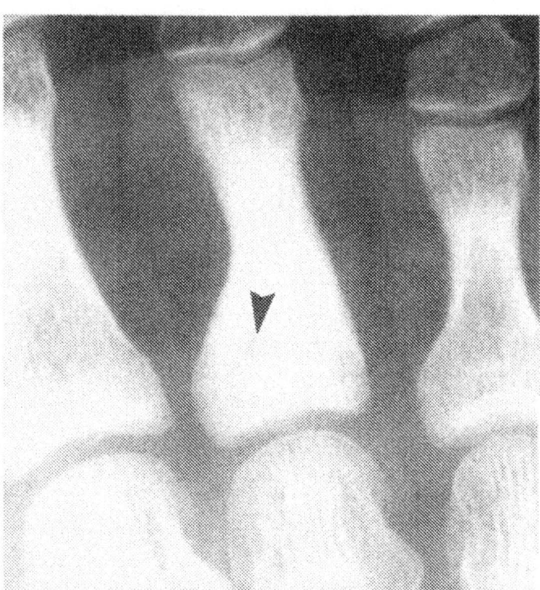

A

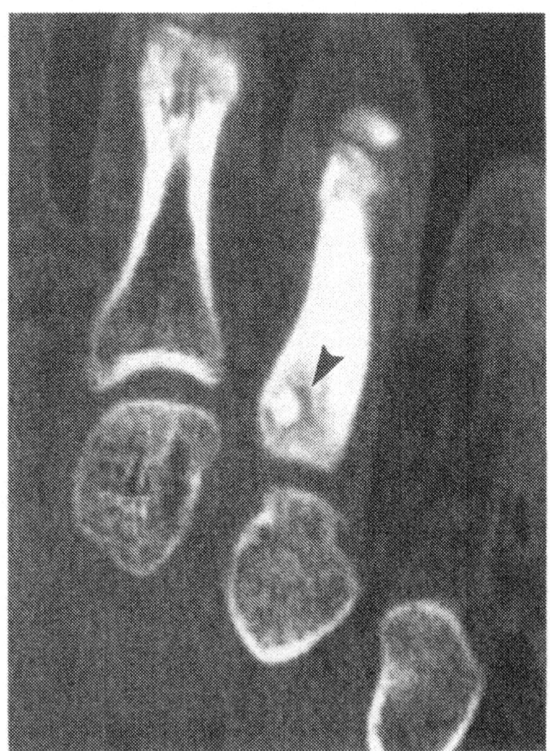

B

Fig. 4–50 Osteoid osteoma, proximal phalanx. (**A**) The entire phalanx is sclerotic (ivory phalanx). Observe the small radiolucent nidus (arrowhead) with a central sclerotic focus. (**B**) On CT examination the nidus is visible (arrowhead), the central calcification is more obvious, and the entire phalanx is homogeneously sclerotic. *Comment:* On bone scan there is avid isotope uptake. The lesion's proximity to the cortex will dictate how much solid periosteal new bone will be found; subperiosteal and cortical lesions will produce a considerable amount, whereas cancellous and intraarticular lesions will produce little to none.

be diagnosed by the fact that it involves simultaneously the metaphysis and epiphysis, coming to lie against the articular surface. The lesion is typically geographic in nature with a sharp zone of transition, endosteal scalloping, and fine internal septations. It is slightly eccentrically placed and exhibits evidence of expansion (Fig. 4–51).

Simple Bone Cyst

Less than 10% of simple bone cysts occur in the foot and ankle.[81] Of these lesions, 80% arise in the calcaneus. The most common calcaneal tumor is a simple bone cyst.[7] These are usually detected in the first two decades of life, often as an incidental finding in trauma (eg, injury during athletic activity) or by causing pathologic fracture.[83]

The predictable location is the junction of the anterior and middle third of the calcaneus. The cysts are purely osteolytic, are round to oval in shape, have sharp margins, can be expansile, and may display light internal septations (Fig. 4–52). Larger lesions can involve the majority of the calcaneus.[83]

Observation, steroid injection, and curettage form the prescribed sequence of treatments.[7,83] There should be clear differentiation from the commonly seen pseudocystic triangle in the calcaneus, which is a normal variant.

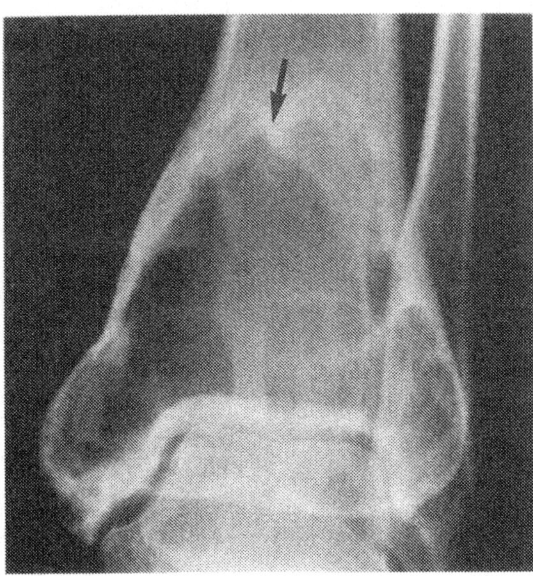

Fig. 4–51 Giant cell tumor, distal tibia. The lesion is typically geographic in nature with a sharp zone of transition (arrow), endosteal scalloping, and fine internal septations. It is slightly eccentrically placed and subarticular and exhibits evidence of expansion. *Comment:* Only about 6% of giant cell tumors are found in the foot and ankle, with more than 90% of these occurring in the distal tibia. The radiographic appearance can be misleading, with benign-looking lesions being malignant.

Enchondroma

These benign, slow-growing cartilage tumors remain asymptomatic until they either pathologically fracture or, in less than 1% of cases, become malignant chondrosarcomas. Less than 10% involve the ankle and foot, with the phalanges being the most singularly common site.[81]

Enchondromas are intramedullary lesions with sharp margins and endosteal scalloping, and in at least 50% of cases they show foci of calcification (Fig. 4–53). Occasionally multiple lesions can be seen even in the same digital ray.

METABOLIC DISORDERS

Paget's Disease

The foot is typically considered an uncommon site of Paget's disease, but it may be involved in up to 20% of patients.[7] The calcaneus is the most common bone of the foot to be involved. The tibia is a frequently involved bone; the fibula is considered a rare site. The majority of Paget's disease involving the foot will be asymptomatic.

The radiographic features are distinctive. Usually the entire bone is involved early, with disease extending from one articular surface to another. The trabecular pattern is coarse, the cortex is thick, and the bone is usually expanded (Fig. 4–54). In the tibia an advancing, tapered, radiolucent interface can often be seen (blade of grass appearance). Isotopic bone scans are characteristically strongly positive.

Complications of Paget's disease include pathologic (banana) fracture, insufficiency fractures, pseudofractures, and avulsion fractures. Malignant degeneration to osteosarcoma or fibrosarcoma occurs in less than 10% of patients.

Osteoporosis

This is a common metabolic disease caused by loss of bone mass. Its etiologies are many and include postmenopausal osteoporosis, senile osteoporosis, endocrine disorders, corticosteroids and heparin, disuse, transient regional osteoporosis, and reflex sympathetic dystrophy syndrome (RSDS).

Postmenopausal Osteoporosis

This is the most common form of skeletal osteopenia. Blood chemistries are normal. Involvement of the foot and ankle is similar to that in other skeletal sites and manifests as thinning of the cortices (pencil-thin cortex) and reduced trabeculae. The calcaneal index has been used to assess the degree of osteoporosis, comparing the Singh index in the hips, but it has an error rate of 25% and is not considered reliable.[84,85]

Disuse Osteoporosis

After immobilization for trauma, there is a rapid loss of bone density over 8 weeks. This can be seen radiographically within a few days. Usually there is a uniform osteopenia of all

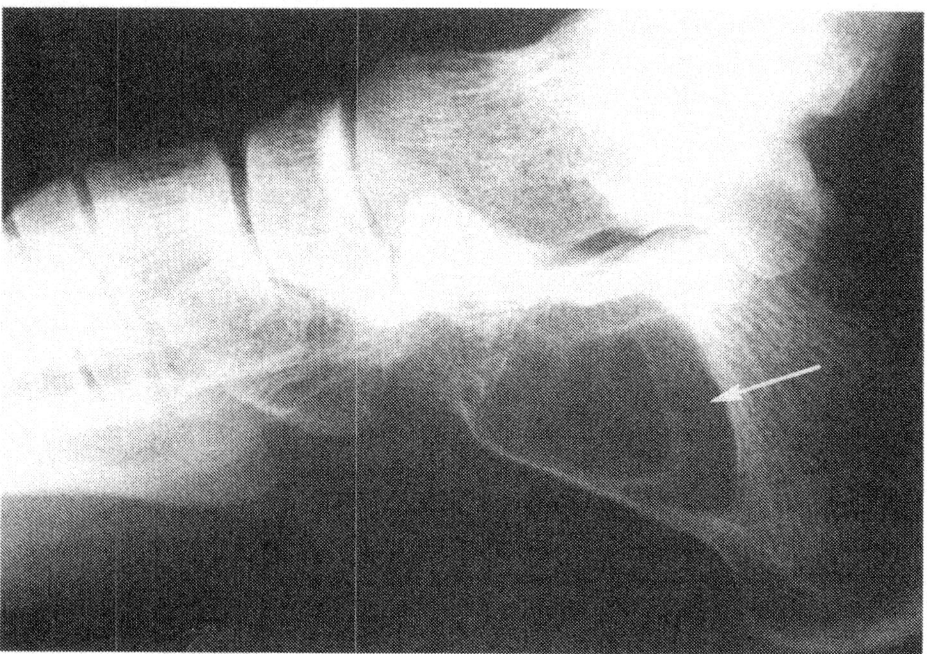

Fig. 4–52 Simple bone cyst, calcaneus. The lesion is purely osteolytic and round to oval in shape. It has sharp margins, is slightly expansile, and displays light internal septations (arrow). *Comment:* Less than 10% of simple bone cysts occur in the foot and ankle, with at least 80% of these arising in the calcaneus. The most common calcaneal tumor is a simple bone cyst.

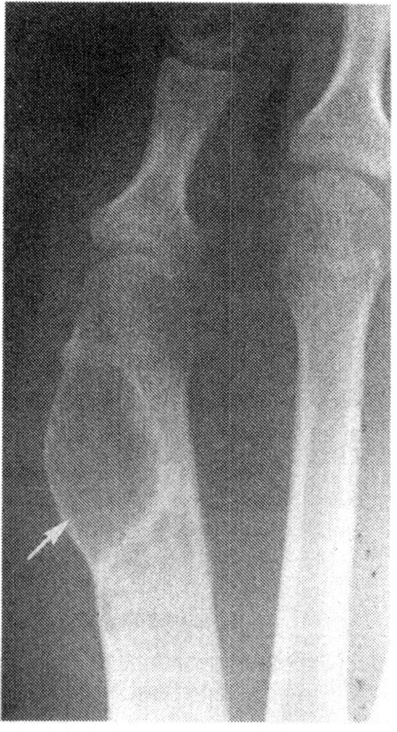

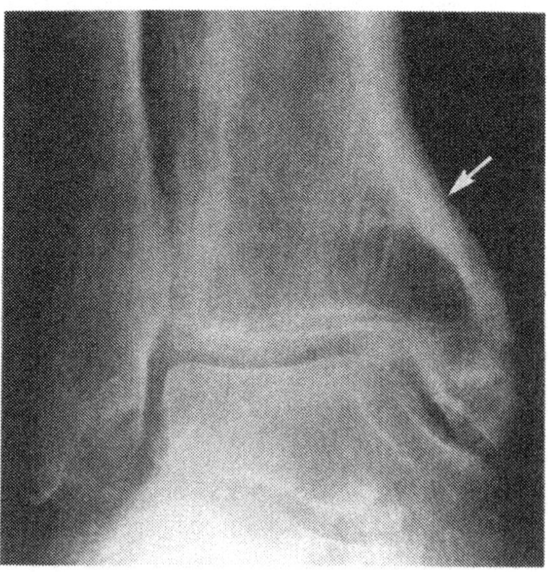

Fig. 4–53 Enchondroma, fifth metatarsal. An expansile, eccentric, geographic lesion is readily appreciated (arrow). No calcification is evident. *Comment:* Less than 10% involve the ankle and foot, with the phalanges being the most common site.

Fig. 4–54 Paget's disease, tibia. The trabecular pattern is coarse, the cortex is thick (arrow), and the bone is expanded. *Comment:* The foot, typically considered an uncommon site of Paget's disease, may be involved in up to 20% of patients. The calcaneus is the most common bone of the foot to be involved. The tibia is a frequently involved bone; the fibula is considered a rare site.

skeletal structures that have been immobilized. Other patterns include prominent juxtaarticular osteopenia and focal areas of radiolucency. Differentiation from early osteomyelitis is difficult.

Reflex Sympathetic Dystrophy Syndrome (RSDS)

Many terms have been used to describe this syndrome, including *Sudek's atrophy, causalgia, shoulder–hand syn-* *drome,* and *posttraumatic osteoporosis.* The accepted term for this symptom complex of pain, swelling, reduced motion, trophic skin changes, and vasomotor instability is *reflex sympathetic dystrophy.* The cause of the syndrome is unknown, and it most commonly complicates even trivial trauma of the foot or ankle. The radiographic features are nonspecific except that the osteopenia can be severe and rapidly progressive (Fig. 4–55).

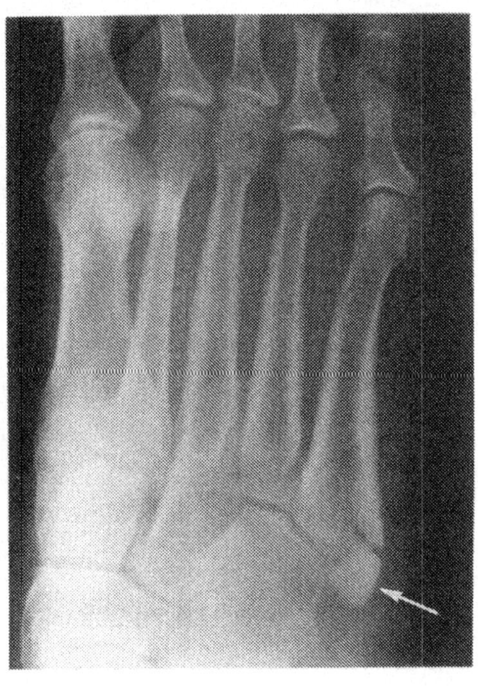

A

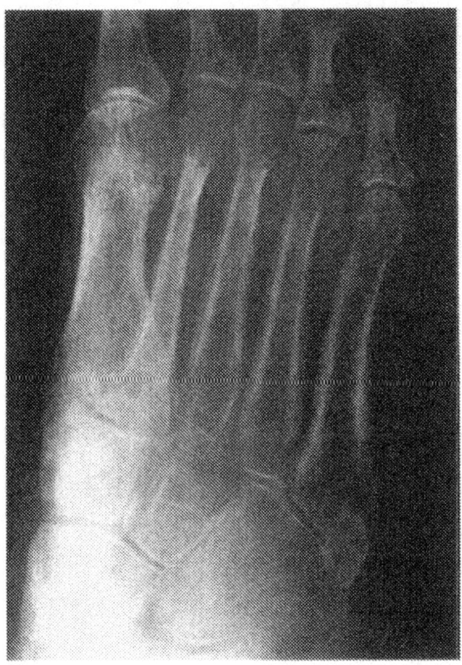

B

Fig. 4–55 Reflex Sympathetic Dystrophy Syndrome. (**A**) This 33-year-old woman had a fracture at the base of the fifth metatarsal (Jones' fracture; arrow). (**B**) At 6 weeks after injury, the foot became swollen and discolored. Radiographically there is generalized osteopenia, and the fracture has not healed well. *Comment:* The accepted term for this symptom complex of pain, swelling, reduced motion, trophic skin changes, and vasomotor instability is *reflex sympathetic dystrophy.* The cause of the syndrome is unknown, and it most commonly complicates even trivial trauma of the foot or ankle.

REFERENCES

1. Ballinger WP. *Merrill's Atlas on Roentgenographic Positioning and Standard Radiologic Procedures* (5th ed). St Louis, Mo: Mosby; 1982.

2. Towbin R, Dunbar JS, Towbin J. Teardrop sign: Plain film recognition of ankle effusion. *AJR.* 1980; 134:985.

3. Olson RW. Ankle arthrography. *Radiol Clin North Am.* 1981,19.255.

4. Frolich H, Gotzen L, Adam D. Evaluation of stress roentgenograms of the upper ankle joint. *Unfallheilunde.* 1980;83:457.

5. Johannsen A. Radiologic diagnosis of lateral ligament lesions of the ankle. A comparison between talar tilt and anterior drawer sign. *Acta Orthop Scand.* 1978;49:259.

6. Brostrom L. Sprained ankles. III. Clinical observations in recent ligament ruptures. *Acta Chirop Scand.* 1965;130:560.

7. Berquist TH. *Radiology of the Foot and Ankle.* New York, NY: Raven; 1989.

8. Rowe LJ, Yochum TR. Radiographic positioning and normal radiographic anatomy. In: Yochum TR, Rowe LJ, eds. *Essentials of Skeletal Radiology.* Baltimore, Md: Williams & Wilkins; 1987; 1:1.

9. Brantigan JW, Pedegana LR, Lippert FG. Instability of the subtalar joint. *J Bone Joint Surg Am.* 1977;59:321.

10. Feist JH, Mankin HJ. The tarsus. I. Basic relationships and motions in the

adult and definition of optimal recumbent oblique projection. *Radiology.* 1962;79:250.

11. Isherwood I. A radiological approach to the subtalar joint. *J Bone Joint Surg Br.* 1961;43:566.

12. Holly EW. Radiography of the tarsal sesamoid bones. *Med Radiogr Photogr.* 1955;31:73.

13. Horsefield D, Murphy G. Stress views of the ankle joint in lateral ligament injury. *Radiography.* 1986;51:224.

14. Ala-Ketola L, Puronen J, Koivisto E, Purepera M. Arthrography in the diagnosis of ligament injuries and classification of ankle injuries. *Radiology.* 1977;125:63.

15. Schweigel JF, Knickerbocher WJ, Cooperberg P. A study of ankle instability utilizing ankle arthrography. *J Trauma.* 1977;17:878.

16. Smith RW, Staple TW. Computerized tomography (CT) scanning technique for the hind foot. *Clin Orthop.* 1983;177:34.

17. Seltzer SE, Weissman BN, Braunstein EM, et al. Computed tomography of the hind foot. *J Comput Assist Tomogr.* 1984;8:488.

18. Solomon MA, Gilula LA, Oloff LM, Oloff J. CT scanning of the foot and ankle: 1. Normal anatomy. *AJR.* 1986;146:1192.

19. Solomon MA, Gilula LA, Oloff LM, Oloff J. CT scanning of the foot and ankle: 2. Clinical applications and a review of the literature. *AJR.* 1986;146:1204.

20. Rosenburg ZS, Feldman F, Singson RD. Peroneal tendon injuries: CT analysis. *Radiology.* 1986;161:743.

21. Fisher MR, Barker B, Amparo EG, et al. MR imaging using specialized coils. *Radiology.* 1985;157:443.

22. Sierra A, Potchen EJ, Moore J, Smith HG. High-field magnetic resonance imaging of aseptic necrosis of the talus. *J Bone Joint Surg Am.* 1986;68:927.

23. Daffner RH, Reimer BL, Lupetin AR, Dash N. Magnetic resonance imaging of acute tendon ruptures. *Skeletal Radiol.* 1986;15:619.

24. Roberts DK, Pomeranz SJ. Current status of magnetic resonance in radiologic diagnosis of foot and ankle injuries. *Orthop Clin North Am.* 1994;25:61.

25. Seldin DW, Heiken JP, Feldman F, Alderson PO. Effect of soft tissue pathology on detection of pedal osteomyelitis in diabetics. *J Nucl Med.* 1985;26:988.

26. D'Ambrosia RD, Shoji H, Riggins RS, Stadalnik RC, DeNardo GL. Scintigraphy in the diagnosis of osteonecrosis. *Clin Orthop.* 1978;130:139.

27. Bassett LW, Gold RH, Wekken MM. Radionuclide bone imaging. *Radiol Clin North Am.* 1981;19:675.

28. Freeman LM, Blaufax MD. Nuclear orthopedics. *Semin Nucl Med.* 1988;18:77.

29. Deutsch AL, Resnick D, Campbell G. Computed tomography and bone scintigraphy in evaluation of tarsal coalition. *Radiology.* 1982;144:137.

30. Shereff MJ. Radiographic analysis of the foot and ankle. In: Jahss MH, ed. *Disorders of the Foot and Ankle.* Philadelphia, Pa: Saunders; 1991:401–427.

31. Perry MD, Mont MA, Einhorn TA, Waller JD. The validity of measurements made on standard foot orthoroentgenograms. *Foot Ankle.* 1992;13:502.

32. Toygar O. Subcutaneous rupture of the Achilles tendon (diagnosis and management). *Helv Chirop Acta* 1947;14:209.

33. Rubin G, Witten M. The talar tilt angle and the fibular collateral ligaments: A method for the determination of talar tilt. *J Bone Joint Surg Am.* 1960;42:311.

34. Christman OD, Snook CA. A reconstruction of lateral ligament tears of the ankle: An experimental study and clinical evaluation of seven patients treated by a new modification of the Elmslie procedure. *J Bone Joint Surg Am.* 1969;51:904.

35. Gould N, Seligson D, Glassman J. Early and late repair of lateral ligaments of the ankle. *Foot Ankle.* 1980;1:84.

36. Resnick DL, Feingold ML, Curd J, et al. Calcaneal abnormalities in articular disorders. Rheumatoid arthritis, ankylosing spondylitis, psoriatic arthritis and Reiter's syndrome. *Radiology.* 1977;125:355.

37. Rowe LJ, Yochum TR. Measurements. In: Yochum TR, Rowe LJ, eds. *Essentials of Skeletal Radiology.* Baltimore, Md: Williams & Wilkins; 1987;1:169–223.

38. Lawson JP. Symptomatic radiographic variants in the extremities. *Radiology.* 1985;157:625.

39. Micheli LJ, Ireland ML. Prevention and management of calcaneal apophysitis in children: An overuse syndrome. *J Pediatr Orthop.* 1987;7:34.

40. Keats TE, Harrison RB. The calcaneal nutrient foremen: A useful sign in the differentiation of true from simulated cysts. *Skeletal Radiol.* 1979;3:239.

41. Sirry A. The pseudocystic triangle in the normal os calcis. *Acta Radiol.* 1951;36:516.

42. Ozonoff MB. The foot. In: Ozonoff MB, ed. *Pediatric Orthopedic Radiology.* Philadelphia, Pa: Saunders; 1979:275–324.

43. Keats TE. *Normal Roentgen Variants That May Simulate Disease* (4th ed). Chicago, Ill: Year Book Medical; 1984.

44. Onitsuka H. Roentgen aspects of bone islands. *Radiology.* 1977;123:607.

45. Hall FM, Goldberg RP, Davies JAK, Fainsurger MH. Scintigraphic assessment of bone islands. *Radiology.* 1980;135:737.

46. Venn-Watson EA. Problems in polydactyly of the foot. *Orthop Clin North Am.* 1976;7:909.

47. Phelps DA, Grogan DP. Polydactyly of the foot. *J Pediatr Orthop.* 1985;54:446.

48. Sartoris DJ, Resnick DL. Tarsal coalition. *Arthritis Rheum.* 1985;28:331.

49. Leonard MA. The inheritance of tarsal coalition and its relationship to spastic flat foot. *J Bone Joint Surg Br.* 1974;56:520.

50. Beckley DE, Anderson PW, Pedegana LR. The radiology of the subtalar joints with special reference to talocalcaneal coalition. *Clin Radiol.* 1975;26:333.

51. Simon RR, Hoffman JR, Smith M. Radiographic comparison of plain films on second- and third-degree ankle sprains. *Am J Emerg Med.* 1986;4:387.

52. Harper MC. Stress radiographs in the diagnosis of lateral instability of the ankle and hindfoot. *Foot Ankle.* 1992;13:435.

53. Larson E. Experimental instability of the ankle: A radiographic investigation. *Clin Orthop.* 1986;204:193.

54. Harsh WN. Effects of trauma upon epiphyses. *Clin Orthop.* 1957;10:140.

55. Salter RB, Harris WR. Injuries involving the epiphyseal plate. *J Bone Joint Surg Am.* 1963;45:587.

56. Arimoto HR, Forrester DM. Classification of ankle fractures: An Algorithm. *AJR.* 1980;135:1057.

57. Berndt AL, Harty M. Transchondral fractures (osteochondritis dissecans) of the talus. *J Bone Joint Surg Am.* 1959;41:988.

58. Hawkins LG. Fractures of the neck of the talus. *J Bone Joint Surg Am.* 1970;52:991.

59. Lance EM, Carey EJ, Wade PA. Fractures of the os calcis: A followup study. *J Trauma.* 1964;4:15.

60. Smith J, Arnoczky SP, Hersh A. The intraosseous blood supply of the fifth metatarsal: Implications of proximal fracture healing. *Foot Ankle.* 1992;13:143.

61. Rogers LF. *Radiology of Skeletal Trauma.* New York, NY: Livingstone; 1992;2.

62. Levy JM. Stress fracture of the first metatarsal. *AJR.* 1978;130:679.

63. Rowe LJ. Metatarsal stress fracture. *ACA Counc Diagn Imag.* 1983:1–5.

64. Smillie IS. Frieberg's infarction (Köhler's second disease). *J Bone Joint Surg.* 1955;37:580.

65. Canale ST, Kelly FB. Fractures of the neck of the talus. *J Bone Joint Surg Am.* 1978;60:143.

66. Lippman HI, Goldin RR. Subcutaneous ossification of the legs with chronic venous insufficiency. *Radiology.* 1960;74:279.

67. Waldvogel FA, Popageogion PS. Osteomyelitis: The past decade. *N Engl J Med.* 1980;303:306.

68. Steinback HL. Infection in bone. *Semin Roentgenol.* 1966;1:337.

69. Dalinka MK, Lally JF, Conwer G. The radiology of osseous and articular infection. *CRC Radiol Nucl Med.* 1975;7:1.

70. Rowe LJ, Yochum TR. Infection. In: *Essentials of Skeletal Radiology.* Baltimore, Md: Williams & Wilkins; 1987;2:921–960.

71. Nguyen VD, London J, Cone RO III. Ring sequestrum: Radiographic characteristics of skeletal fixation pin tract osteomyelitis. *Radiology.* 1986;158:129.

72. Miller WB, Murphy WA, Gilula LA. Brodie's abscess. Reappraisal. *Radiology.* 1979;132:15.

73. Rowe LJ, Yochum TR. Arthritis. In: *Essentials of Skeletal Radiology.* Baltimore, Md: Williams & Wilkins; 1987;2:539–698.

74. Stiles RG, Resnick DL, Sartoris DJ. Radiologic manifestations of arthritides involving the foot. *Clin Podiatr Med Surg.* 1988;5:1.

75. Karasick D, Wapner KL. Hallux rigidus deformity: Radiologic assessment. *AJR.* 1991;157:1029.

76. Taylor JAM, Sartoris DJ, Huang GS, Resnick DL. Painful conditions affecting the first metatarsal sesamoid bones. *RadioGraphics.* 1993;13:817.

77. Rubin G, Witten M. Plantar calcaneal spurs. *Am J Orthop.* 1963;5:38.

78. Katzman B, Young S, Shavelson D. The heel spur syndrome: A report of 46 patients with 61 painful heels. *Curr Podiatr Med.* 1987;36:23.

79. Schneider R, Goldman AB, Bohne WHO. Neuropathic injuries to the lower extremity in children. *Radiology.* 1978;128:713.

80. Rowe LJ. Psoriatic arthropathy. *ACA Counc Diagn Imag.* 1980:1–5.

81. Dahlin DC, Unni KK. *Bone Tumors: General Aspects and Data on 8,542 Cases.* Springfield, Ill: Thomas; 1986.

82. Shereff MJ, Cullivan OPA, Johnson KA. Osteoid osteoma of the foot. *J Bone Joint Surg Am.* 1983;65:638.

83. Rowe LJ, Brandt JR. Simple bone cysts in athletes. *Chirop Sports Med.* 1988;2:33.

84. Aggarwal ND, Singh GD, Aggarwal R, et al. A survey of osteoporosis using the calcaneum as an index. *Int Orthop.* 1986;10:147.

85. Cockshott WP, Occleshaw CJ, Webber C, et al. Can a calcaneal morphologic index determine the degree of osteoporosis? *Skeletal Radiol.* 1984;12:119.

Chapter 5

Passive Motion Palpation

Passive motion palpation (PMP) is best defined as the motion palpation challenge of an articulation without the influence of weight bearing. PMP should not be confused with motion palpation, developed by Henri Gillet[1] and widely used throughout the profession. Motion palpation of the lower extremity, as taught today, is limited to general range of motion rather than specific palpation.

Motion palpation is performed with the patient standing for the sacroiliac joints or sitting for the spine and rib cage. This places a weight-bearing stress on the joints being palpated. Any distortion below the area being palpated will alter the findings as long as weight bearing is maintained. If the range of motion seems restricted or painful or feels odd, or if specific ligaments are suspect, PMP of the individual articulations may be performed.

Radiographic examination is necessary to prove or disprove the presence of pathology, but it cannot show function. Even if gross distortions and pathology are present, if the articulations are functioning the foot may be relatively symptom free.

Hiss[2] has stated that comfort varies directly with function. Many times over the years, patients have presented with feet that I could not imagine would be able to bear the body weight, much less function normally. Many of these, after a thorough examination, needed only manipulation of specific joints for restoration of normal function, and the patient walked out of the office pain free.

With an understanding of anatomy and a knowledge of muscle testing on the part of the examiner, PMP is the most effective means of determining the problems of the foot. By specific palpation in the directions of normal joint movement, it is possible to test for restrictions and hypermobility. If fixations are present, they can be adjusted accurately, and the muscles involved can be evaluated for dysfunction. If pain is present and/or instability is detected, additional radiographs with the X-ray beam directed to the specific articulation may be of benefit in arriving at a diagnosis.

The PMP techniques described in this chapter are based upon the work of Raymond T. Broome, DC.[3] Broome credits Mennell[4] and Gillet[1] for the basis of his work. Broome's PMP allows the practitioner to challenge each segment of the ankle and foot in each direction of movement without affecting the adjacent articulations. Broome's contribution to the examination of the foot is a major accomplishment and should be recognized as such. Although the methods described below may not be exactly as shown by Broome, they are based on the principles of his work.

A plastic model of the foot and ankle is invaluable in learning anatomy, PMP, and adjusting positions. The number of articulations, bony differences, and angles make the use of a model necessary in the evaluation process. There should be no hesitation in using a model in one's examination and treatment. I find one useful for determining radiographic angles as well as for a reminder of all the complexities of the foot.

PMP is best performed in the supine position. It is important to explain to the patient what is taking place and that if at any time pain is felt he or she should let it be known immediately. The patient must be relaxed. Most patients will react by contracting the musculature upon contact. Even the seemingly relaxed leg and foot will relax further when the patient is instructed to do so. This is necessary not only for PMP but also for the adjusting procedures.

Contact with the patient's foot must be positive yet without gripping or probing with pressure enough to cause pain. Palpation around the fibulocalcaneal ligaments, even in an old sprain case, may be painful. Specific pressure is applied with movement of each bone in the direction in which it normally moves. If pain is elicited, the examiner must then determine whether the pain is from lack of movement, excessive movement, ligamental damage, contusion, edema of the articulation, or a combination thereof. Some gross distortions, obvious range of motion problems, and the like may be helped with general mobilization techniques, but most cases with foot symptoms require specific analysis and specific adjusting.

My own foot was an extreme case in point proving the value of specific motion palpation. While traveling in Europe, I fractured the three middle metatarsals at the base and sustained two chip fractures on the first metatarsal base and the first cuneiform. In Greece, the three metatarsals were rebroken 5 weeks later. Upon my arrival in Great Britain with the freshly refractured foot, Broome adjusted every articulation in the foot except the three metatarsal bases with the cuneiforms without pain. My foot and lower leg were placed in a cast, where they remained for 6 weeks. Since then (1986) I have walked the 13-km gorge on Crete and the Kathrine gorge in Northern Territory, Australia without problems of any kind. Today, many years later, the healed fractures of the metatarsals are barely visible on plain films.

In PMP, as the joints are moved upon each other one should feel a spring or end play at the limits of the range of motion. If a fixation is present there will be no end play, and the sensation of bone against bone will be felt. A loss of joint play, or fixation, has many possible causes, including intrinsic trauma (the unexpected movement of an articulation within an overall normal movement). Immobilization from wearing ill-fitting shoes because of style or necessity (eg, high heels at work) or the abuse of wearing old, worn out, "comfortable" shoes can cause fixations. Hyperextension of the great toe when kneeling for a long time can distort and fix joints. Residuals from old injuries, the aging process, and postural stresses from other distortions all can cause fixations in the feet.

THE ANKLE JOINT AND HINDFOOT

The talus (Fig. 5–1), having no muscle attachments, is subject to the pressures applied to it from adjacent structures and is restrained by its ligaments. The trochlea of the talus is gripped by the tibia with its medial malleolus and by the fibula (Fig. 5–2). The trochlea is wider anteriorly than posteriorly and, with dorsiflexion, exerts pressure laterally and medially. The facetal facing of the fibula allows for slight lateral rotation during dorsiflexion as well as movement proximally.

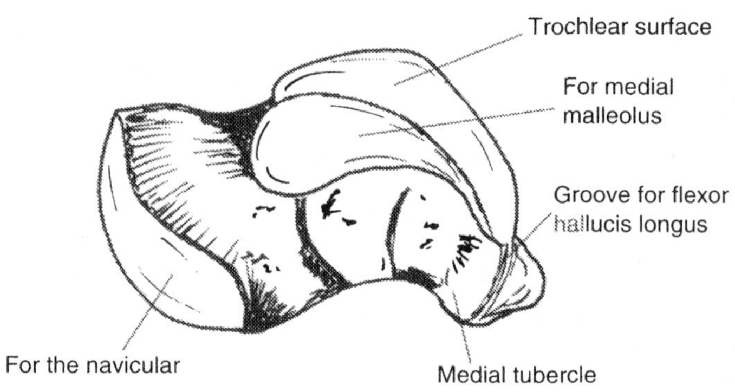

Fig. 5–1 Right talus, medial view.

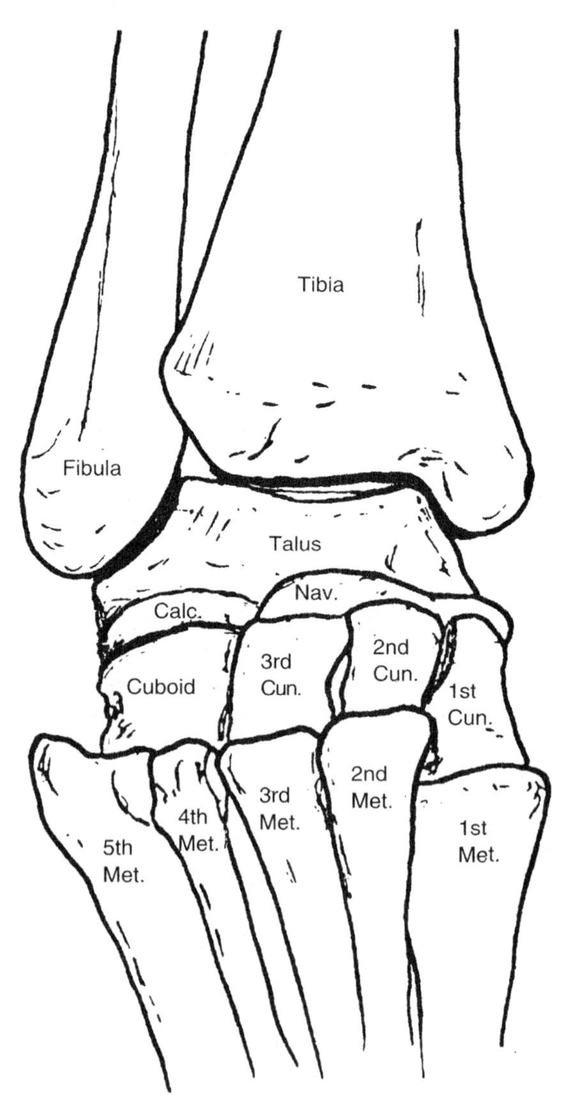

Fig. 5–2 Right ankle and foot, anterior view with forefoot flexed.

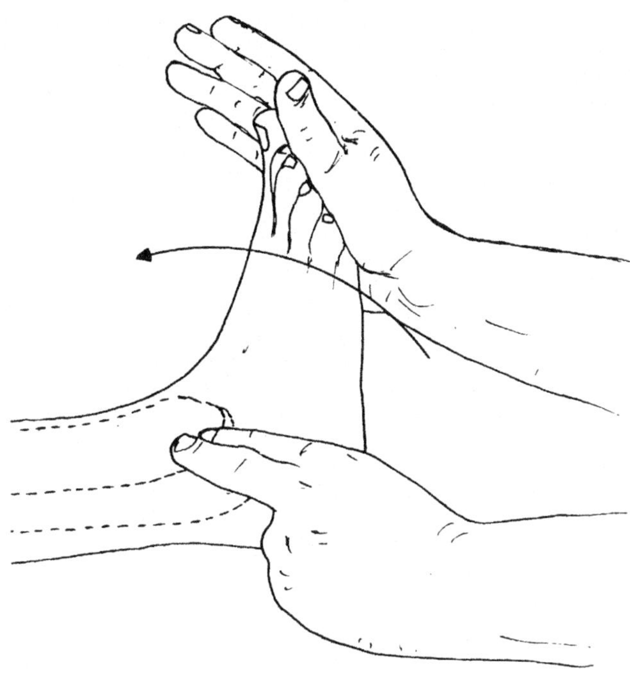

Fig. 5–3 Palpation of fibular movement during dorsiflexion of the ankle.

For PMP of the fibulotibial articulation during dorsiflexion of the ankle, beginning with the ankle in slight plantar flexion, move the ankle into dorsiflexion while palpating the anterior surface of the fibulotibial joint (Fig. 5–3). With dorsiflexion, the anterior fibula should separate slightly from the tibia, rotate laterally, and glide proximally. Repeat dorsiflexion, and palpate the proximal end of the fibula at the knee (Fig. 5–4). Movement should correspond with the movement felt distally.

Movement of the fibular head on the tibia is governed by its location on the posterolateral surface of the tibia, where the condyle begins to narrow, and by its muscle attachments. The fibula can move anteriorly/inferiorly (by actions of the peroneus longus, peroneus tertius, extensor hallucis longus, and extensor digitorum longus muscles) and superiorly (by action of the biceps femoris when the knee is extended). It moves posteriorly (by action of the biceps with knee flexion past 90° and inferiorly by action of the flexor hallucis longus, peroneus brevis, and extensor digitorum longus muscles). Fibular movement at the ankle and the knee may be altered as a result of muscle spasms or weakness. For instance, if the fibula is fixed superiorly as a result of a contracted biceps and there is a weakness of the everters and dorsiflexors of the foot (originating on the fibula), no movement will be felt.

THE TALUS

Normal movement of the talus is necessary for complete dorsal and plantar movement of the whole foot.

Anterior Glide of the Talus under the Tibia

Support the foot with the outside hand, gripping immediately behind the fibula and tibia on the posterior surface of the talus (Fig. 5–5). With the inside hand in full pronation, use the thumb web to grip the anterior surface of the foot just below the tibia, and apply pressure anteriorly.

Posterior Glide of the Talus on the Tibia

With the outside hand, support the distal end of the tibia (Fig. 5–6). With the inside hand, grasp the medial longitudinal

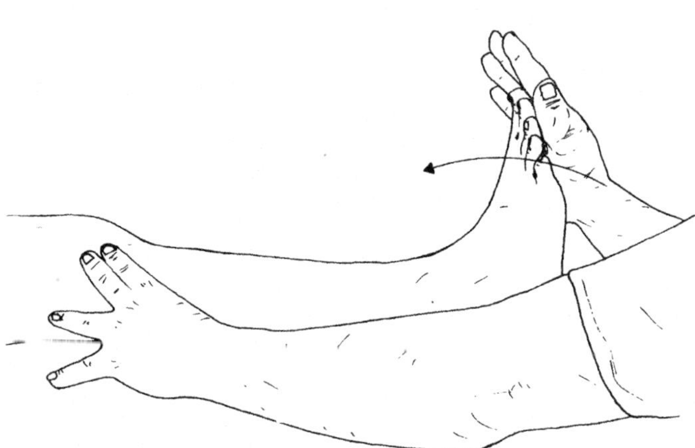

Fig. 5–4 Palpation of the fibular head during dorsiflexion.

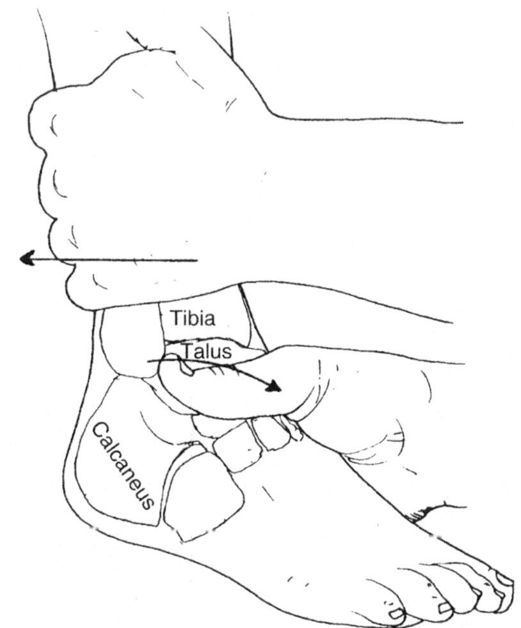

Fig. 5–5 Test for anterior glide of the talus under the tibia.

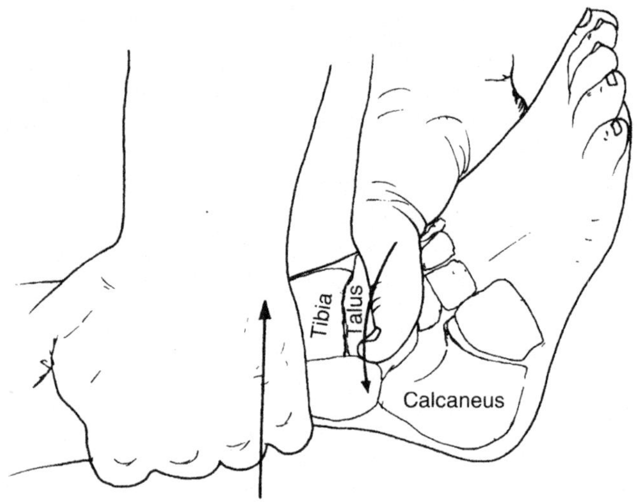

Fig. 5–6 Test for posterior glide of the talus under the tibia.

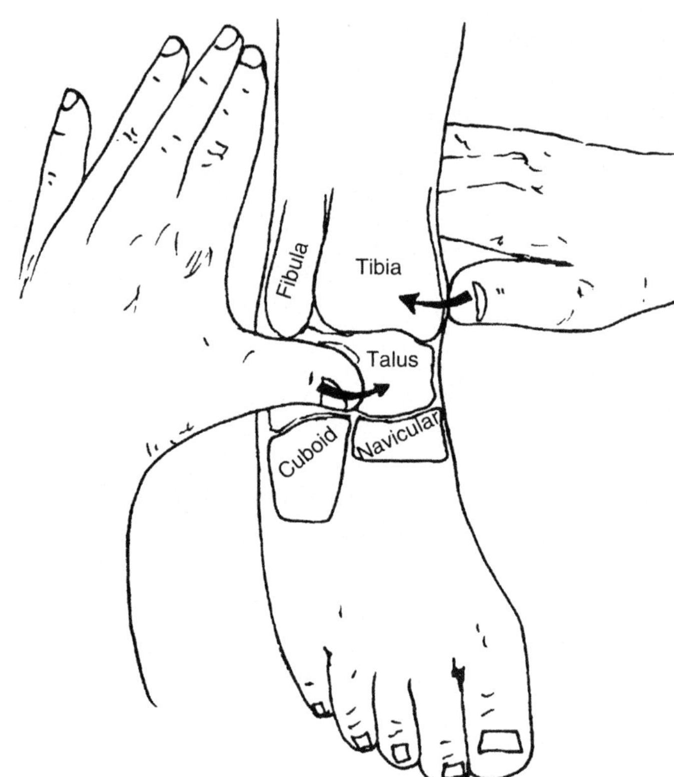

Fig. 5–7 Test for medial movement of the talus under the tibia.

arch, dorsiflexing the arch of the foot to make it rigid without dorsiflexing the ankle. Grip the navicular bone with the thumb on the dorsal surface and the index finger wrapping around the bone to the plantar surface. Using the rigid foot, apply pressure posteriorly on the navicular, which in turn applies direct pressure on the talus posteriorly.

Besides the dorsiflexion–plantar flexion movement, the talus has some mediolateral movement as well.

For efficiency in the examination, the next test should be for anterior glide on the calcaneus, but this is dealt with later in the chapter.

Medial Movement of the Talar Head on the Tibia

Support the tibia with the heel of the inside hand, or use the thumb pad against the tibia (Fig. 5–7). The elbow should be in line, directly medial to the joint. Use the pad (not the tip) of the outside thumb on the lateral surface of the talar head (just over the sulcus). Apply pressure medially on the talar head against resistance from the opposite direction.

Lateral Movement of the Talar Head on the Tibia

Reverse the procedure for medial glide, providing resistance with the outside hand (Fig. 5–8). The medial side of the talar head is usually a sensitive area. Applying pressure laterally, by using the pad of the inside thumb, will be more comfortable to the patient. Anterior to posterior movement of the talocalcaneal (subtalar) articulation is minimal compared with the talotibial articulation.

A review of the calcaneal facets shows their relationship (Fig. 5–9). Most of the body weight is shifted onto the larger posterior facet, allowing movement anterior to posterior and medial to lateral and from plantar flexion to dorsiflexion. Pres-

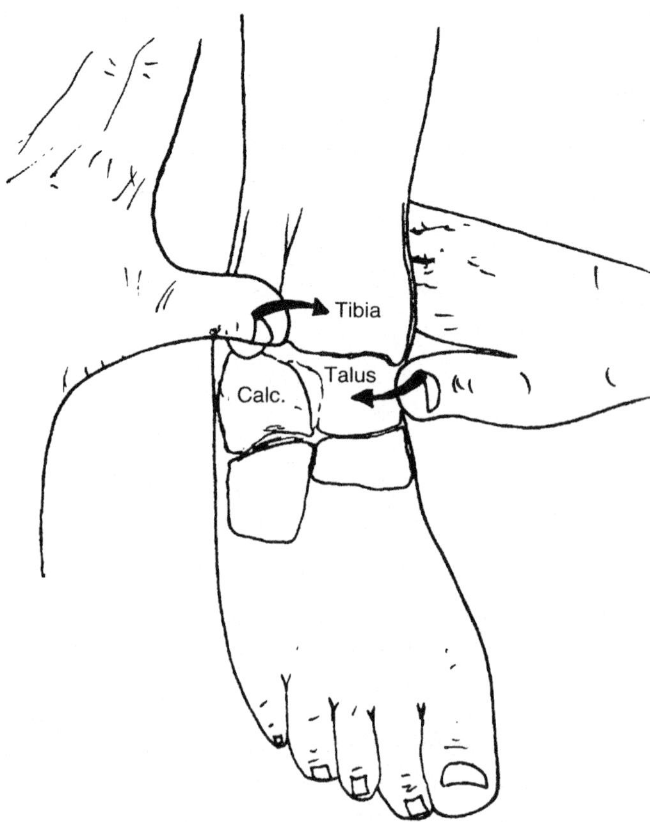

Fig. 5–8 Test for lateral movement of the talus under the tibia.

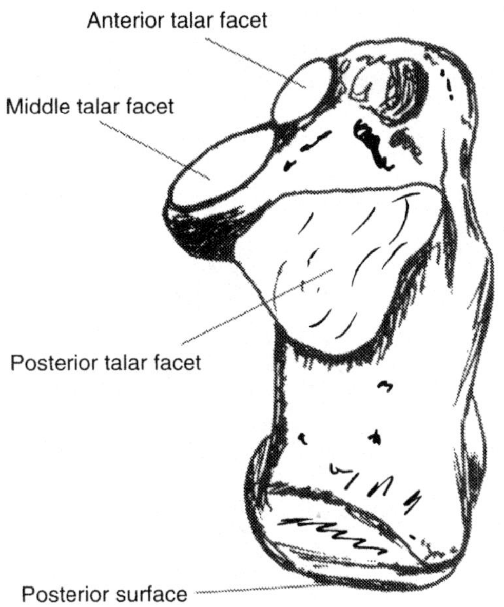

Fig. 5–9 Right calcaneus from above.

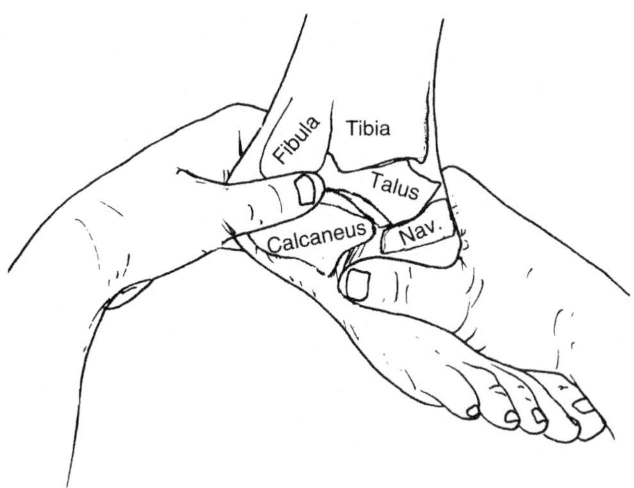

Fig. 5–10 Test for medial spring of the talocalcaneal joint.

surc may bc applied to the talocalcaneal articulation to determine whether the normal springy end feel is present.

Test for Medial Spring

Grasp the foot with the inside hand over the dorsum, index finger around the talar head, and thumb over the cuboid (Fig. 5–10). Grasp the heel with the outside hand, and allow the thumb access to the talocalcaneal joint. Supinate and abduct the forefoot slightly to provide a rigid lever. Apply pressure along the line of articulation (Fig. 5–11), under and around the lateral malleolus. If the spring is absent, further investigation is necessary.

Test for Lateral Spring

Grasp the tarsal arch with the outside hand, index finger over the calcaneocuboid articulation (Fig. 5–12). Adduct and slightly pronate the foot to tighten the lateral longitudinal arch and stiffen the foot. Grasp the heel with the inside hand, and place the thumb pad over the subtalar articulation. Apply pressure in several places along the articulation (Fig. 5–11), and note the presence or absence of spring.

Posterior Glide of the Talus on the Calcaneus

Support the heel with the outside hand. Using the web of the inside hand, apply pressure posteriorly (Fig. 5–13).

Anterior Glide of the Talus on the Calcaneus

Use two fingers on the inside hand to support the posterior surface of the talus level with the tip of the fibula (Fig. 5–14).

With the outside hand, palm up, grasp the heel and apply pressure posteriorly against the resistance from the support hand.

Most of the mediolateral movement of the talus on the calcaneus takes place anteriorly. In the normal resting foot, the talar head is superior to the calcaneus anteromedially. Posterolaterally, however, it lies next to the calcaneus and cuboid in approximately the same 45° plane as the cuboidocuneiform angle. The position of the talar head prohibits much movement laterally (Fig. 5–15). Upon weight bearing, the talar head and navicular move medially.

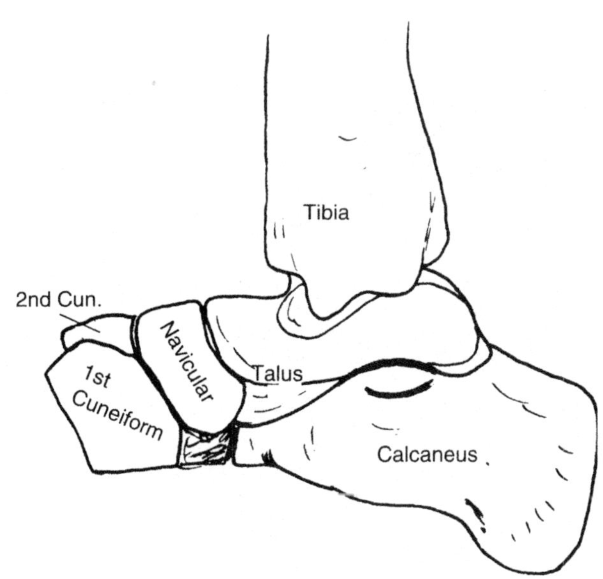

Fig. 5–11 Contour of the talocalcaneal articulation.

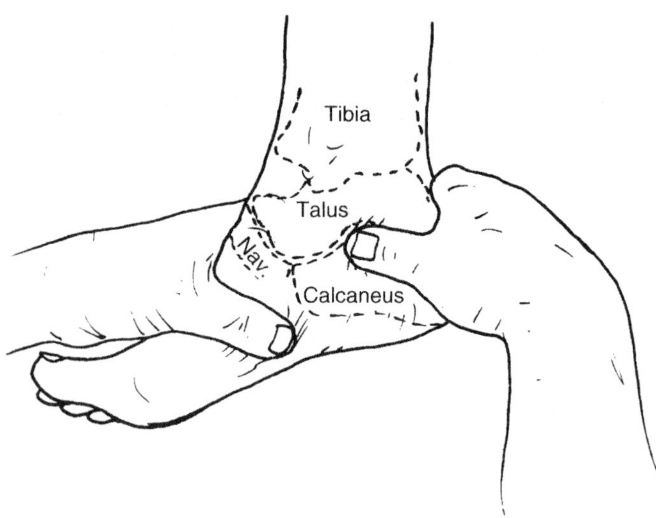

Fig. 5–12 Test for lateral spring: talocalcaneal articulation.

Test for Lateral Glide of the Talar Head on the Calcaneus

To test for lateral glide of the talar head on the calcaneus, use the outside hand thumb pad on the anterior calcaneus (Fig. 5–16). With the thumb pad of the inside hand, apply lateral pressure on the talar head just in front of the medial malleolus.

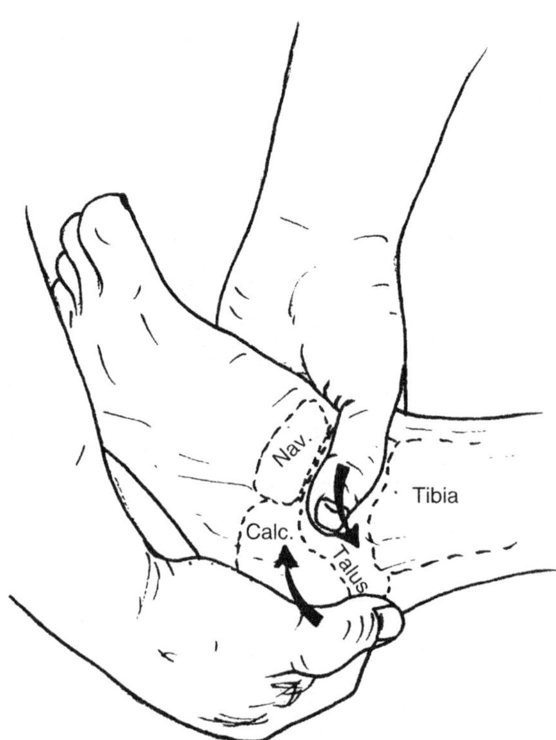

Fig. 5–13 Test for posterior glide of the talus on the calcaneus.

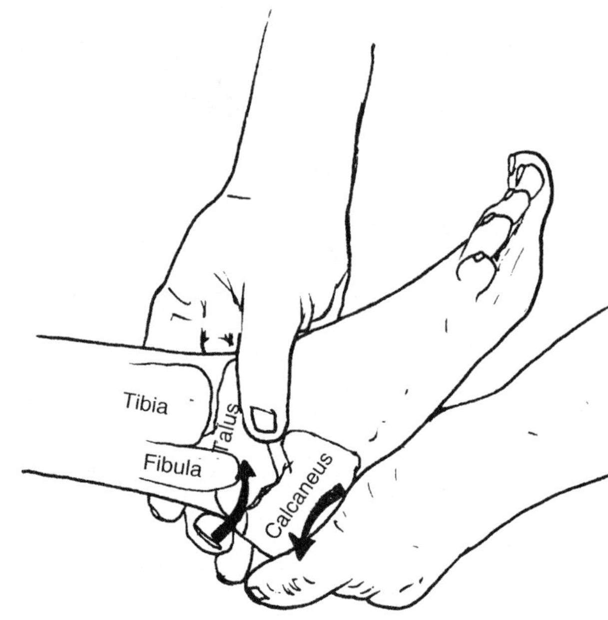

Fig. 5–14 Test for anterior glide of the talus on the calcaneus.

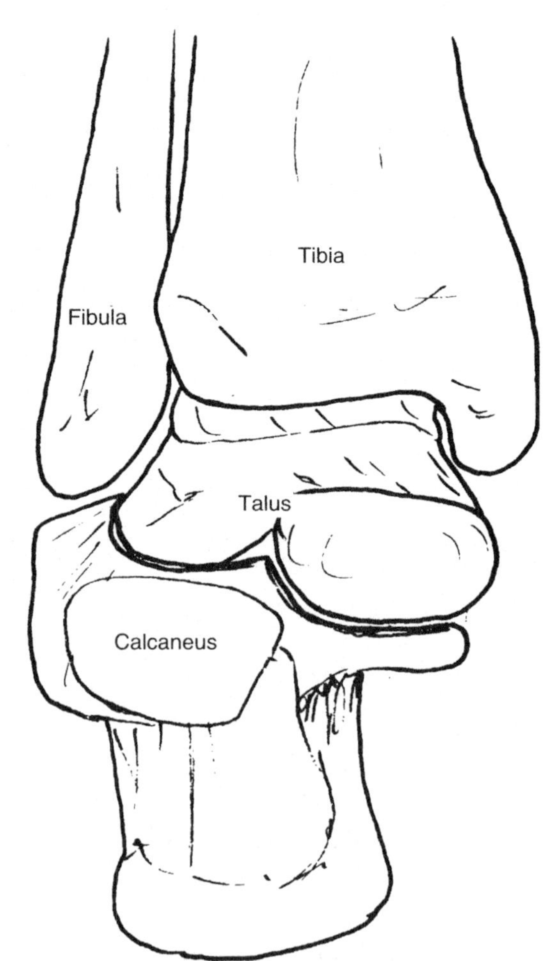

Fig. 5–15 Right ankle, anterior view.

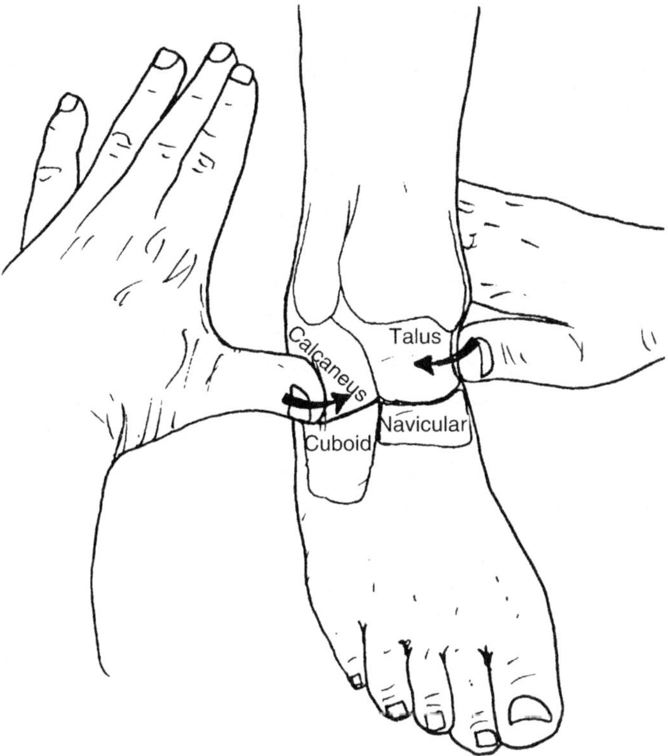

Fig. 5–16 Test for lateral glide of the talus on the calcaneus.

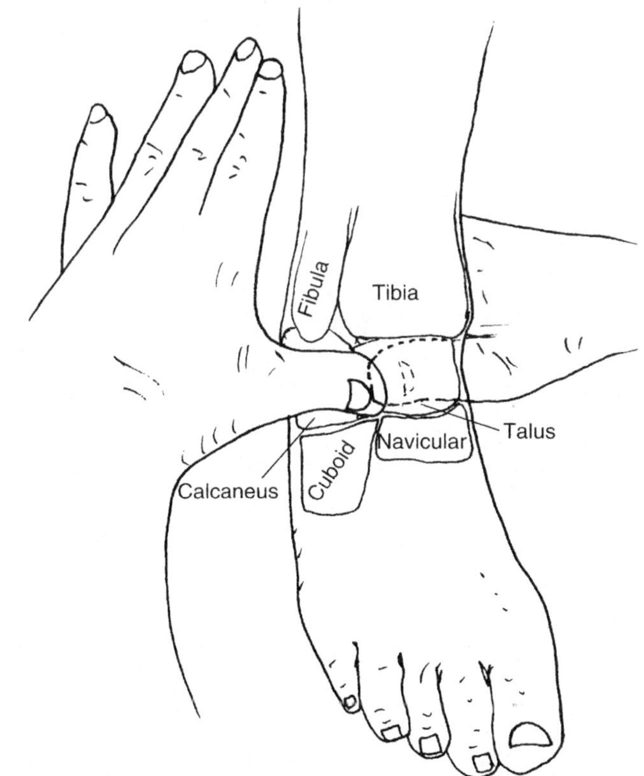

Fig. 5–17 Test for medial glide of the talar head on the calcaneus.

For added security, the outside hand may support the heel during the test.

Test for Medial Glide of the Talar Head on the Calcaneus

To test for medial glide of the talar head on the calcaneus, support the heel with the inside hand, thumb pad on the medial surface of the calcaneus (Fig. 5–17). With the thumb pad of the outside hand, apply medial pressure on the lateral surface of the talar head (immediately over the sulcus).

Mobilization Testing of the Calcaneus

Movement at the subtalar joint consists of the above movements as well as their combination. Mobilization techniques may be used as a screening method (Fig. 5–18). With the inside hand, grasp the foot, the index finger around and under the medial malleolus and the thumb over the area of the third cuneiform, navicular, and lateral talar head. Slightly supinate the foot to make the medial longitudinal arch rigid. This contact allows the greatest possible restriction of the talus yet permits movement of the calcaneus. With this contact, the examiner can evaluate all movements of the calcaneus.

Move the calcaneus through a dorsiflexion–plantar flexion rocking action (Fig. 5–18), through inversion-eversion (Fig. 5–19), and through abduction-adduction (Fig. 5–20). After directional testing, test overall flexibility with circumduction or gross mobilization in all directions. In these tests, look for mobility, smoothness of movement, pain, and a normal end feel.

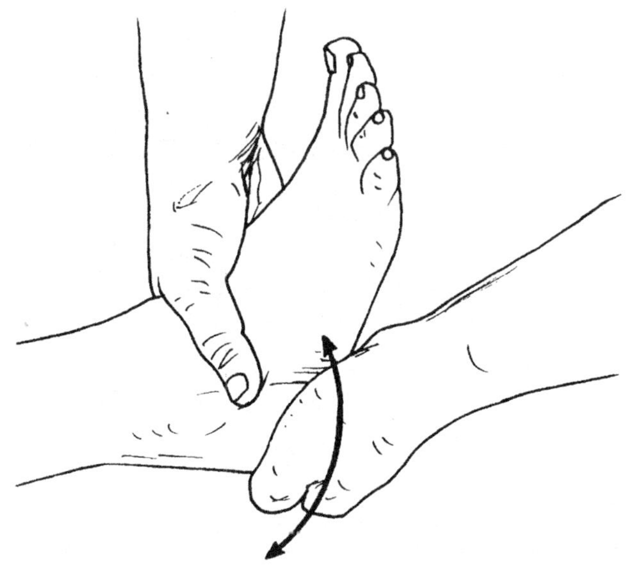

Fig. 5–18 Mobilization of the calcaneus: plantar flexion–dorsiflexion.

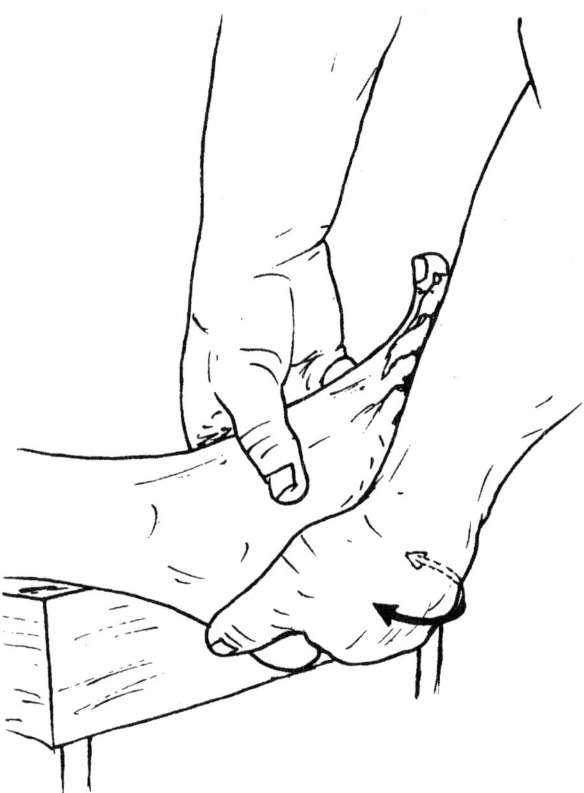

Fig. 5–19 Mobilization of the calcaneus: inversion-eversion.

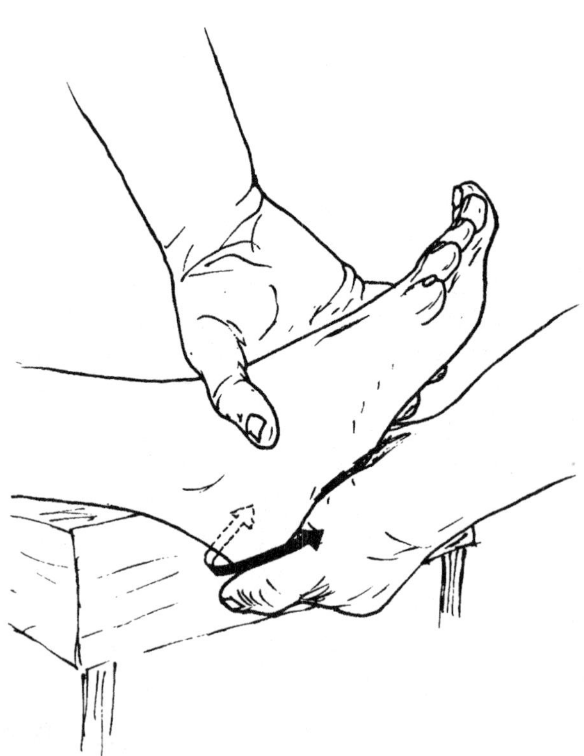

Fig. 5–20 Mobilization of the calcaneus: adduction-abduction.

THE TARSAL ARCH

For the purpose of efficiency, the tarsals are divided into three segments:

1. the cuboid and its articulations
2. the navicular and its articulations
3. the first cuneiform and its articulations

The Cuboid

The cuboid has mediolateral and dorsal-plantar movement with the calcaneus (Fig. 5–21) as well as dorsal-plantar movement and rotation with the fourth and fifth metatarsals. The cuboid has dorsal-plantar movement at a 45° angle with the third cuneiform and sometimes with the navicular (Fig. 5–22).

Medial Movement of the Cuboid on the Calcaneus

Grasp the heel with the inside hand. Place the thumb on the medial surface of the anterior tubercle of the calcaneus to provide resistance (Fig. 5–23). Apply medial pressure on the lateral surface of the cuboid (just behind the overhang of the fifth metatarsal).

Lateral Movement of the Cuboid on the Calcaneus

Place the inside hand palm down over the dorsum of the foot and the thumb on the sulcus just proximal to the groove for the peroneus longus to provide resistance (Fig. 5–24). Grasp the heel with the outside hand and apply medial pressure on the lateral surface of the anterior calcaneus.

Tests for Plantar Movement of the Cuboid

The next several tests of plantar movement of the cuboid are best done by securing the cuboid on the plantar surface. Pres-

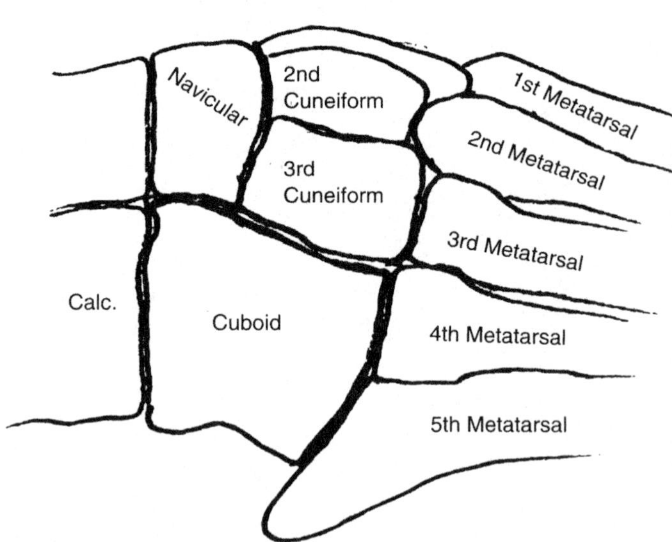

Fig. 5–21 Right foot viewed 45° lateral and superior.

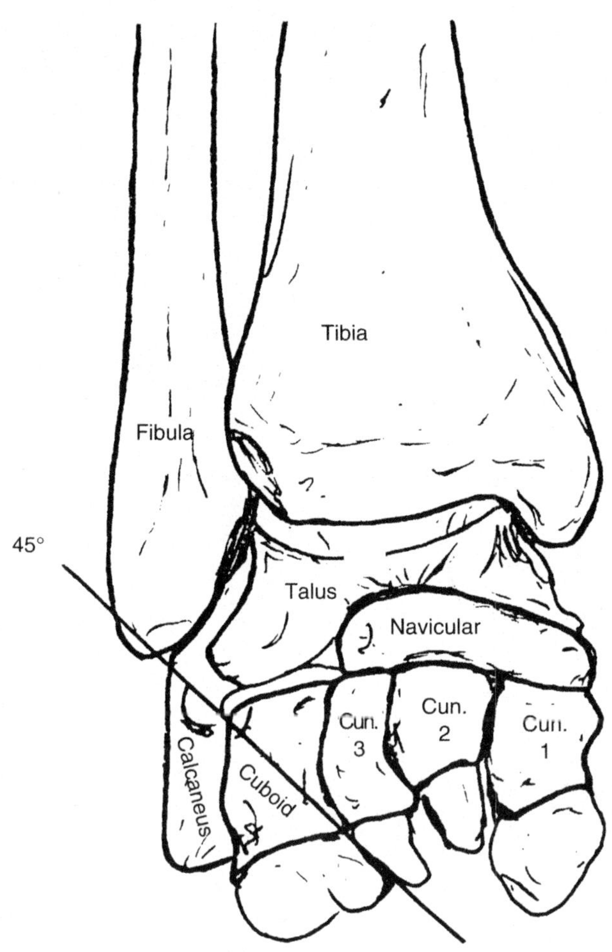

Fig. 5–22 Right foot from the front showing the angle of articulation with the third cuneiform.

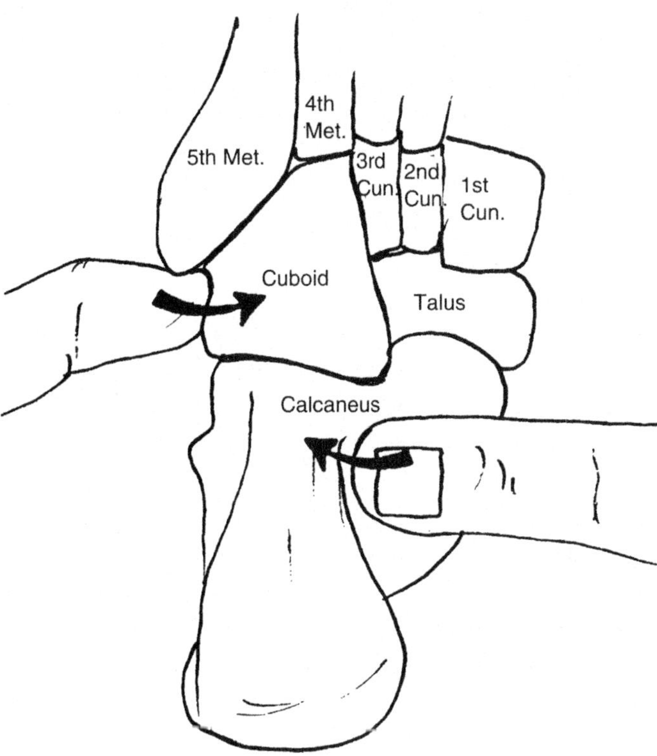

Fig. 5–23 Right foot, plantar view showing finger placement for testing medial movement of the cuboid on the calcaneus.

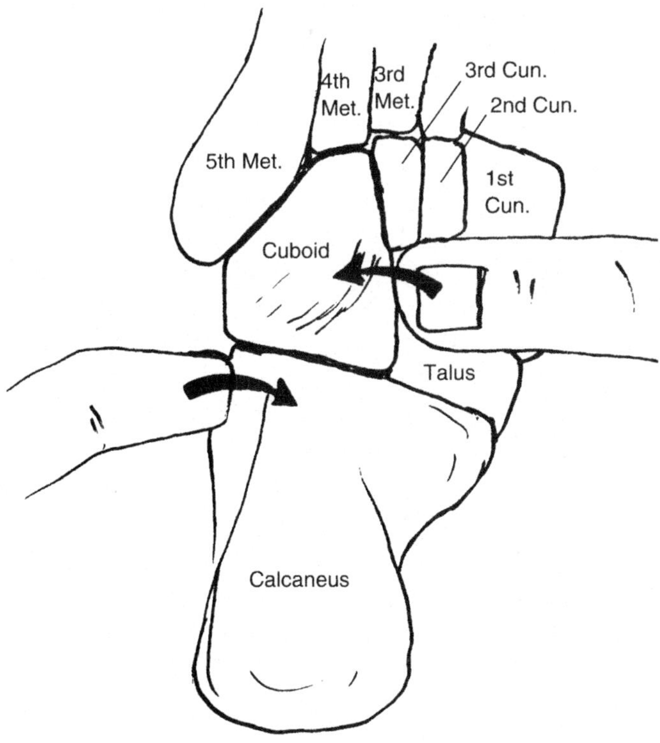

Fig. 5–24 Test for lateral movement of the cuboid on the calcaneus.

sure may then be applied inferiorly on the adjacent structures to test for fixation. Move to the side of the table and rotate the foot and ankle medially for these tests. Place the fingers of the outside hand under the heel with the thumb pad under the cuboid to provide resistance. Testing is best accomplished by rotating the inside hand over with the thumb toward the outside of the foot (Fig. 5–25). This allows the proximal portion of the thumb pad to be used to apply pressure.

Test for plantar glide of the calcaneus on the cuboid. Apply plantar pressure opposite the cuboid resistance (Fig. 5–25). Each articulation is different; therefore, pressure should be tested in several degrees to accommodate the individual articulation shape.

Test for plantar movement of the navicular on the cuboid. The direction of pressure must be altered to accommodate the 45° angle of the articulation (Fig. 5–26).

Test for plantar movement of the third cuneiform on the cuboid. Again, the direction of pressure must be altered to accommodate the 45° angle of the articulation (Fig. 5–27).

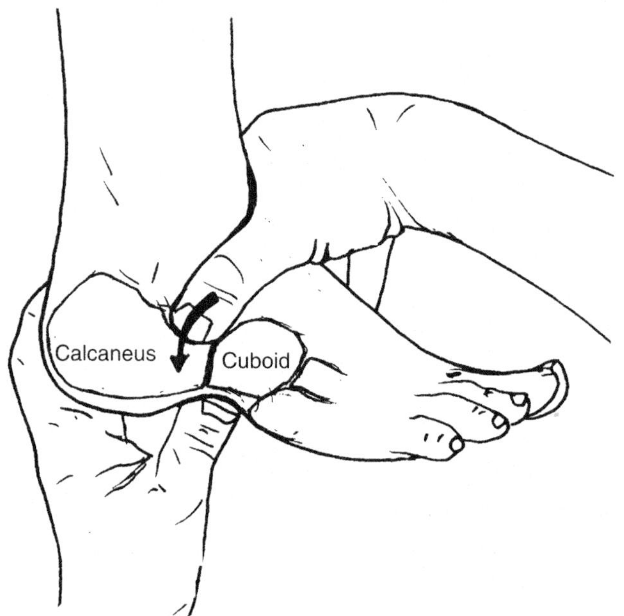

Fig. 5–25 Test for plantar movement of the calcaneus on the cuboid.

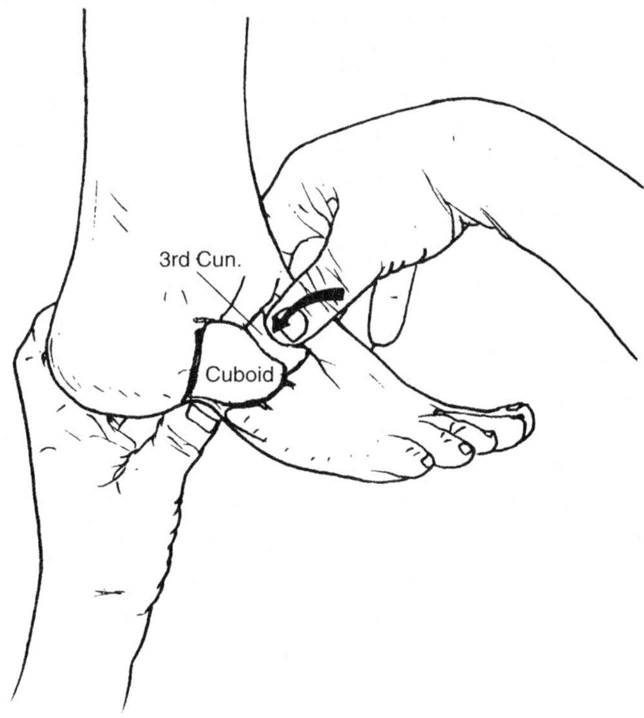

Fig. 5–27 Test for plantar movement of the third cuneiform on the cuboid.

Test for fourth metatarsal plantar movement on the cuboid. Figure 5–28 illustrates positioning and movement for this test.

Test for fifth metatarsal plantar movement on the cuboid. Plantar pressure may be applied to the fifth metatarsal and then still further on the lateral surface of the tuberosity for some rotation movement (Fig. 5–29).

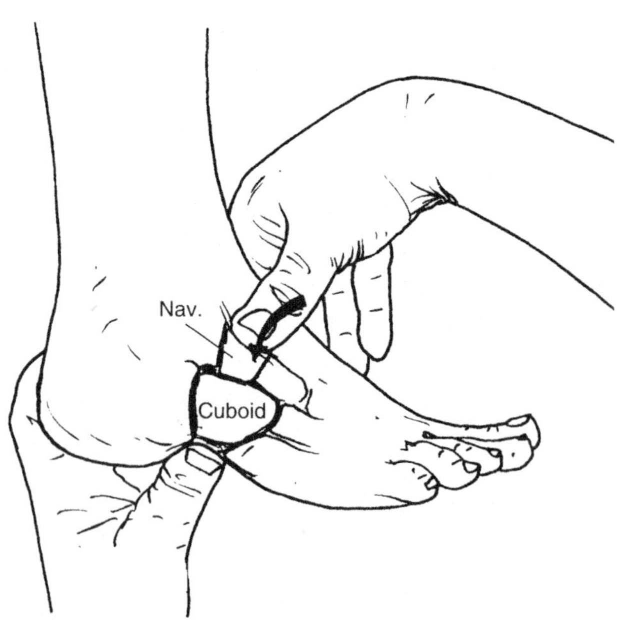

Fig. 5–26 Test for plantar movement of the navicular on the cuboid.

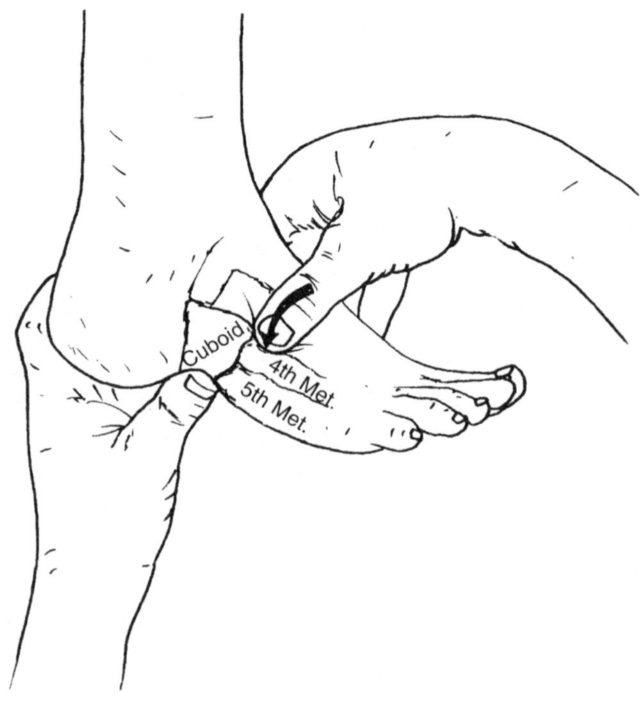

Fig. 5–28 Test for plantar movement of the fourth metatarsal on the cuboid.

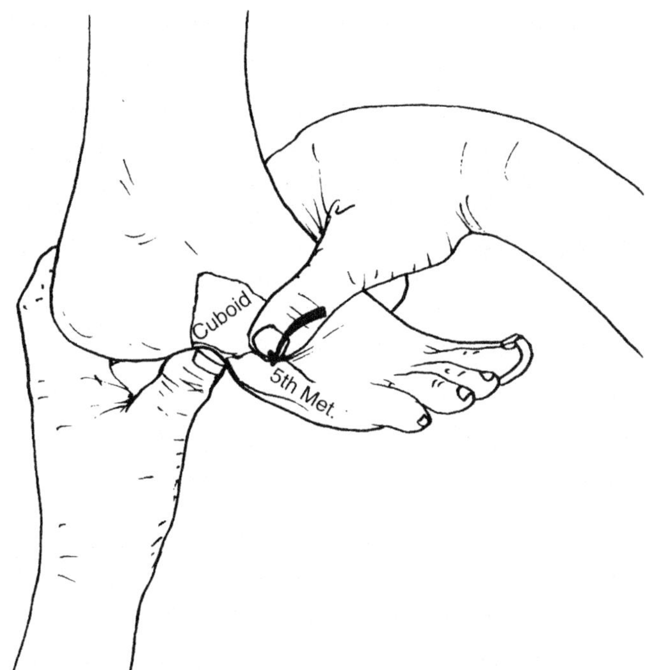

Fig. 5–29 Test for plantar movement of the fifth metatarsal on the cuboid.

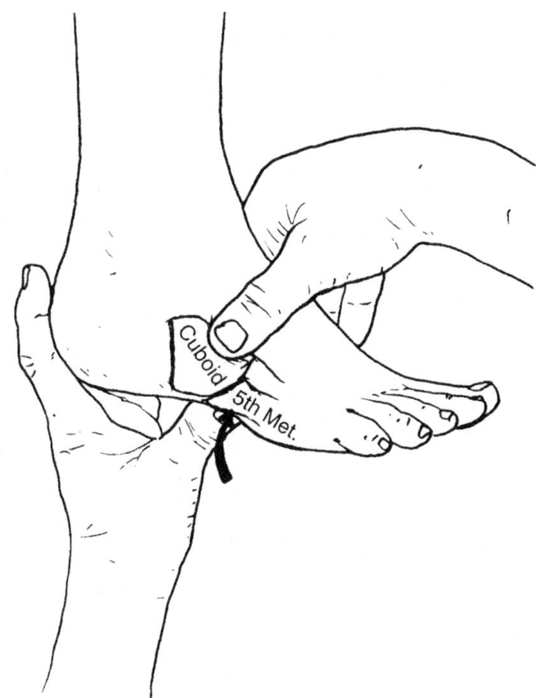

Fig. 5–30 Test for dorsal movement of the fifth metatarsal on the cuboid.

Tests for Dorsal Movement of the Cuboid

When testing for dorsal movement of the other bone structures with the cuboid, maintain the same hand position and rotate the foot even farther medially. With the inside thumb, apply pressure to the dorsal surface of the cuboid to provide resistance while applying dorsal pressure to the other bone structures. Pressure may now be applied on each segment to test for dorsal movement with the cuboid. This is accomplished in a manner opposite that for the plantar movement tests.

To test for dorsal movement of the fifth metatarsal on the cuboid (Fig. 5–30), apply pressure on the tuberosity of the fifth metatarsal for rotation and on the base for dorsal movement.

The plantar surface of the third cuneiform is narrow and sometimes difficult to locate (Fig. 5–31). By following the ridge on the underside of the cuboid next to the peroneal groove, the examiner can palpate the third cuneiform just as the ridge ends. Keep in mind the 45° angle at this articulation.

The Navicular

The navicular articulates with the talus posteriorly and has mediolateral, dorsal-plantar, and rotational mobility. Anteriorly, it articulates with the three cuneiforms. The second and third cuneiforms display minimal dorsal-plantar movement because of their triangular shape. The first cuneiform has minimal mediolateral and dorsal-plantar mobility. As noted above, the navicular also articulates occasionally with the cuboid (Fig. 5–32).

Lateral Movement of the Navicular on the Talus

With the outside hand proximal thumb pad, contact the lateral surface of the talar head just in front of the tibia (Fig. 5–33).

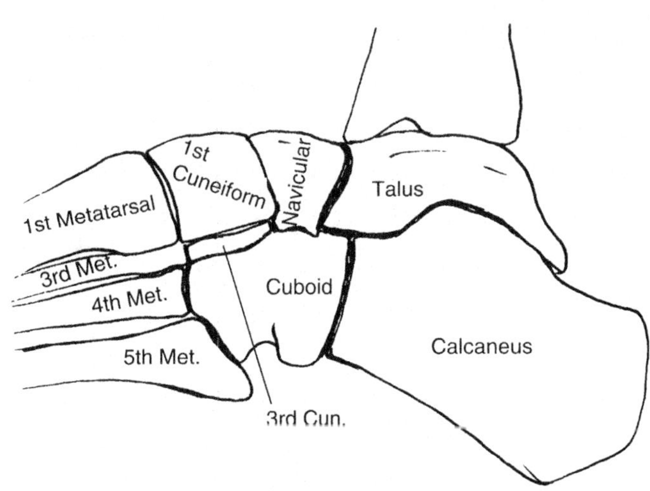

Fig. 5–31 Right foot, plantar-medial view showing cuboid relationships.

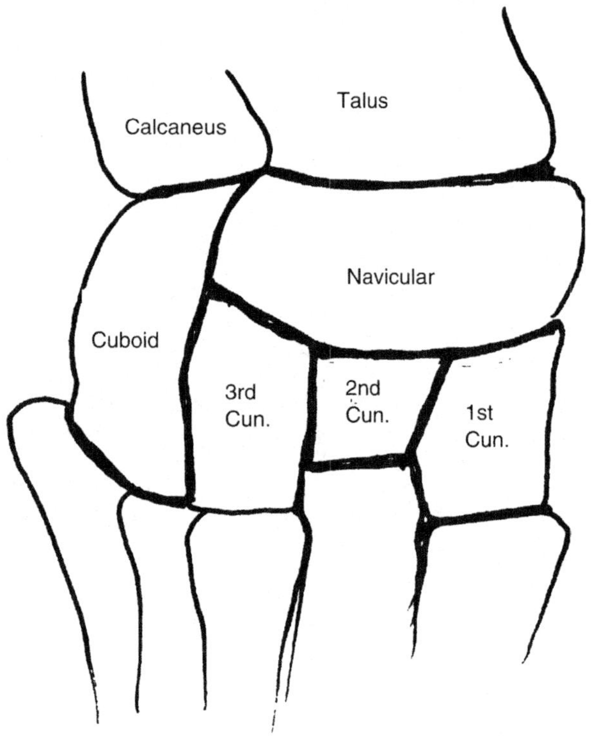

Fig. 5–32 Right foot from above showing the navicular and its articulations.

With the outside thumb providing resistance, apply lateral pressure on the tubercle of the navicular.

Medial Movement of the Navicular on the Talus

With the hands remaining in the same place, reverse the thumb contacts. Place the thumb pad of the outside hand on the lateral surface of the navicular, and apply pressure laterally on the talar head (Fig. 5–34). When testing for plantar movement of the other bone structures with the navicular, place the foot and leg into a few degrees of lateral rotation and the foot into slight plantar flexion for greater exposure of the medial arch.

Test for Plantar Movement of the Talus on the Navicular

With the inside hand, grasp the heel and apply dorsal pressure on the inferior surface of the navicular to provide resistance (Fig. 5–35). With the outside thumb, apply plantar pressure on the superior surface of the talar head.

Test for Plantar Movement of the Second Cuneiform on the Navicular

The second cuneiform is the flat spot on the dorsal surface and may sometimes be mistaken for the first cuneiform which is narrow on the dorsal surface (Fig. 5–36).

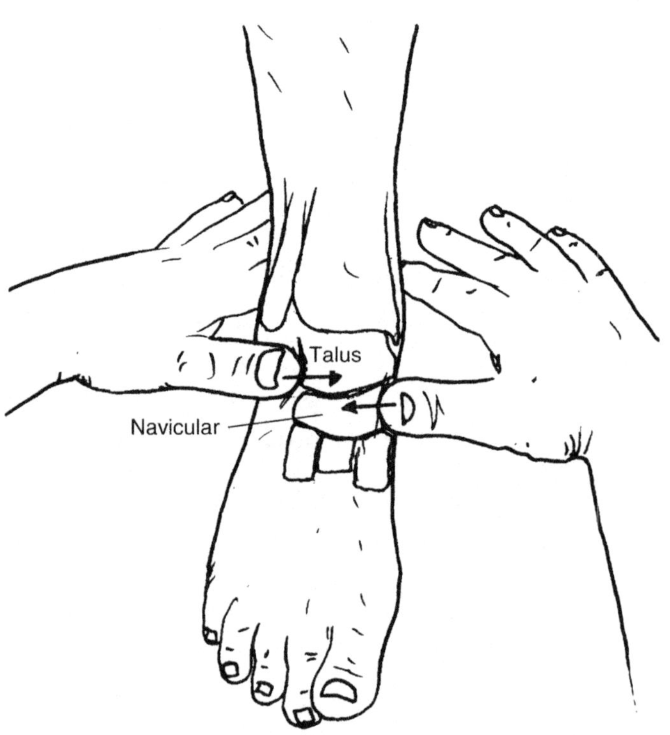

Fig. 5–33 Test for lateral movement of the navicular on the talus.

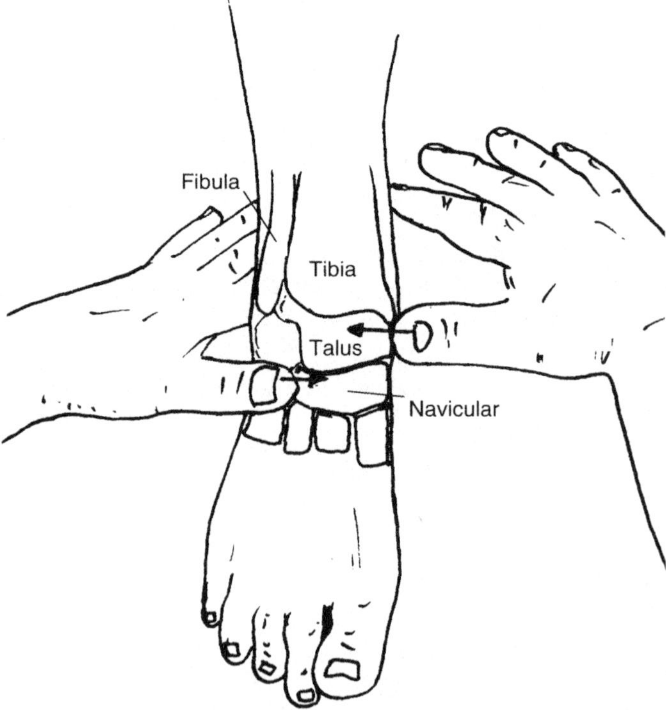

Fig. 5–34 Test for medial movement of the navicular on the talus.

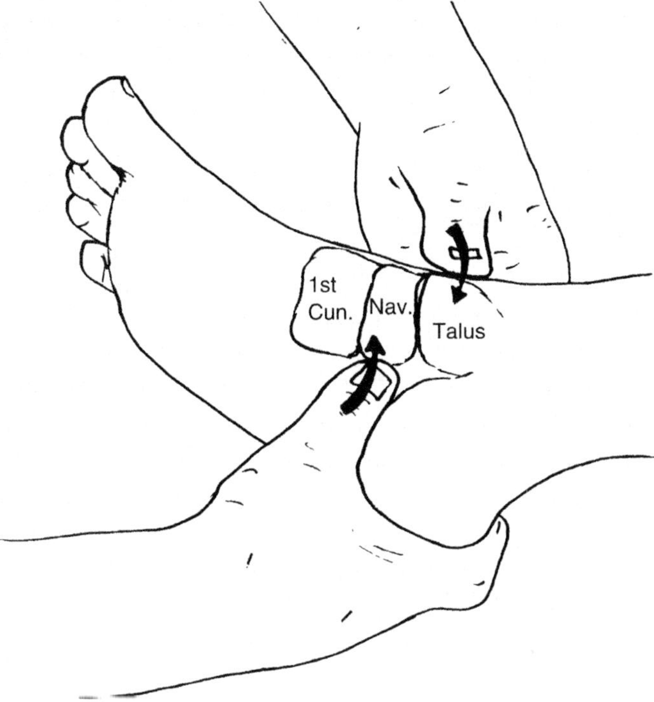

Fig. 5–35 Test for inferior movement of the talus on the navicular.

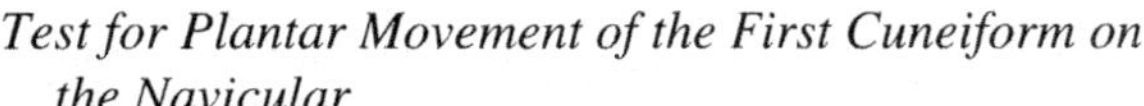

Test for Plantar Movement of the First Cuneiform on the Navicular

The first cuneiform is usually the most prominent structure on the dorsum of the foot, but it is narrow at the top and slopes quickly plantar-medially. To make contact, use a larger expanse of the thumb pad (Fig. 5–37).

Dorsal Movements on the Navicular

To test for dorsal movement of the other bone structures on the navicular, place the foot and leg into greater lateral rotation to expose the plantar surface of the foot. With the heel resting on the fingers of the outside hand, place the thumb pad on the dorsal surface of the navicular to provide resistance.

Test for dorsal movement of the first cuneiform on the navicular. With the inside thumb, apply dorsal pressure on the inferior surface of the first cuneiform (Fig. 5–38).

Test for dorsal movement of the second and third cuneiforms on the navicular. The plantar surfaces of the second and third cuneiforms are difficult to distinguish. The third is usually the most prominent and may be found by following the ridge just proximal to the peroneal groove on the cuboid until it seems to drop off (Fig. 5–39). No test is shown for the second and third cuneiforms.

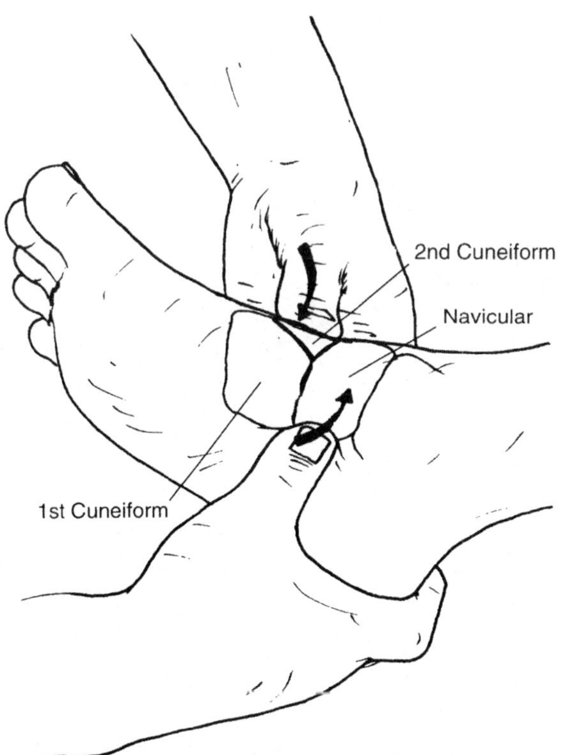

Fig. 5–36 Test for plantar movement of the second cuneiform on the navicular.

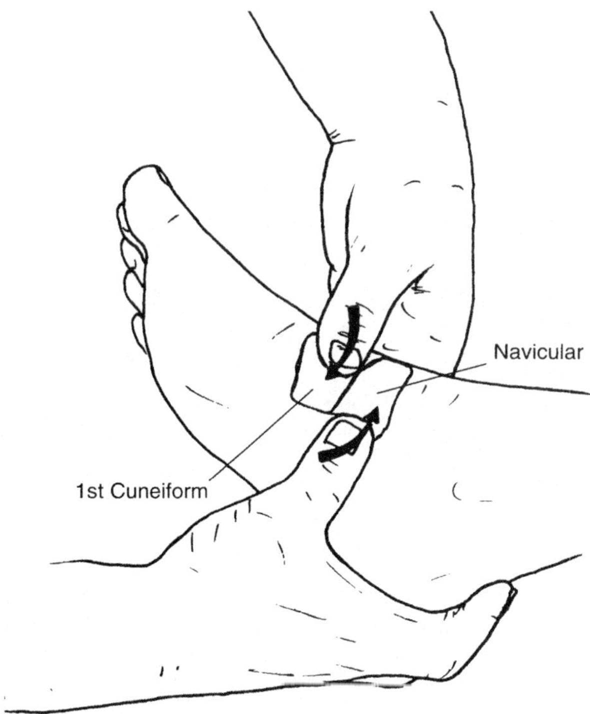

Fig. 5–37 Test for plantar movement of the first cuneiform on the navicular.

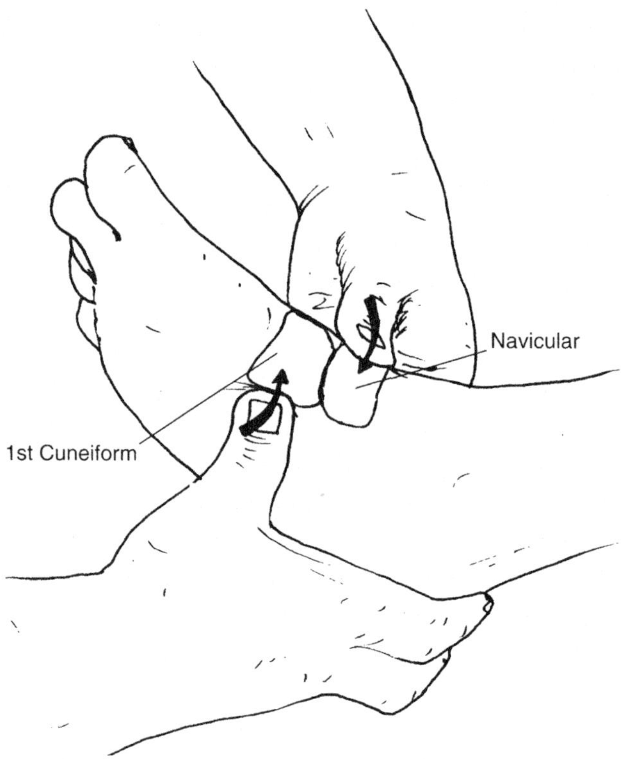

Fig. 5–38 Test for dorsal movement of the first cuneiform on the navicular.

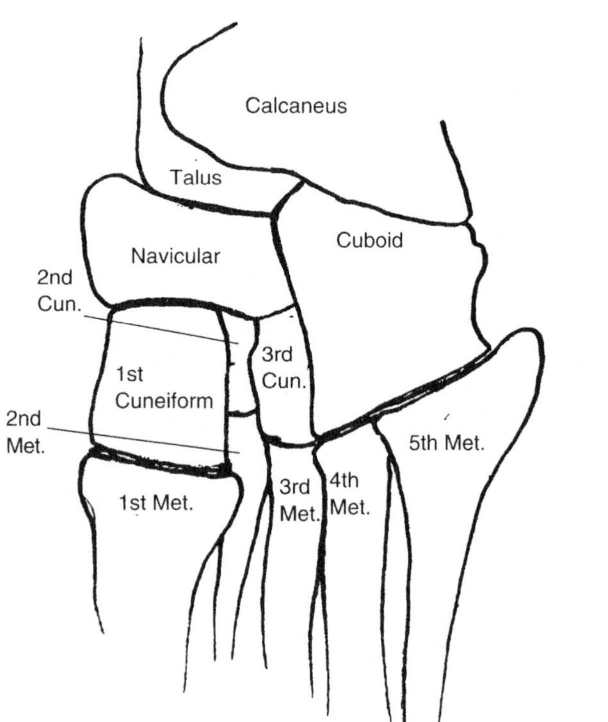

Fig. 5–39 Right foot from below showing the navicular and its articulations.

Test for dorsal movement of the talus on the navicular. Apply plantar resistance on the navicular while moving the talus dorsally (Fig. 5–40).

The First Cuneiform

The large first cuneiform is the most prominent structure on the plantar surface of the medial arch (Fig. 5–41). To test for plantar movement of the other bone structures on the first cuneiform, place the foot in lateral rotation and restrain the heel with the inside hand. Apply pressure on the plantar surface of the first cuneiform with the inside thumb to provide resistance (Fig. 5–42).

Test for Plantar Movement of the First Metatarsal on the First Cuneiform

Figure 5–42 illustrates this test.

Test for Plantar Movement of the Second Metatarsal on the First Cuneiform

The second metatarsal head is next to the distal half of the first cuneiform (Fig. 5–41). The head has a flat surface similar to that of the second cuneiform (Fig. 5–43).

Test for Plantar Movement of the Second Cuneiform on the First Cuneiform

The second cuneiform is easily located next to the prominent first cuneiform. The dorsal surface is flat and extends along the proximal half of the first cuneiform (Fig. 5–44).

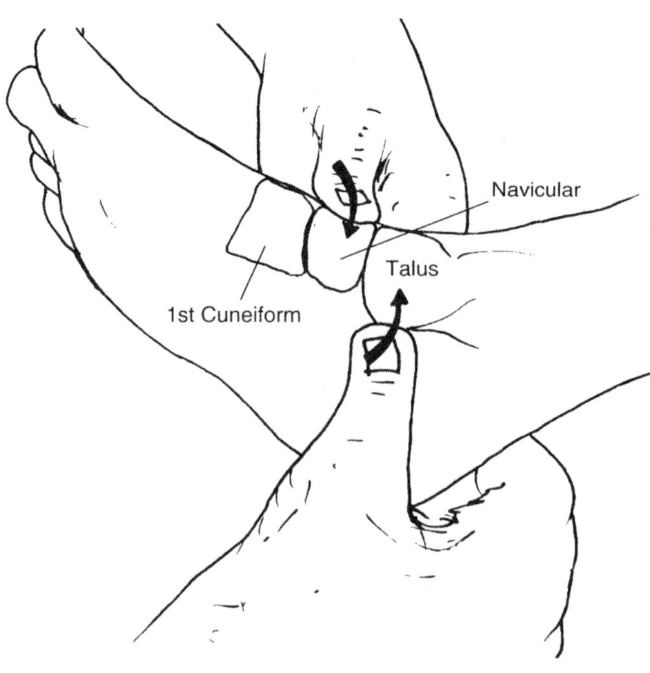

Fig. 5–40 Test for dorsal movement of the talus on the navicular.

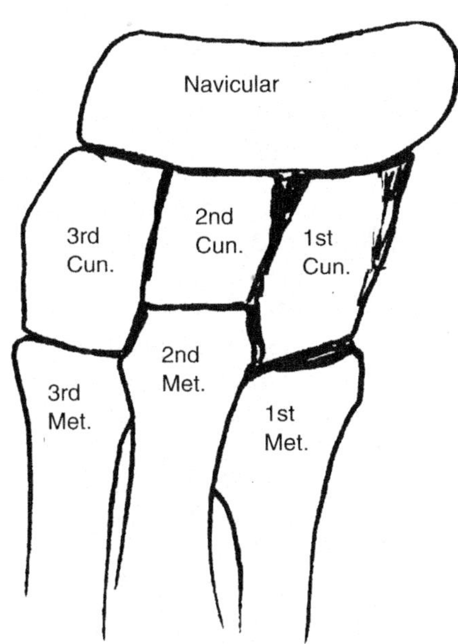

Fig. 5–41 Dorsal surface of the right foot showing the cuneiform relationships.

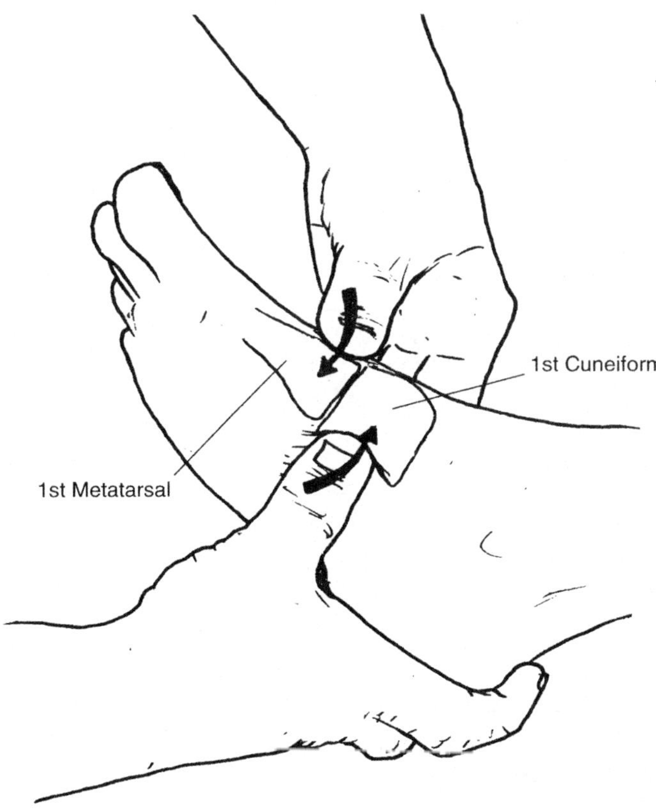

Fig. 5–42 Test for plantar movement of the first metatarsal on the first cuneiform.

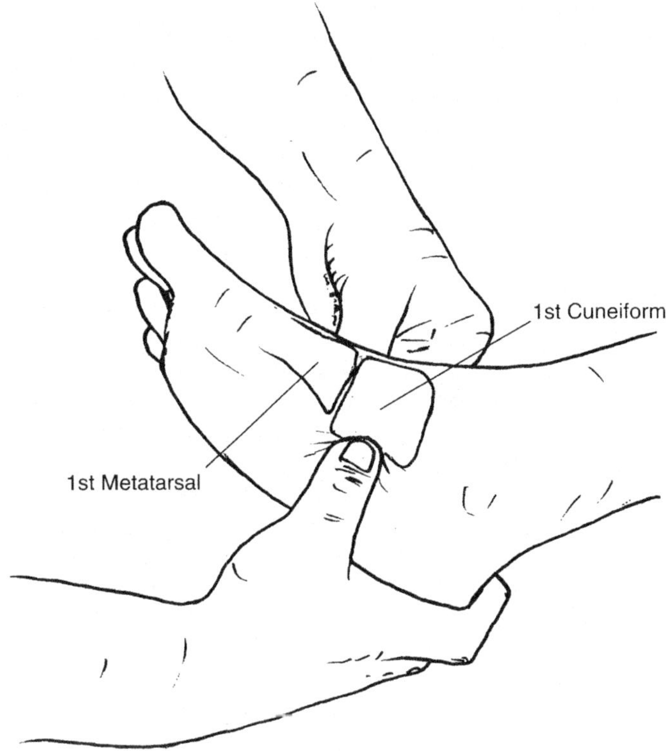

Fig. 5–43 Test for plantar movement of the second metatarsal on the first cuneiform.

Tests for Dorsal Movements on the First Cuneiform

In testing for dorsal movements of the other bone structures on the first cuneiform, keep the foot and leg rotated laterally and the foot resting in the fingers of both hands. A broad contact must be used on the first cuneiform because of its shape, as noted before.

To test for dorsal movement of the first metatarsal on the first cuneiform (Fig. 5–45), apply dorsal pressure on the plantar surface of the first metatarsal base.

The second metatarsal base is wedged between the base of the third and the first cuneiforms. Pressure applied immediately lateral to the plantar surface of the first cuneiform will indicate the mobility of the two.

To test for the second and third cuneiforms, refer to Figure 5–39 for the contacts, and use the same procedures described for the first cuneiform.

The tests for navicular movement with the cuneiforms were described earlier.

THE METATARSALS

Hiss[2] determined that by securing the talus, calcaneus, and navicular dorsiflexion and plantar flexion of each metatarsal, with its corresponding tarsal bone, produces a set ratio of movement.

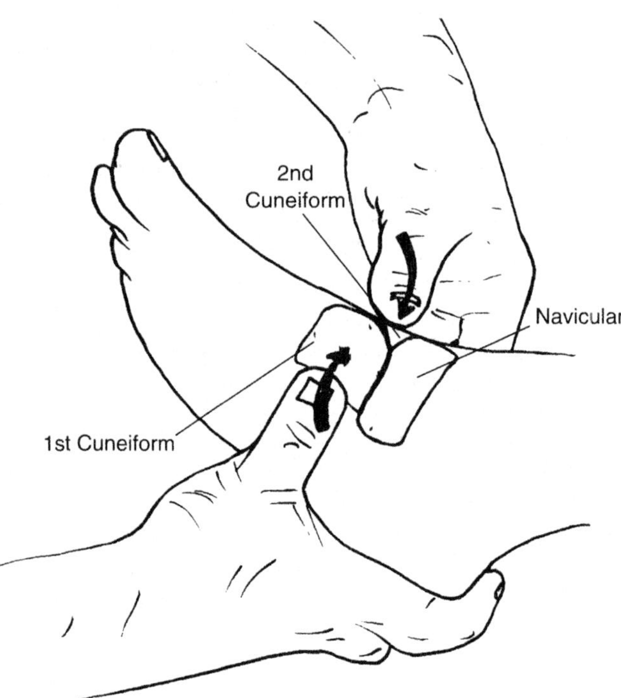

Fig. 5–44 Test for plantar movement of the second cuneiform on the first cuneiform.

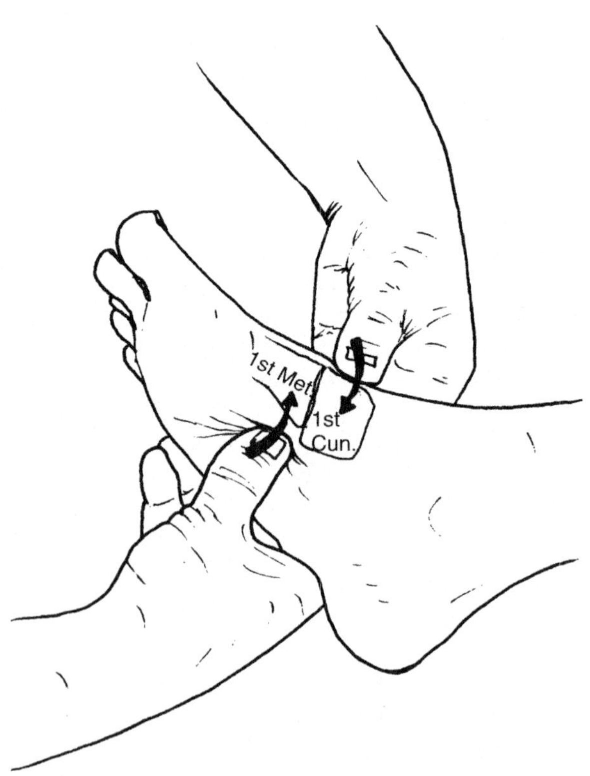

Fig. 5–45 Test for dorsal movement of the first metatarsal on the first cuneiform.

As shown in Figure 5–46, the first three metatarsals of the medial longitudinal arch show no movement at their respective cuneiform articulations. All the movement occurs at the cuneiform-navicular articulation. The second cuneiform shows the least movement, so that it becomes the standard (1:1) for comparison. The first and third cuneiforms have a ratio of 2:1 with the second cuneiform.

At the fourth and fifth metatarsals, little or no movement may occur at the calcaneocuboid articulation. All the movement takes place at the metatarsocuboid joints. When tested, the fourth and fifth metatarsals show 4:1 and 5:1 ratios, respectively, compared with the second metatarsal.

With the inside hand, secure the plantar surface of the calcaneus with the thumb and the naviculotalar joint with the index finger while gripping the heel with the hand (Fig. 5–47). With the outside hand, move the metatarsal unit, checking for the amount of mobility. Restrictions of mobility at any of the metatarsotarsal units indicate the possibility of a fixation.

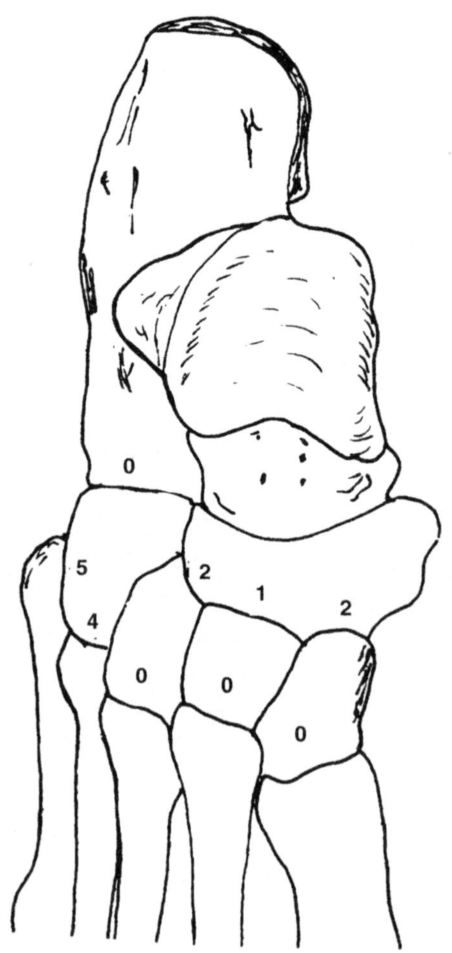

Fig. 5–46 Ratios of metarsotarsal movement with the talus and calcaneus blocked.

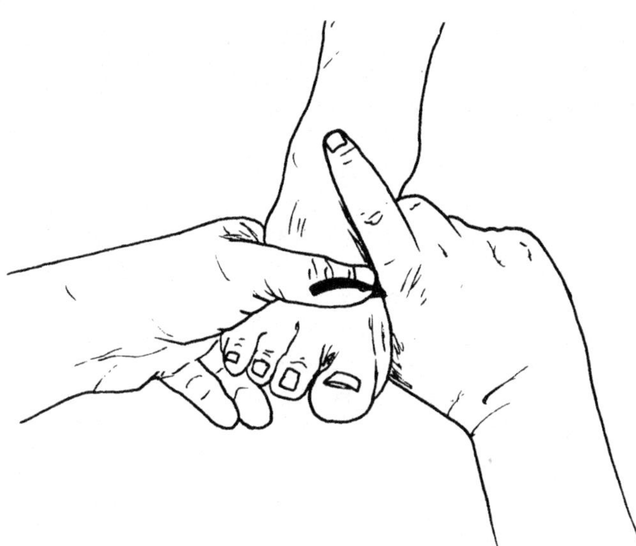

Fig. 5–47 Test for medial rotation of the first metatarsal on the first cuneiform.

Medial Rotation of the First Metatarsal on the First Cuneiform

Some rotation of the first metatarsal head occurs with the first cuneiform. With the finger of the inside hand, apply resistance to the medial surface of the first cuneiform (Fig. 5–47). With the outside thumb, apply pressure medially on the base of the first metatarsal.

Rotation of the Fourth and Fifth Metatarsals on the Cuboid

Secure the cuboid with the outside hand. By gripping the metatarsal with the thumb and index finger of the inside hand, the ability to rotate may be tested (Fig. 5–48). The fifth metatarsal should rotate more than the fourth.

Rotation of the Medial Longitudinal Arch

The medial longitudinal arch plays the major part in adapting to terrain and maintaining body balance. To achieve this with the lateral arch planted on the ground, the arch must be elevated and dropped as needed and must rotate at each segment. Testing for rotational ability may help in finding subtle fixations not noted during motion palpation. More important, it gives the examiner a gauge of the flexibility and therefore the adaptability of the foot.

With the foot and leg rotated laterally, grasp the heel with the inside hand and secure the talus with the thumb. With the outside hand palm down, grasp the metatarsals and test for the amount of rotation. If the amount of rotation seems normal, no

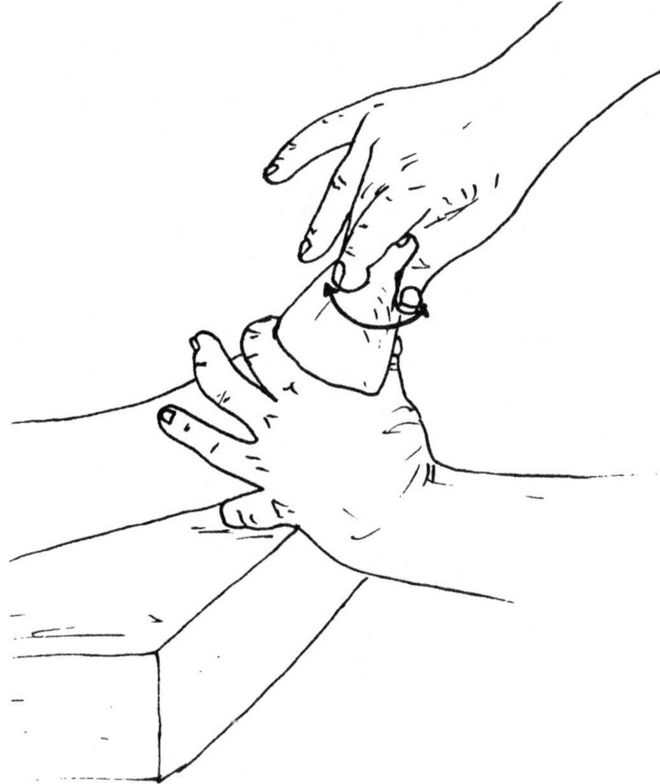

Fig. 5–48 Rotation of the fourth and fifth metatarsals on the cuboid.

further testing is necessary. If restricted, specific pressure may be brought to bear on each of the segments. The navicular on the talus may be tested clockwise and then counterclockwise by hooking the thumb under the navicular.

Mobility of the Metatarsal Heads with Each Other

Grasp the head of the first metatarsal with the index finger and thumb of the inside hand (Fig. 5–49). Grasp the head of the second metatarsal with the outside hand. Plantar and dorsal movement with respect to each other may now be compared. This procedure may then go on to the fifth metatarsal. Mobility is usually restricted most between the second and third, with about twice as much mobility at the first and second and at the third and fourth and the most mobility at the fourth and fifth. Restrictions may be due to overall immobility, specific dysfunctions, or pathology. Hypermobility often results from strain of the interosseous structures.

Test for Dorsal-Plantar Glide of the Metatarsophalangeal Joints

The metatarsophalangeal joints of the four lesser digits may be palpated for dorsal-plantar glide and rotation. By securing the metatarsal heads with the finger and thumb of the outside

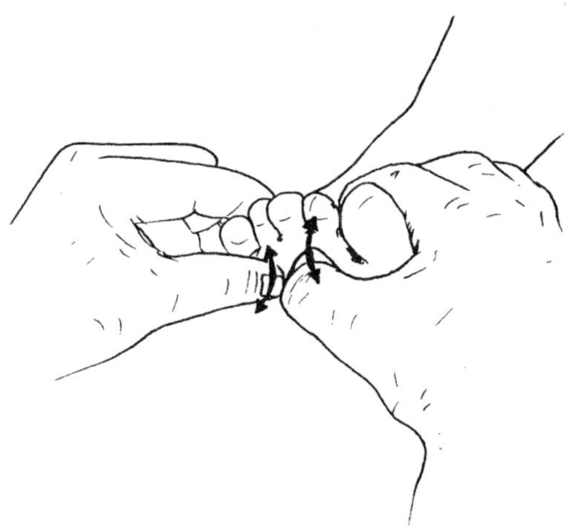

Fig. 5–49 Test for mobility of the metatarsal heads with respect to each other.

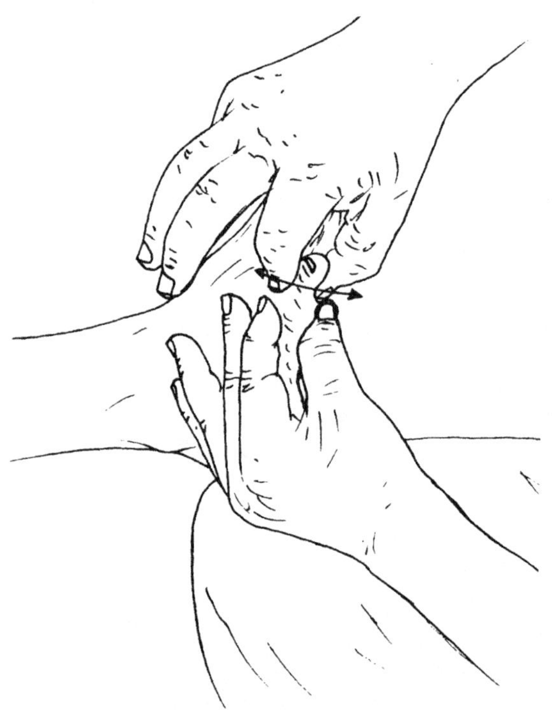

Fig. 5–50 Test for dorsal-plantar glide of the metatarsophalangeal joints.

hand and by using the index finger and thumb of the inside hand, the appropriate pressure may be applied (Fig. 5–50).

Test for Dorsal-Plantar, Mediolateral, and Rotation Movement of the First Metatarsophalangeal Joints

Grasp the first metatarsal at the head with the thumb and finger of the outside hand (Fig. 5–51). By gripping the proxi-

mal phalanx of the great toe with the index finger and thumb of the inside hand, pressure may be applied dorsal-plantarly, mediolaterally, and in rotation.

CONCLUDING REMARKS

At first the thought of PMP of the entire foot structure may seem complicated and time consuming. As with all techniques, it takes a knowledge of anatomy and a great deal of practice to become proficient. By practicing on a real foot with a plastic model handy for reference, it is not difficult. With practice, three things become apparent:

1. It takes little time to do the task efficiently after a few times through.
2. Fixations may be found that cannot be found in any other way.
3. The appropriate technique for the correction of fixations becomes readily apparent.

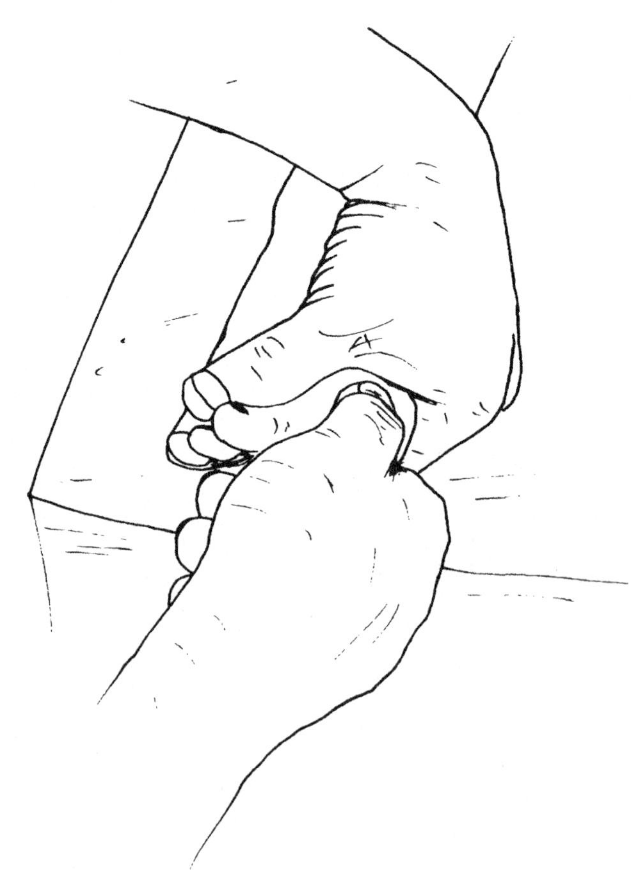

Fig. 5–51 Test for dorsal-plantar and mediolateral movement of the phalanx on the first metatarsal.

REFERENCES

1. Gillet H. *Bulletin.* Bruxelles, Belgium: European Chiropractic Association; 1978:28–30.

2. Hiss JM. *Functional Foot Disorders.* New York, NY: Oxford University Press; 1949.

3. Broome R. *The Foot and Ankle* [videotape]. Bournemouth, England: Anglo-European College of Chiropractic; 1987.

4. Mennell JM. *Foot Pain.* Boston, Mass: Little, Brown; 1969.

Chapter 6

Adjustive Techniques

Egyptologists suggest that the Egyptians were using manipulative techniques before the time of Christ. Other cultures that used manipulation in one form or another include the Greeks, the natives of the Americas, the Eastern Europeans, and the Japanese.

Andrew Still linked manipulation to the principles of osteopathy, starting the first osteopathic school in 1874 at Kirksville, Missouri. D.D. Palmer in 1895 founded the principles of chiropractic. He did not claim the discovery of manipulation. He did claim to be the first to use the spinous and transverse processes of the vertebrae as levers, making it possible specifically to adjust vertebrae. Palmer founded the first chiropractic college in 1897 in Davenport, Iowa.

Palmer referred to adjusting the 300 articulations of the body, which included the extremities as well as the spine and pelvis. Over the years the philosophy of some schools and some political entities have placed restrictions on the areas to be manipulated. The profession as a whole, however, encompasses manipulation of all the articulations as accepted practice.

When dysfunction exists in an extremity that may be related to a fixation of the spine or pelvis, all fixations of the spine and pelvis should be corrected before the extremity problem is addressed.

Many of the adjustive techniques in this text are based on those developed by D. Metzinger (personal communications, 1949–1957) and taught to me by C.G. Crawford (personal communications, 1955–1956) and Metzinger. The short lever techniques in this text are based on those developed by Broome.[1] They were designed to adjust specifically each articulation of the foot and ankle without affecting the surrounding structures. Broome's short lever techniques may be used on a fixation even though pathology may exist in an adjacent articulation. An example of short lever technique application was the adjustment of my foot with five fractures present (described in Chapter 5).

There are many adjustive techniques in chiropractic, each with its own success. Each practitioner must choose the technique suitable to his or her physical abilities and to the patient being treated. All adjustive techniques, regardless of their origin, must stand up to scrutiny to determine whether they are anatomically correct and effective and do no harm to the patient. With each fixation described in the following, the technique shown first is the one that I prefer for the usual patient. Alternative techniques, both long lever and short lever, are shown where appropriate. Each technique is described and illustrated where possible.

LONG LEVER TECHNIQUES

Most of the long lever techniques are accomplished by making a specific contact on the most distal bone of the articulation. Instruct the patient to relax the musculature as much as possible. Move the distal bone on the proximal one by finding the point of resistance (where the thrust is to be made), relax, then move smoothly to the point of resistance and without hesitation accelerate the thrust using the utmost speed.

Long lever techniques are usually quicker to execute, making them the preferred technique where possible. When pathology is detected or suspected, the short lever techniques should be used.

SHORT LEVER TECHNIQUES

In using the short lever techniques as introduced by Broome,[1] it is essential to be accurate in the contacts (to confine the force to the one articulation) and precise in the direction of thrust. It is also important that the adjuster maintain a correct body position to maintain tension on the articulation. The execution of the thrust is explosive.

To make a specific short lever contact and to allow the maximum pressure to be exerted during the thrust, the middle finger is used. Reinforcing the middle finger with the index finger is the most efficient use of the hand. In some areas reinforcement with the index finger may not be possible, but the same principle applies as in the following example (Fig. 6–1).

If the cuboid is dorsally fixed in its relationship with the calcaneus (ie, fails to move plantarly), contact is made with the middle finger on the dorsal surface of the cuboid. Place the index finger over the middle finger to give additional support. Contact should be specific and confined to the one bone structure.

Using the same type of finger placement and being specific, contact the plantar surface of the anterior calcaneus (Fig. 6–2; note that the index finger reinforcement is omitted to illustrate the contact). With both contacts in place, it is possible to exert maximum pressure with the thrust affecting only the one articulation (Fig. 6–3).

With the contacts in direct opposition, place your elbows against your rib cage (Fig. 6–4). This enables you to have complete control. Place the patient's foot with the contacts on your sternum. Apply slight traction on the foot by moving your torso forward and then footward. Take up all the slack in

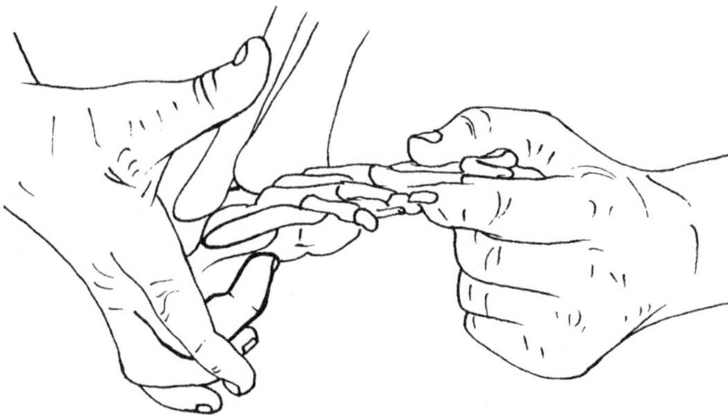

Fig. 6–2 Short lever contact for dorsal fixation of the cuboid on the calcaneus, ending position.

the contact. A quick, explosive thrust is made by pulling sharply posterior on your elbows and shoulders. This is best accomplished by attempting to bring the scapulae together (Fig. 6–5). The thrust should be made in equal and opposite directions.

The short lever technique is not easy to learn. I suggest that the practitioner use subjects with feet that are easy to work with in developing the skill necessary to execute this technique. Each of the short lever techniques may be modified to suit the adjuster and/or the patient. As long as the adjuster understands the anatomy and the direction necessary for correction, a technique may be improvised.

Not all feet are alike. Not all adjusters are alike. The small adjuster with small hands certainly will have greater difficulty in adjusting a large foot. The necessity of knowing the anatomy and of understanding what must be accomplished cannot be overemphasized. Once both are known, the adjustment is usually easy.

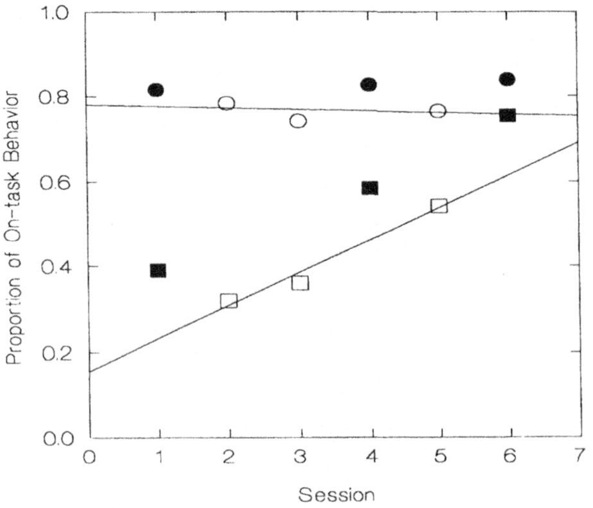

Fig. 6–1 Short lever contact for dorsal fixation of the cuboid on the calcaneus, beginning position.

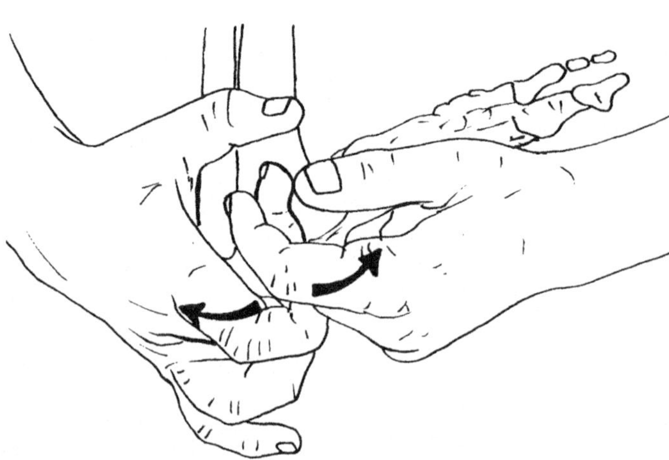

Fig. 6–3 Short lever contact for dorsal fixation of the cuboid on the calcaneus, both hands.

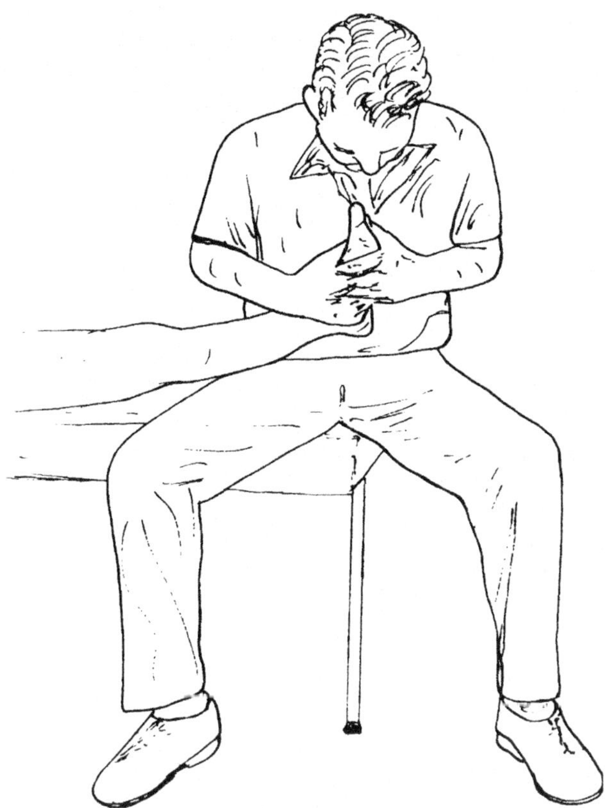

Fig. 6–4 Body position for short lever technique.

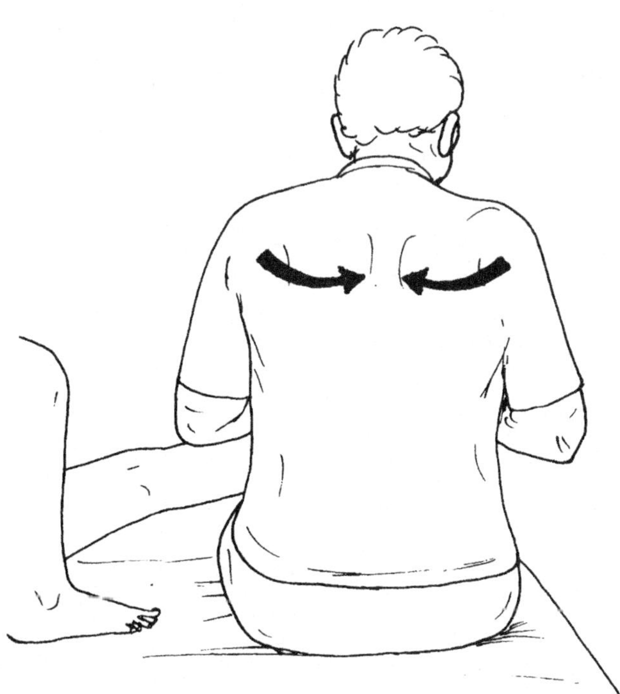

Fig. 6–5 Short lever body position from the back.

THE ANKLE

Posterior Fibula Head

Place the patient in the prone position with the knee flexed to 90° and the ankle resting against your shoulder (Fig. 6–6). Use a hook pisiform contact with the outside hand at the fibula head reinforced with the support hand. Rotate the fibula head anterolaterally and thrust with a sharp, shallow pull. (Take care not to pinch the lateral head of the gastrocnemius muscle.)

Alternative Technique 1

With the patient in the prone position and the leg extended, slightly rotate the leg laterally (Fig. 6–7). Stabilize the leg with the support hand, using a pisiform contact on the posterior aspect of the fibula head. The thrust is quick and shallow and follows the articular plane anterolaterally.

Alternative Technique 2

With the patient supine, stabilize the ankle by grasping it between your knees and applying mild traction (Fig. 6–8). With the inside hand, grasp the patient's medial and anterior knee structures to prevent anterior movement. With the outside hand, use an index finger hook behind the fibular head and the rest of the fingers around the fibula. The thrust is a sharp pull anterolaterally.

Superior Fibula Head

A superior fibula head results from a hypertonic biceps femoris muscle and/or weakness of the foot muscles attached to the fibula (peroneus longus, brevis, and tertius; flexor

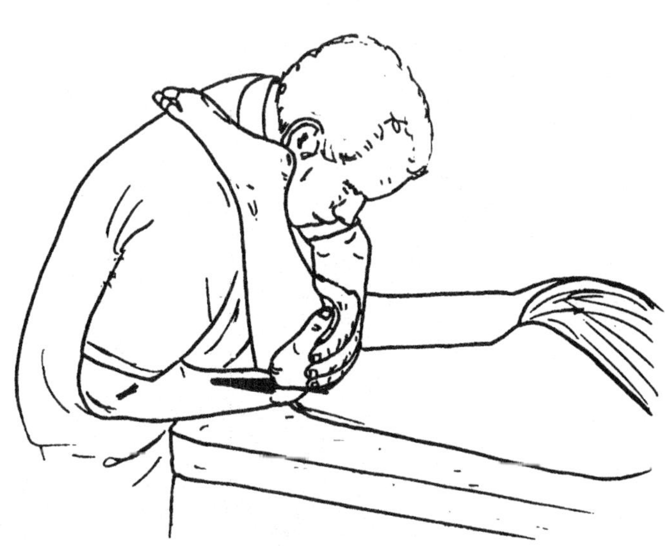

Fig. 6–6 Adjustment for posterior fibula head.

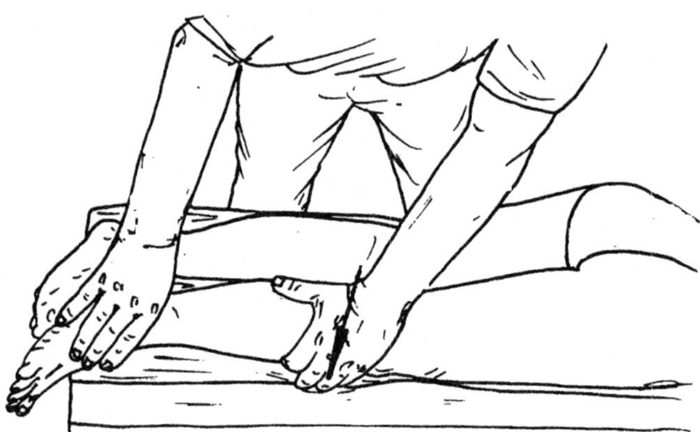

Fig. 6–7 Adjustment for posterior fibula head, alternative technique.

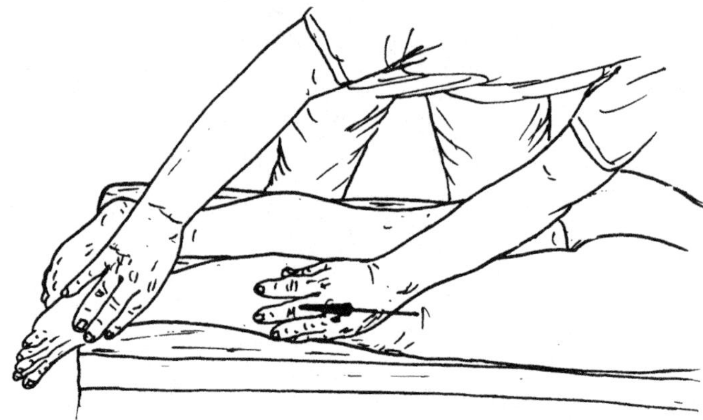

Fig. 6–9 Adjustment for superior fibula head.

hallucis longus; extensor hallucis longus; extensor digitorum longus; soleus; and posterior tibialis). With the patient in the prone position, medially rotate the leg by rotating the foot out with the support hand. From the opposite side of the table, contact the fibula head with a pisiform contact on the headward hand. The thrust is shallow and as inferior as possible (Fig. 6–9).

Anterior Fibula Head

With the patient in the supine position, support the ankle with the footward hand. Use a pisiform contact on the anterior fibula head and thrust posteriorly (Fig. 6–10).

Inferior Fibula Head

With the patient in the prone position and the knee flexed, dorsiflex the ankle using your chest. While applying dorsiflexion, contact the fibula head with both thumbs. The

thrust is made by using your body weight to dorsiflex the ankle farther while thrusting with both thumbs toward the table (Fig. 6–11).

Anterior Fixation of the Talus on the Tibia

With the patient supine and the heel off the edge of the table, grasp the tibia underneath with the middle finger of the outside hand. Grasp the medial foot with the inside hand thumb and index finger, securing the navicular. Bring the foot to 90° of flexion and thrust toward the floor (Fig. 6–12). By grasping the navicular and the other tarsals, pressure is applied through the navicular and its broad articular surface with the talus. The thrust should be shallow and quick.

Posterior Fixation of the Talus on the Tibia

With the patient supine, cradle the calcaneus with the inside hand. The index finger should contact the posterior talus. Con-

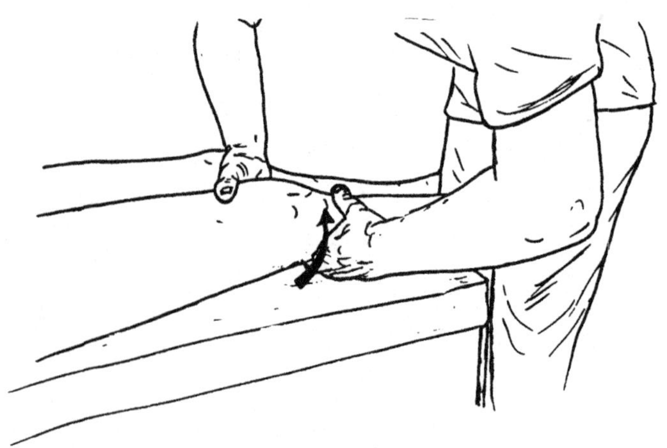

Fig. 6–8 Adjustment for posterior fibula head, alternative technique.

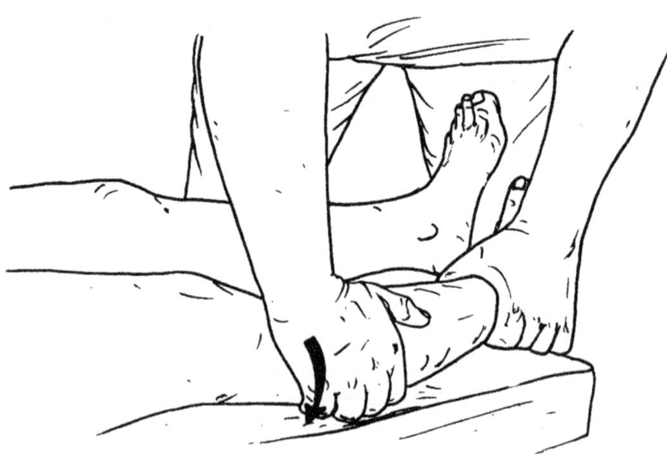

Fig. 6–10 Adjustment for anterior fibula head.

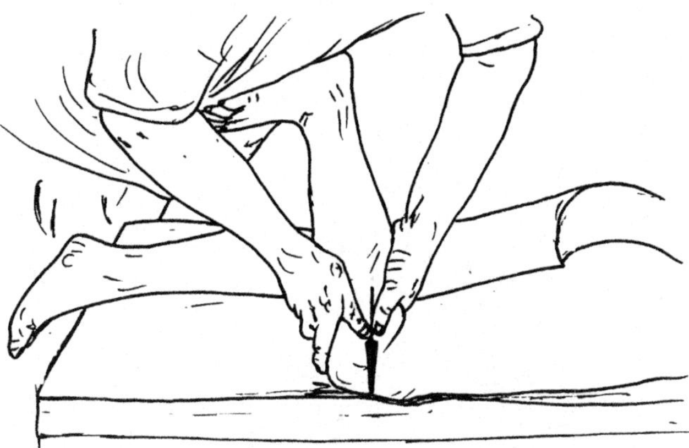

Fig. 6–11 Adjustment for inferior fibula head.

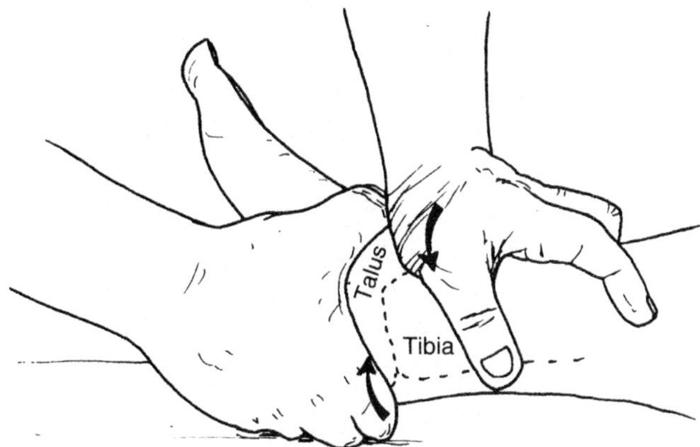

Fig. 6–13 Adjustment for posterior fixation of the talus on the tibia.

tact the anterior surface of the tibia with the heel of the outside hand. Thrust toward the floor with the outside hand. The thrust should be shallow and quick (Fig. 6–13).

Alternative Short Lever Technique

With the patient supine, sit on the table facing the medial side of the affected ankle. Contact the posterior talus with the distal hand. With the proximal hand, contact the anterior tibia. Apply traction by flexing forward and turning slightly footward, and thrust (Fig. 6–14).

Posterior Fixation of the Talus on the Calcaneus

With the patient supine and the heel off the end of the table, grasp the posterior talus with the fingers of the inside hand. Grasp the plantar surface of the calcaneus with the outside hand. Thrust is made with the outside hand toward the floor (Fig. 6–15).

Anterior Fixation of the Talus on the Calcaneus

With the patient supine, hold the heel with the outside hand. The inside hand should grasp the medial arch with the index finger and thumb holding the navicular. Rotate the navicular laterally without influencing the cuboid. (If the cuboid is contacted, the thrust will include the calcaneus.) Thrust posteriorly

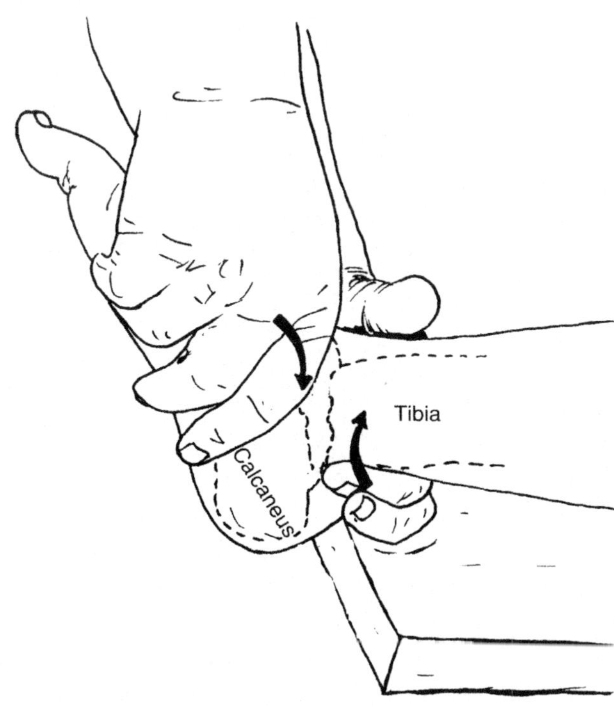

Fig. 6–12 Contacts for anterior fixation of the talus on the tibia.

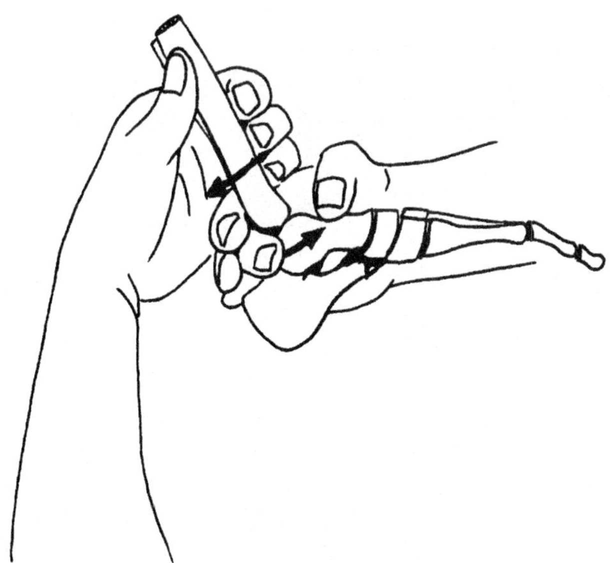

Fig. 6–14 Short lever contacts for posterior fixation of the talus on the tibia.

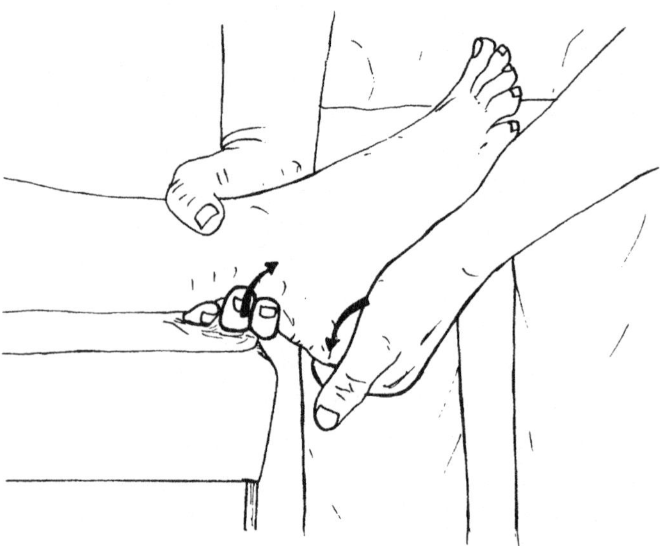

Fig. 6–15 Contacts for posterior fixation of the talus on the calcaneus.

with the inside hand, exerting pressure through the navicular to the talus using its broad articular surface (Fig. 6–16).

Lateral Fixation of the Talar Head on the Tibia

Place the middle finger of the inside hand on the lateral surface of the talar head, loosely grasping the foot (Fig. 6–17). With the outside hand under the ankle, grasp the tibia on the medial surface (Fig. 6–18). The thrust may be made as a short

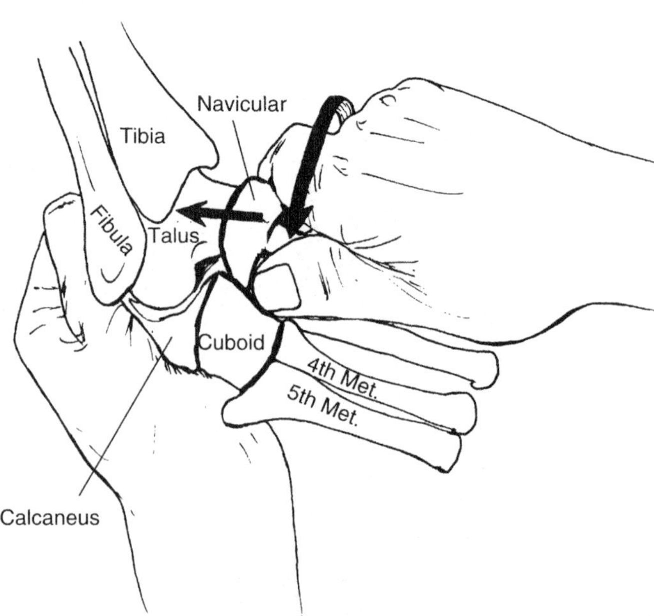

Fig. 6–16 Contacts for anterior fixation of the talus on the calcaneus.

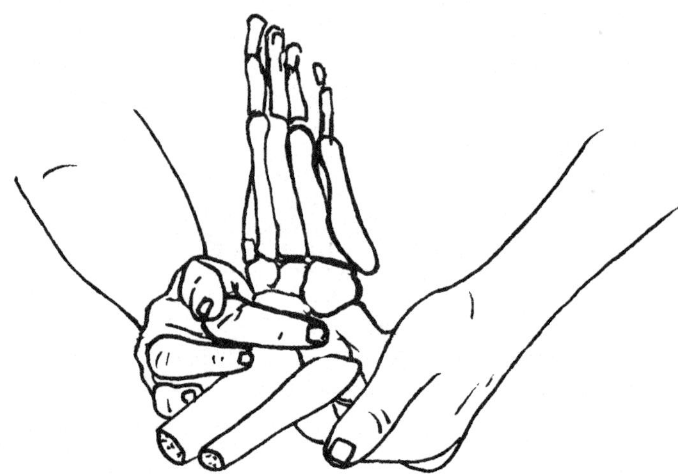

Fig. 6–17 Contacts for lateral fixation of the talar head on the tibia.

lever or long lever technique. The short lever technique uses a slight traction with the foot against your chest and the short lever style thrust. For the long lever technique, apply traction and pull-thrust with both hands simultaneously.

Medial Fixation of the Talar Head on the Tibia

With the patient supine, place the inside hand under the distal leg with the middle and index fingers contacting the lateral

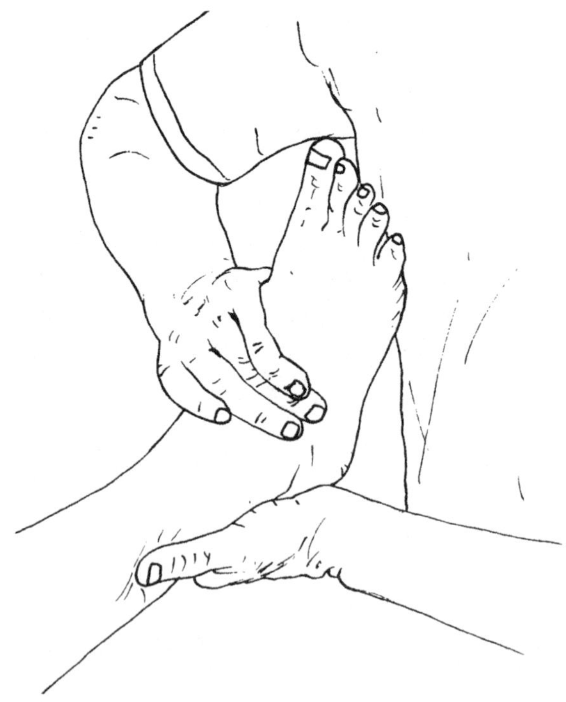

Fig. 6–18 Contacts for lateral fixation of the talar head on the tibia.

surface of the tibia. With the outside hand over the talar arch, contact the medial surface of the talar head with the middle finger. The thumb will be under the arch (Fig. 6–19). The thrust may be made with a long lever technique using traction and speed or as a short lever technique.

Lateral Fixation of the Talar Head on the Calcaneus

With the patient supine, grasp the calcaneus with the outside hand. Place the thenar pad on the posterolateral surface of the calcaneus with the middle and ring fingers grasping the anteromedial surface of the calcaneus. With the middle finger of the inside hand over the ankle, contact the lateral surface of the talar head. The thrust may be made as a long lever or short lever technique (Fig. 6–20).

Medial Fixation of the Talar Head on the Calcaneus

With the patient prone, grasp the ankle with the outside hand. The middle finger should contact the medial talar head (Fig. 6–21). Place the inside hand over the bottom of the heel, and contact the lateral surface of the calcaneus with the middle and index fingers as far anterior as possible (Fig. 6–22). The thrust may be made as a long lever or short lever technique (Fig. 6–23).

Medial Calcaneus on the Talus (Posterior Aspect)

With the patient prone, use the inside hand to grasp the tarsal arch of the foot with the index finger over the talar head. Slightly dorsiflex the foot on the ankle. Grasp the calcaneus

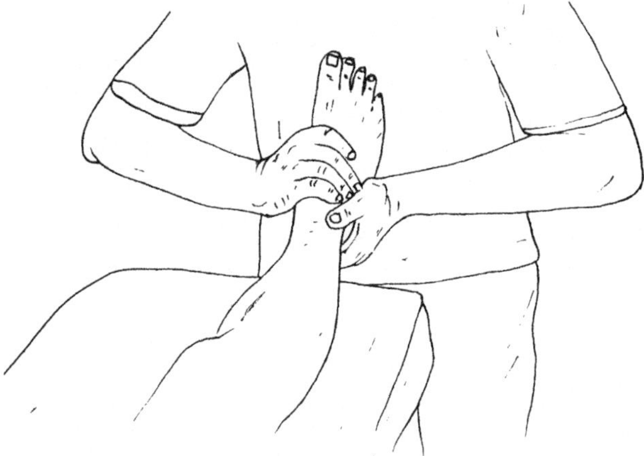

Fig. 6–20 Contacts for lateral fixation of the talar head on the calcaneus.

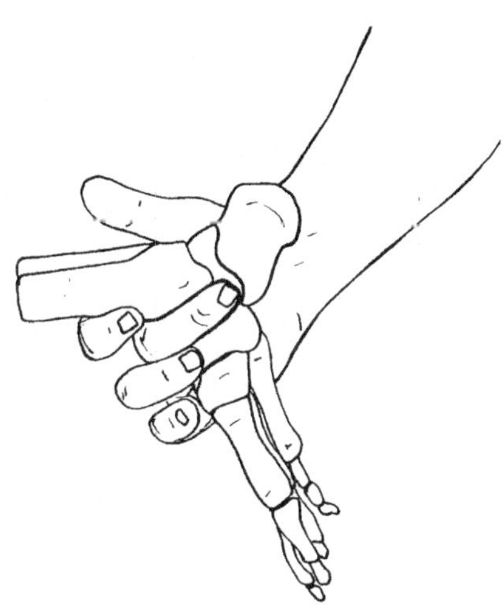

Fig. 6–21 Contact for medial fixation of the talar head on the calcaneus.

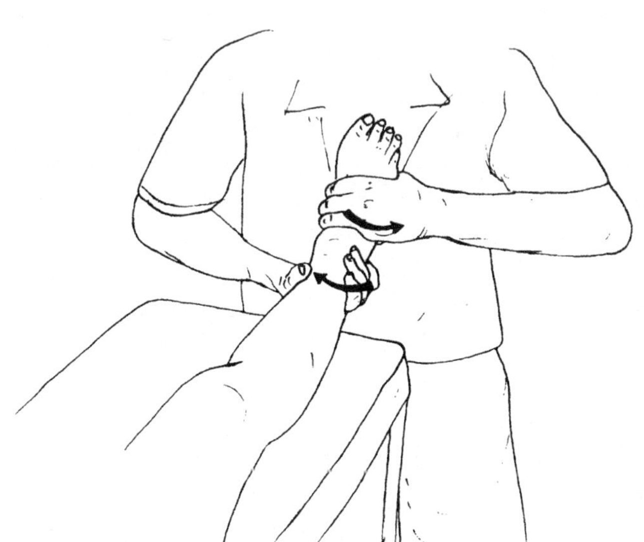

Fig. 6–19 Contacts for medial fixation of the talar head on the tibia.

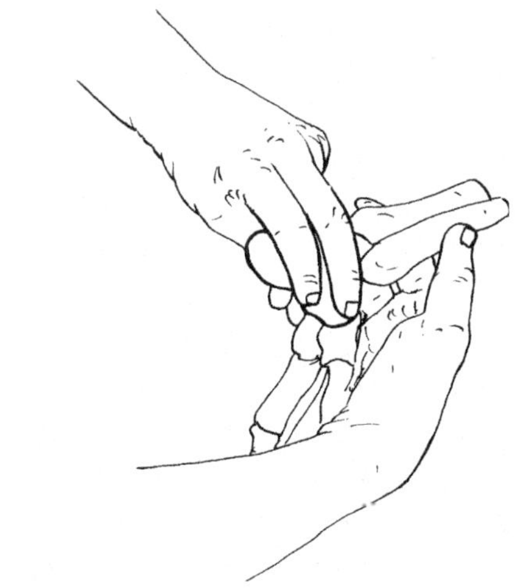

Fig. 6–22 Inside hand contact for medial fixation of the talar head on the calcaneus.

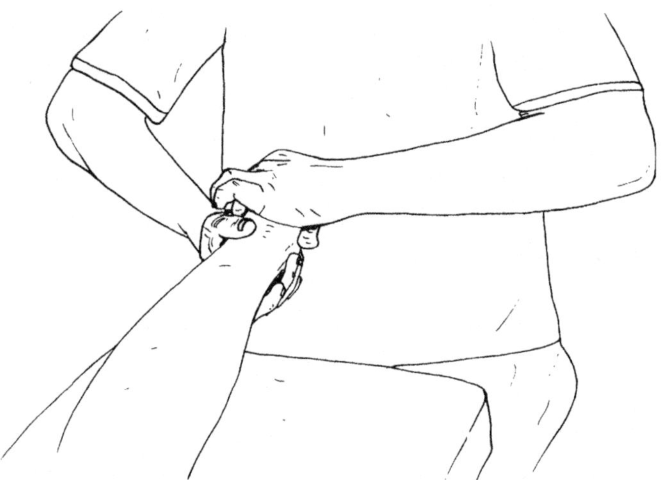

Fig. 6–23 Contacts and thrust for medial fixation of the talar head on the calcaneus.

---

with the outside hand firmly. Place your elbows directly opposite each other, and maintain your wrists rigid (Fig. 6–24A). With slight traction, thrust by bringing your elbows toward the floor while maintaining rigid wrists. The thrust should be spontaneous and fast (Fig. 6–24, B and C).

THE FOOT

Fixations of the Cuboid

Lateral Fixation of the Calcaneus on the Cuboid

The point of contact is just below the fibula and slightly anterior. Palpation will reveal the peroneal trochlea, and contact should be made just distal to the trochlea (Fig. 6–25). With the thenar eminence of the outside hand, grasp the heel, contacting the anterolateral surface of the calcaneus. Make sure that none of the thumb web is over the fibula. Place the inside hand over the tarsal arch and use an index finger contact on the plantar surface of the medial cuboid (Fig. 6–26). The adjustment is made by stepping forward on the outside foot, flexing the knee, and applying slight traction with the inside hand. Drop the outside elbow to the level of the articulation. Thrust medially with the outside hand while providing resistance at the cuboid with the inside hand. This move is made as one smooth action with a rapid increase in speed at the point of resistance.

Alternative technique. With the patient prone, contact the lateral surface of the anterior calcaneus. Use the base of the index finger of the outside hand. Hold the cuboid with the thumb (Fig. 6–27). Support the heel gently with the inside hand. Thrust medially with great speed.

Alternative short lever technique 1. With the patient supine, lean forward to make the contacts as well as the thrust. Place

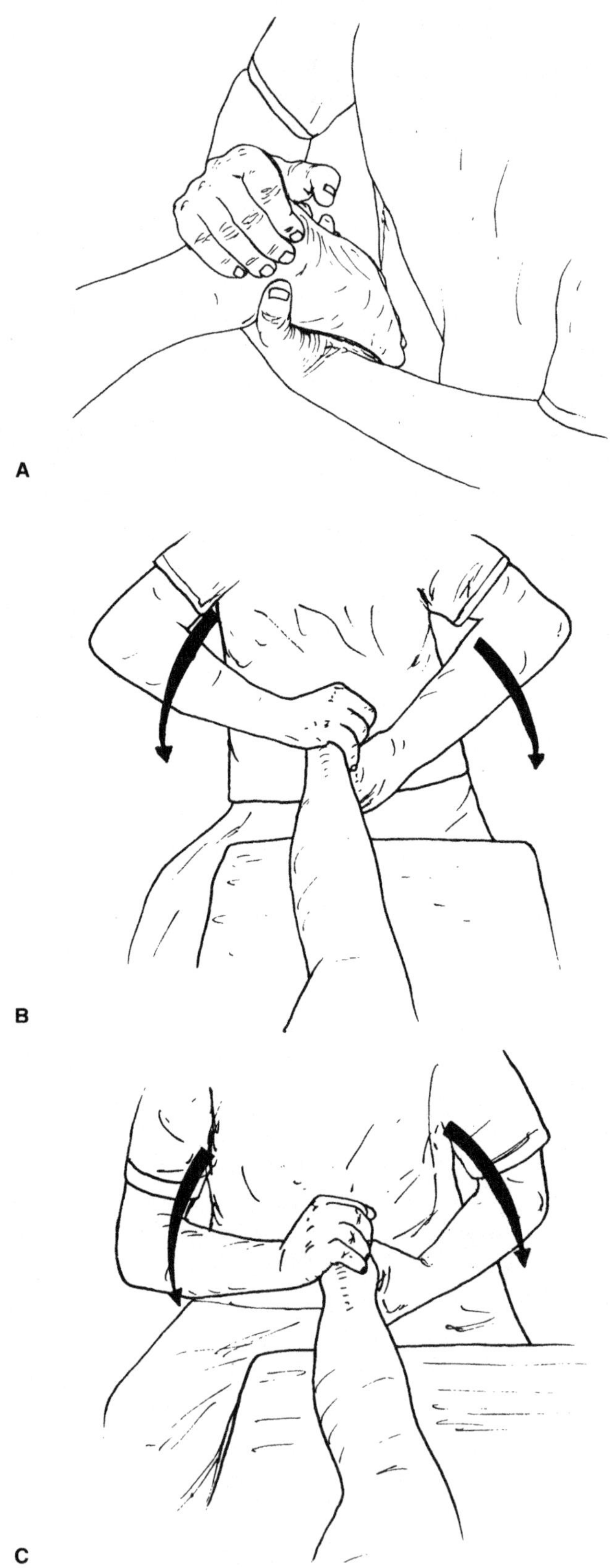

Fig. 6–24 (A) Contacts for medial fixation of the calcaneus on the talus (posterior view). **(B)** Start of thrust. **(C)** End of thrust.

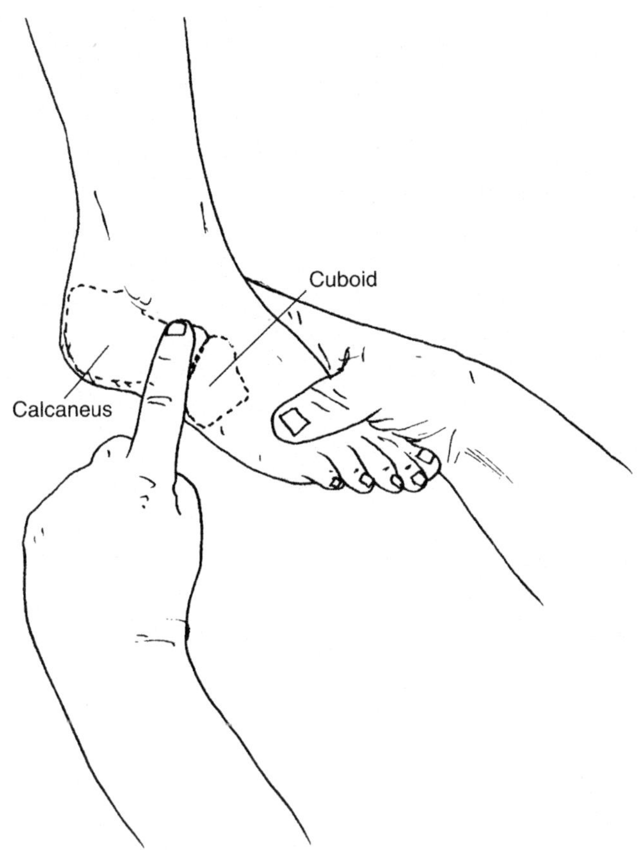

Fig. 6–25 Point of contact for lateral fixation of the calcaneus on the cuboid.

the distal thumb pad of the inside hand on the medial-plantar surface of the cuboid. The middle finger extends over the tarsal arch and hooks the lateral surface of the anterior calcaneus (Fig. 6–28A). With the outside hand, grasp the heel and use the thenar eminence to reinforce the middle finger contact of the inside hand (Fig. 6–28B). The thrust is made with slight traction. Thrust medially with the outside hand while pulling with the middle finger of the inside hand. Simultaneously, a lateral thrust is made with the thumb of the inside hand on the cuboid bone.

Alternative short lever technique 2. Sit on the table facing footward. With the middle finger of the inside hand, grasp the anterior calcaneus on the lateral surface from underneath. With the outside hand, hook the middle finger on the medial side of the cuboid (Fig. 6–29). Thrust is a short lever type with equal and opposite pressure.

Medial Fixation of the Calcaneus on the Cuboid

With the patient supine, sit on the table facing forward. Cup the heel with the outside hand, taking a middle finger contact on the medial surface of the anterior calcaneus (Fig. 6–30). With the inside hand over the top of the foot, take a middle

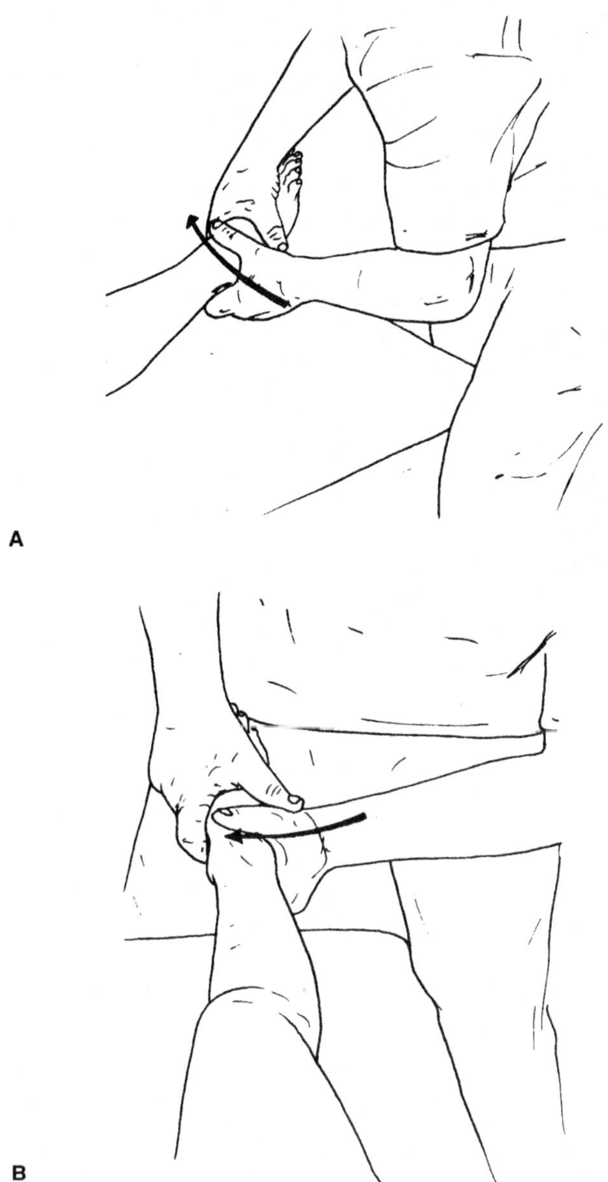

Fig. 6–26 **(A)** Contacts for lateral fixation of the calcaneus on the cuboid. **(B)** Direction of thrust.

finger contact on the lateral surface of the cuboid (Fig. 6–31). Take up the tension and, using a short lever technique, thrust in equal and opposite directions.

Plantar Fixation of the Calcaneus on the Cuboid

Sit on the side of the table. With the footward hand underneath the foot, hook the middle finger on the dorsal surface of the cuboid (Fig. 6–32). With the headward hand, take a middle finger contact on the plantar surface of the anterior calcaneus (Fig. 6–33). With the foot placed on your sternum, lean for-

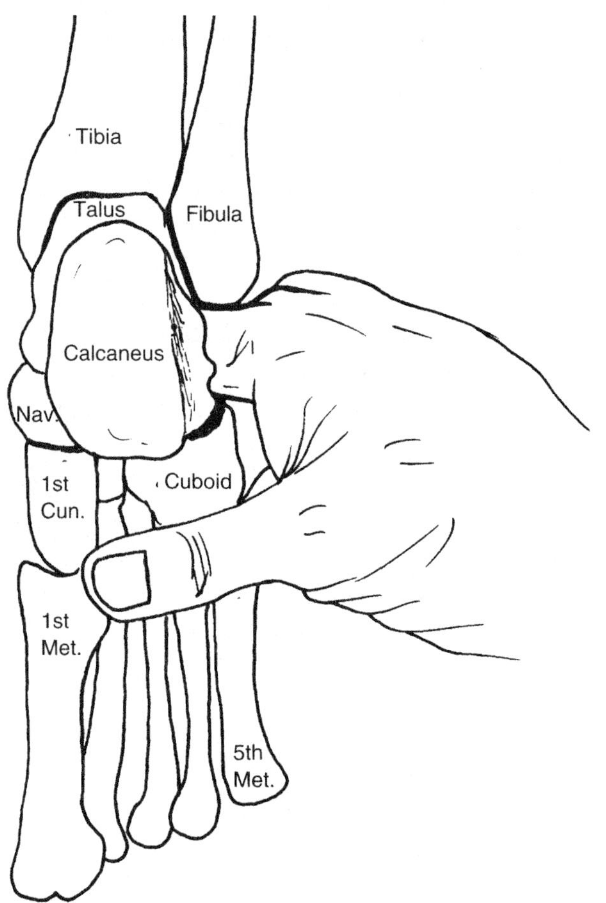

Fig. 6–27 Contact for lateral fixation of the calcaneus on the cuboid, prone technique.

---

ward and turn footward to apply traction. Thrust with a short lever technique.

Dorsal Fixation of the Calcaneus on the Cuboid

Reverse the contacts for the plantar fixation and use the same short lever technique.

Dorsal Fixation of the Navicular or Third Cuneiform on the Cuboid

Sit on the side of the table with the patient in the supine position. With the headward hand, hook the middle finger under the cuboid. With the footward hand over the dorsum of the foot, contact the navicular or the third cuneiform with a middle finger contact. Lean forward and footward to apply slight traction, and use a short lever thrust. The 45° angle of the articulation must be kept in mind during the thrust.

Plantar fixations of the navicular or third cuneiform seldom occur because of the 45° angle of the articulations.

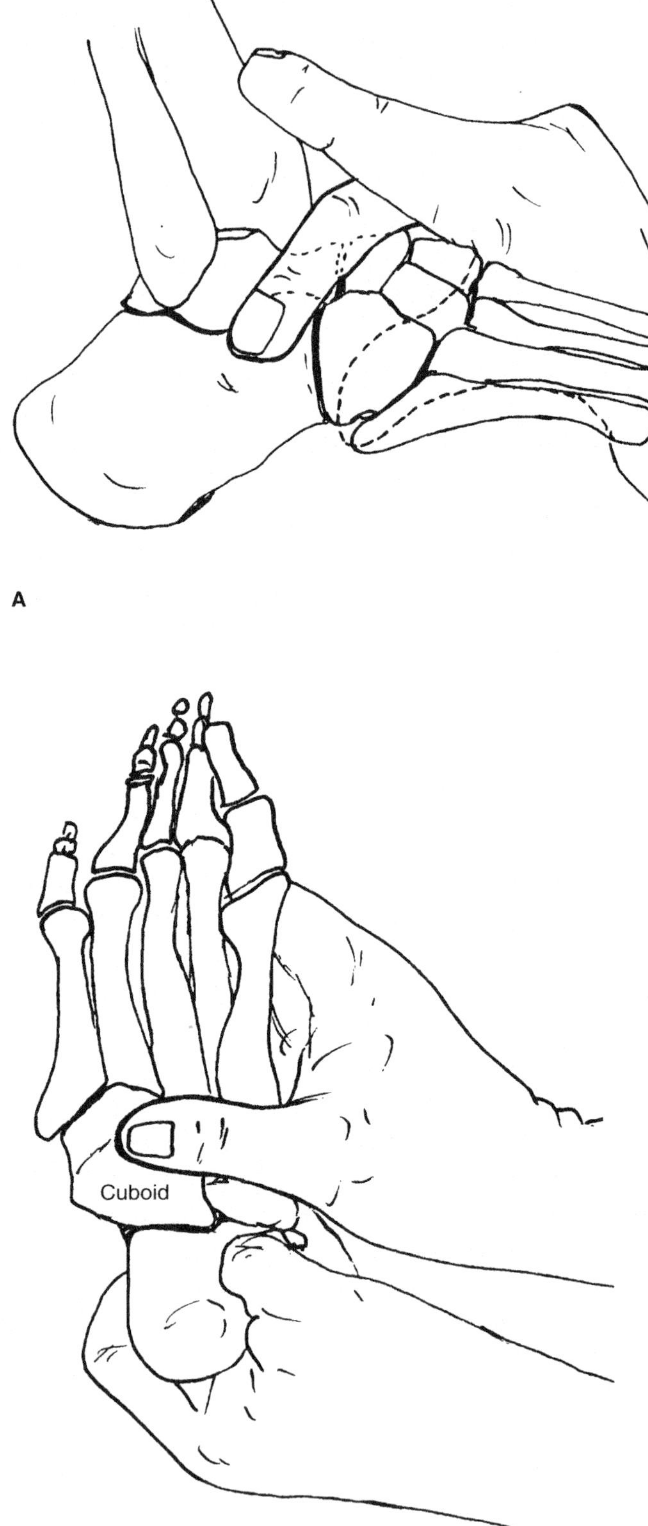

Fig. 6–28 **(A)** Lateral fixation of the calcaneus on the cuboid, middle finger placement. **(B)** Thumb contact for short lever technique.

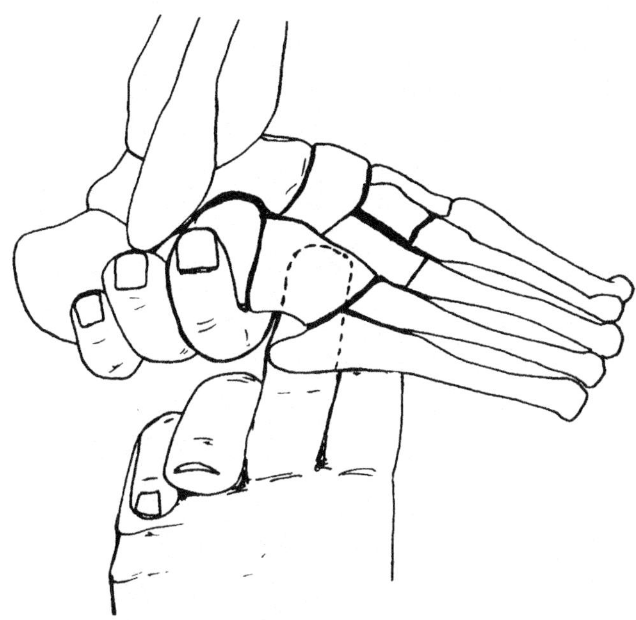

Fig. 6–29 Alternative short lever contacts for lateral fixation of the calcaneus on the cuboid.

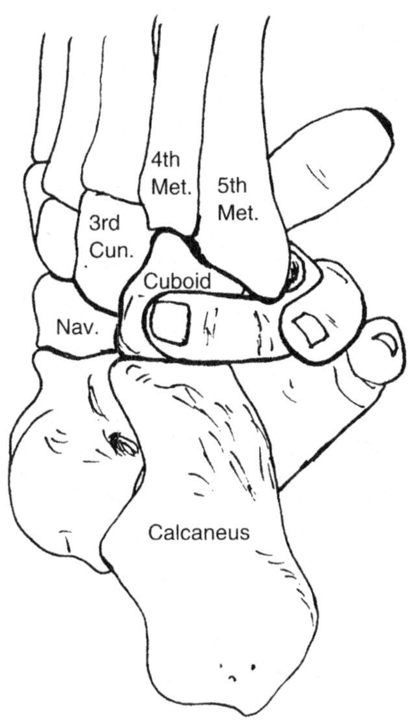

Fig. 6–31 Second contact for medial fixation of the calcaneus on the cuboid.

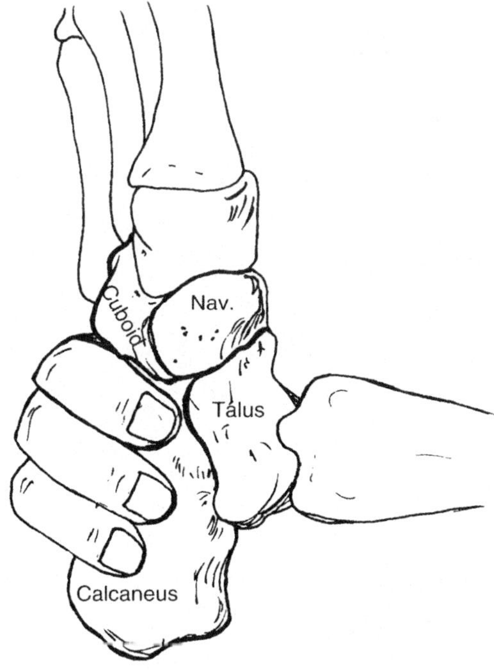

Fig. 6–30 First contact for medial fixation of the calcaneus on the cuboid.

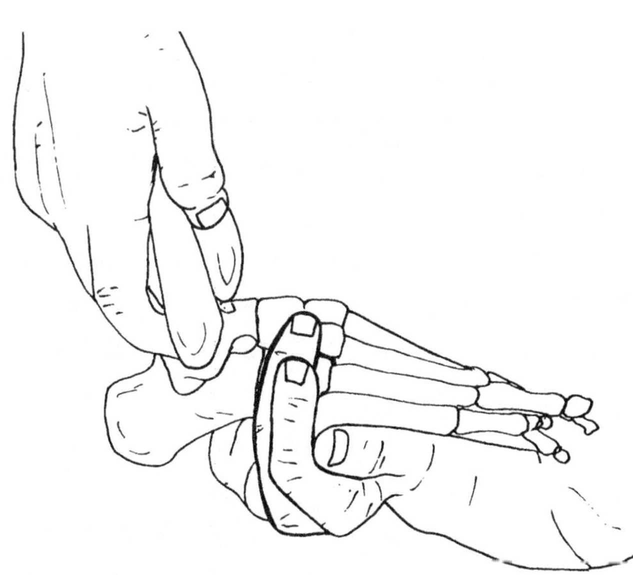

Fig. 6–32 First contact for plantar fixation of the calcaneus on the cuboid.

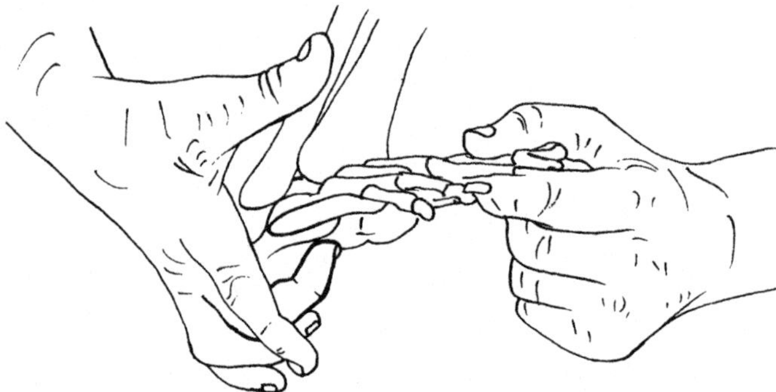

Fig. 6–33 Second contact for plantar fixation of the calcaneus on the cuboid.

Dorsal Fixation of the Fourth and Fifth Metatarsals on the Cuboid

With the patient in the supine position, sit on the side of the table. With the headward hand, hook the middle finger under the cuboid. The footward hand under the metatarsals hooks the dorsal surface of the fourth or fifth metatarsal head with the middle finger (Fig. 6–34). Lean forward and footward to apply slight traction, and use a short lever thrust.

Plantar Fixation of the Fourth and Fifth Metatarsals on the Cuboid

Reverse the contacts for the dorsal fixation technique.

Fixations of the Navicular

Medial Fixation of the Talus on the Navicular

With the patient supine, grasp the dorsum of the ankle with the outside hand. Use a middle finger contact on the medial surface of the talar head while grasping the calcaneus with the thumb on the plantar surface. With the inside hand, use a middle finger contact on the lateral surface of the navicular (Fig. 6–35). Either a long or a short lever technique may be used.

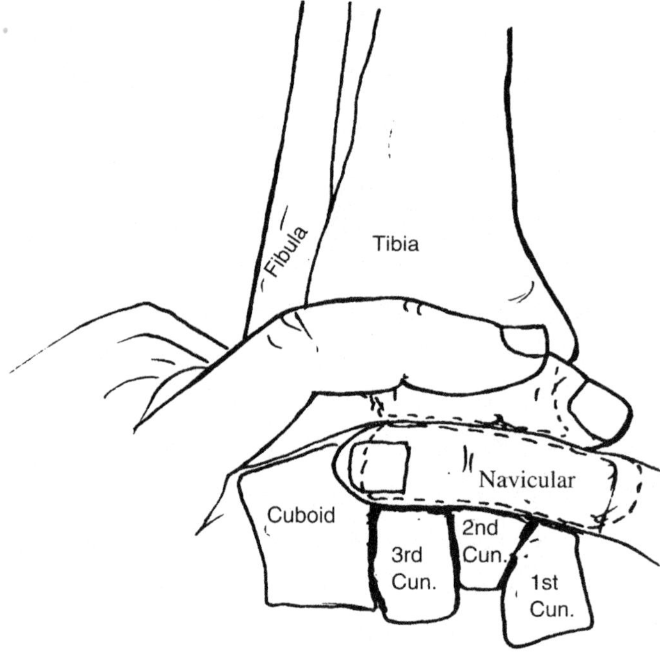

Fig. 6–35 Contacts for medial fixation of the talus on the navicular.

Lateral Fixation of the Talus on the Navicular

Reverse the contacts for the medial fixation technique.

Dorsal Fixation of the Talar Head on the Navicular

With the patient supine, sit facing the lateral side of the foot to be adjusted. With the footward hand, use a middle finger contact on the dorsal surface of the talus. With the headward hand, hook the middle finger around and contact the plantar surface of the navicular (Fig. 6–36). Use the short lever technique.

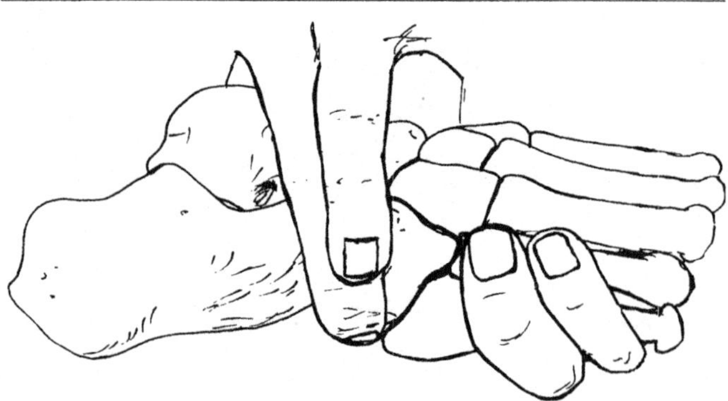

Fig. 6–34 Contacts for dorsal fixation of the fourth and fifth metatarsals on the cuboid.

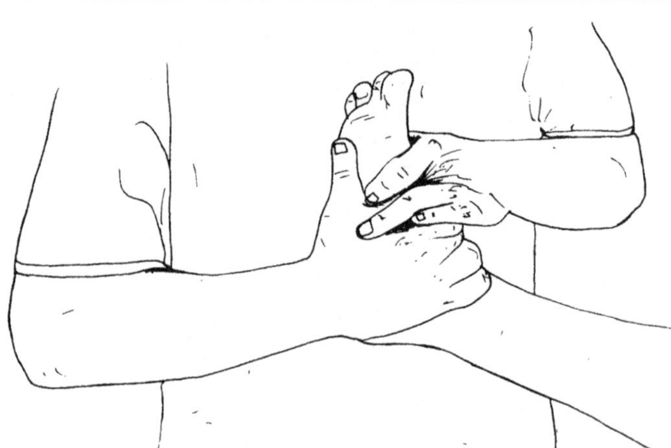

Fig. 6–36 Contacts for dorsal fixation of the talar head on the navicular.

Plantar Fixation of the Talar Head on the Navicular

The short lever technique may be used by reversing the contacts for the dorsal fixation (above).

Alternative long lever technique. With the inside hand, contact the dorsal surface of the navicular with the first pad of the middle finger (nearest the metacarpal; Fig. 6–37A). With the outside hand, reinforce the contact (Fig. 6–37B) and place both thumbs on the plantar surface of the metatarsals (Fig. 6–38A). Utmost speed is necessary for this thrust. The direction is straight plantar (Fig. 6–38B).

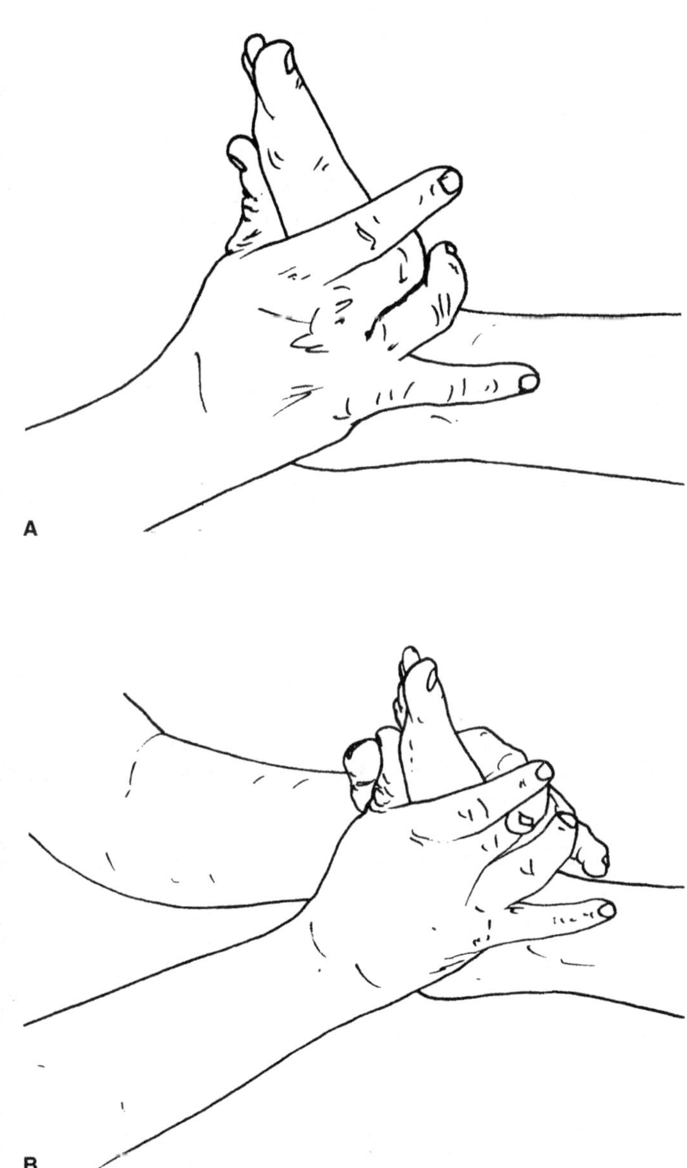

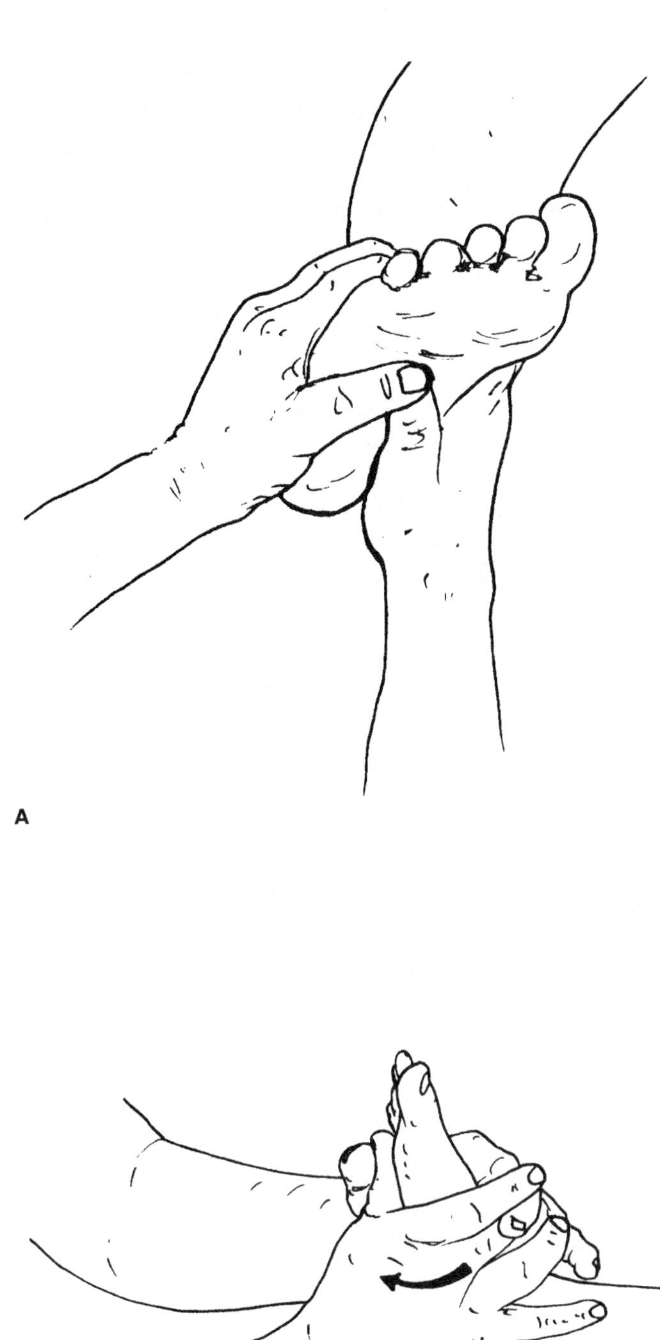

Fig. 6–37 (A) Inside hand contact for plantar fixation of the talar head on the navicular. **(B)** Reinforcement of contact with the outside hand.

Fig. 6–38 (A) Thumb contacts for plantar fixation of the talar head on the navicular, alternative technique. **(B)** Thrust.

Superiority of the Talonavicular Articulation

Occasionally the talus will dorsiflex and the navicular will be fixed with it, palpating as a superiority of both. When this occurs, use the same hand positions as in the preceding technique, but place the contact over the articulation. Apply distal traction, and thrust plantarly with a scooping move (Fig. 6–39).

Dorsal Fixation of the First, Second, and Third Cuneiforms on the Navicular

Using the first pad of the middle finger of the inside hand, contact the appropriate cuneiform. Reinforce the contact with the outside hand, and place the thumbs on the plantar surface of the metatarsals (Fig. 6–40). Utmost speed is called for with this long lever technique.

Alternative short lever technique. With the patient supine, sit facing the lateral side of the foot. With the headward hand, contact the plantar surface of the navicular. With the footward hand, contact the appropriate cuneiform. The thrust is made in equal and opposite directions (Fig. 6–41).

Plantar Fixation of the First, Second, and Third Cuneiforms on the Navicular

For a short lever technique, reverse the contacts of the preceding technique.

Alternative long lever technique. With the patient prone, place the foot in the palm of your outside hand. Place the middle finger of the outside hand around the medial arch on the plantar surface of the appropriate cuneiform (Fig. 6–42A). Turn and face the outside of the foot. With the inside hand, take a pisiform contact over the other finger for reinforcement (Fig. 6–42B).

Care must be taken with this technique. Do not plantar flex the ankle more than a few degrees. Move the foot toward the

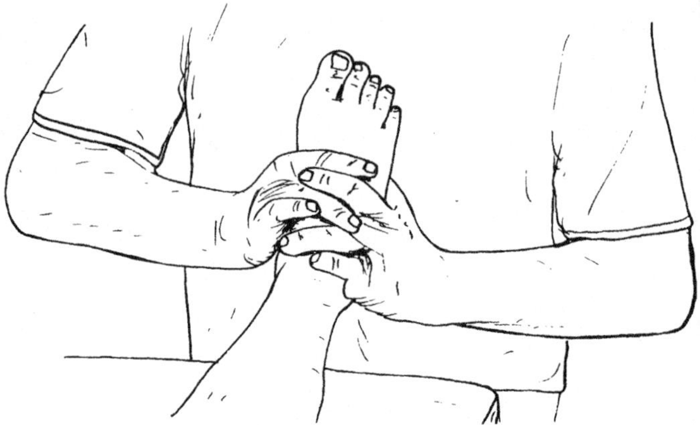

Fig. 6–40 Contacts for dorsal fixation of the first, second, and third cuneiforms on the navicular.

outside of the table to provide dorsal movement of the medial arch and for the patient's comfort during the thrust. The thrust is made with the inside hand; it is sharp, quick, and shallow while the outside hand restrains the foot (Fig. 6–42C).

This technique may be used for a plantar fixation of the navicular on the talus and a plantar fixation of the first metatarsal on the first cuneiform. The navicular articulation with the cuboid was discussed earlier.

Fixations of the First Cuneiform

The first cuneiform articulates with the navicular, as already discussed. It also articulates with the second cuneiform, the second metatarsal, and the first metatarsal (Fig. 6–43).

Dorsal Fixation of the Second Cuneiform on the First Cuneiform

With the patient supine, sit facing the lateral side of the foot. With the footward hand, place the middle finger over the navicular and contact the dorsal surface of the second cuneiform.

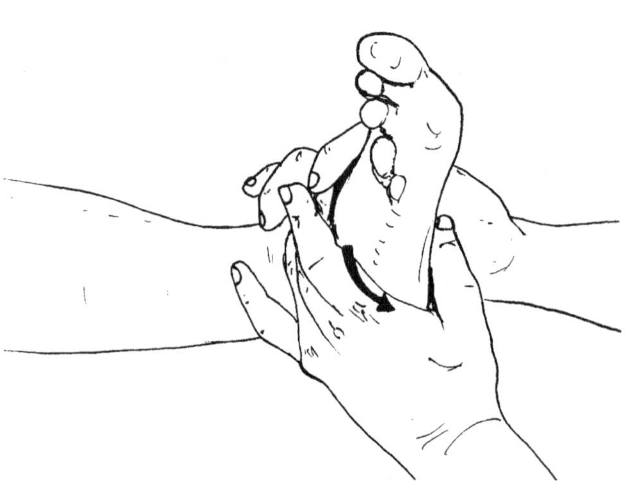

Fig. 6–39 Thrust for superior talonavicular articulation.

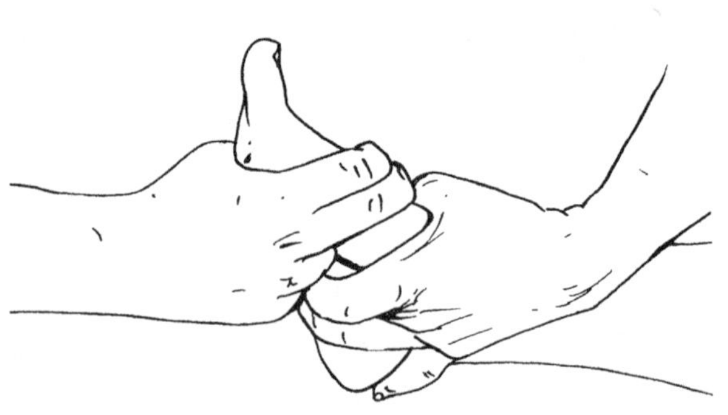

Fig. 6–41 Short lever contacts for dorsal fixation of the first, second, and third cuneiforms on the navicular.

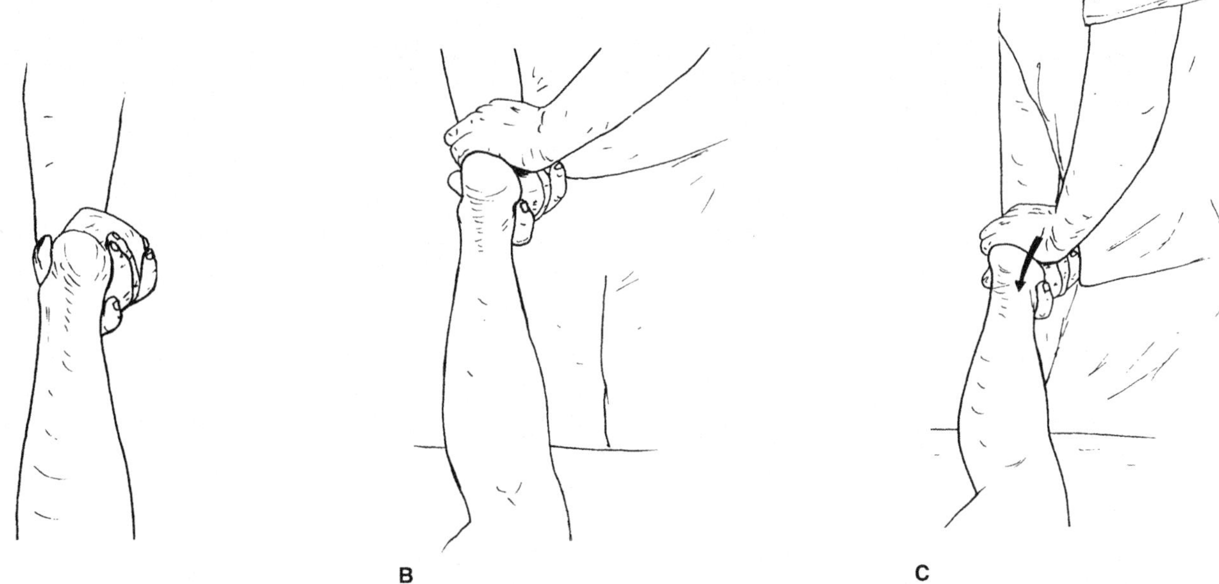

A   B   C

Fig. 6–42 (A) Plantar surface contact for dorsal fixation of the first, second, and third cuneiforms on the navicular, alternative technique. **(B)** Thrusting hand contact. **(C)** Thrust.

With the headward hand, contact the plantar surface of the first cuneiform (Fig. 6–44). Use the short lever technique.

Plantar Fixation of the Second Cuneiform on the First Cuneiform

Reverse the above contacts. The plantar surface of the second cuneiform is difficult, if not impossible, to contact. Contact is made indirectly on the plantar surface of the third cuneiform, which takes advantage of the 45° angle of the second and third articulations (Fig. 6–45).

Dorsal Fixation of the First or Second Metatarsal on the First Cuneiform

Short lever technique. With the patient supine, sit facing the lateral side of the foot. With the headward hand, contact the plantar surface of the first cuneiform with the middle finger. With the footward hand, contact the second or first metatarsal head with the middle finger (Fig. 6–46). Apply traction and thrust.

Long lever technique. With the patient supine, contact either the first or second metatarsal head with the first pad

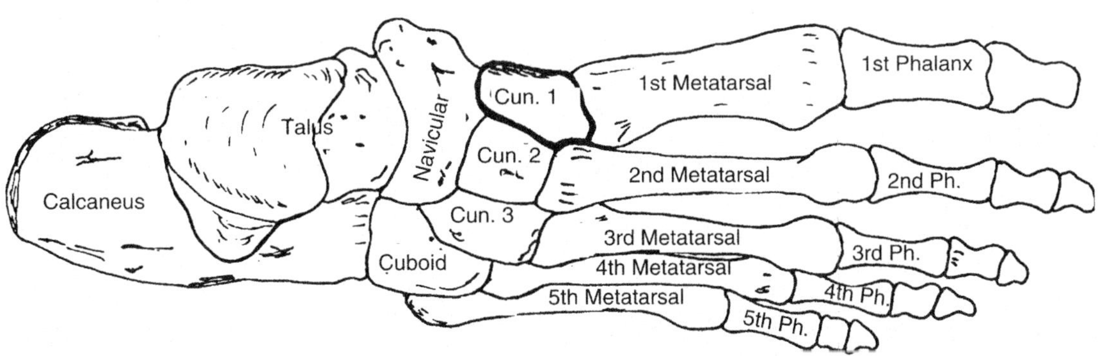

Fig. 6–43 Right foot from above.

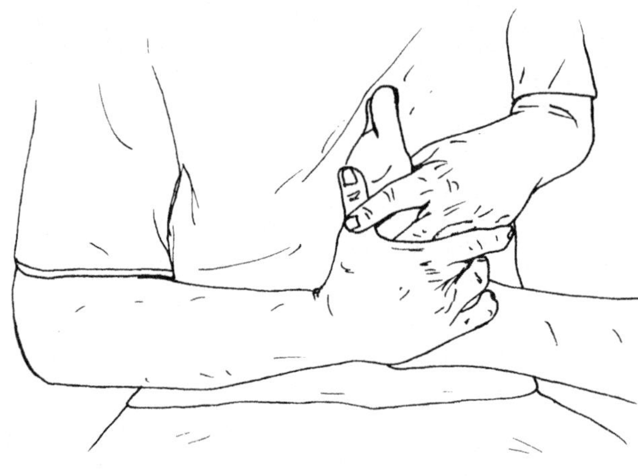

Fig. 6–44 Contacts for dorsal fixation of the second cuneiform on the first cuneiform.

(proximal) of the middle finger of the inside hand. Reinforce the contact with the outside hand. Place the thumbs on the plantar surface of the distal metatarsals. Apply traction and thrust quickly and smoothly using the long lever technique (Fig. 6–47). This technique may be used for a dorsal fixation of the third and sometimes the fourth metatarsal heads.

Plantar Fixation of the First Metatarsal on the First Cuneiform

With the patient prone, place the foot in the palm of the outside hand. Wrap the middle finger of the outside hand around to contact the plantar surface of the first metatarsal (Fig. 6–48A). Turn and face the outside of the foot. With the inside hand, take a pisiform contact over the other finger for reinforcement (Fig. 6–48B).

Care must be taken with this technique. Do not plantar flex the ankle more than a few degrees. Move the foot toward the outside of the table to provide dorsal movement of the medial

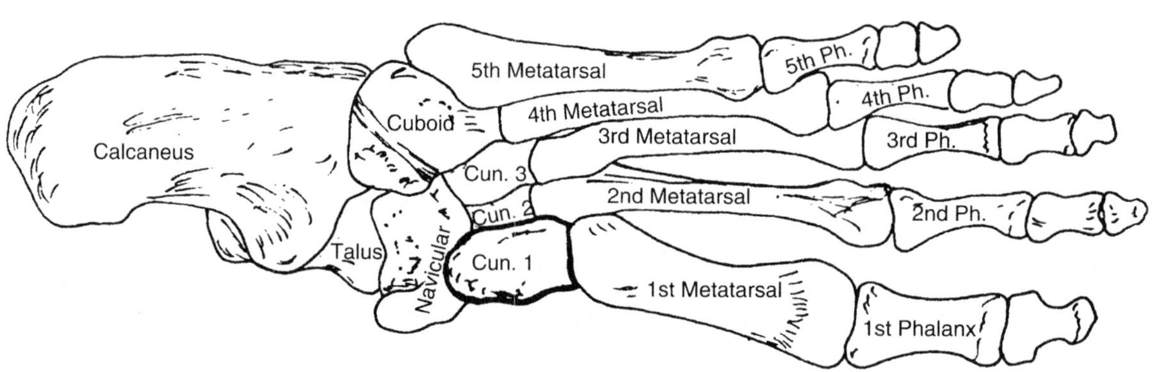

Fig. 6–45 Right foot from below.

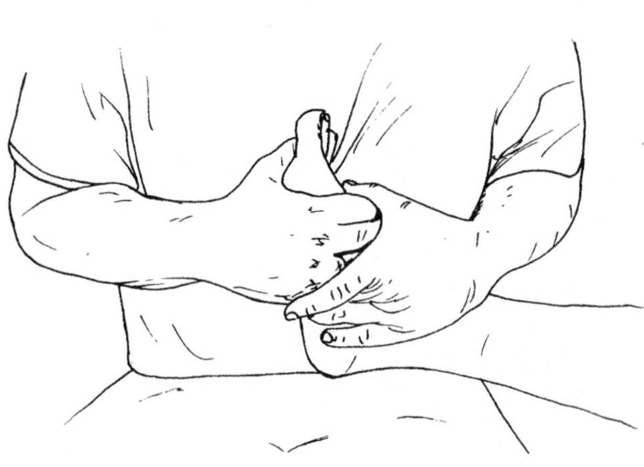

Fig. 6–46 Short lever contacts for dorsal fixation of the first or second metatarsal on the first cuneiform.

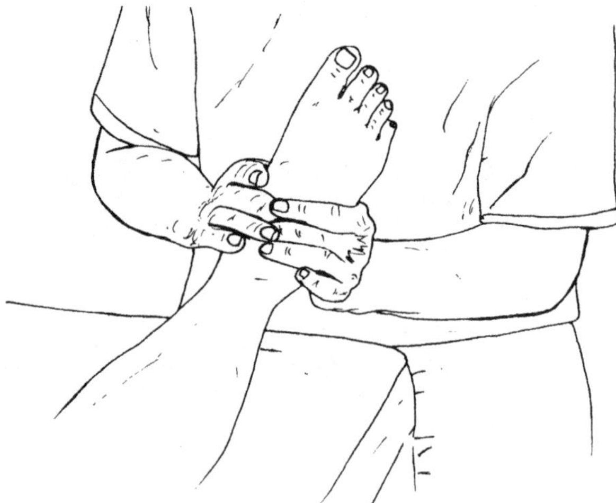

Fig. 6–47 Long lever technique for dorsal fixation of the first or second metatarsal on the first cuneiform.

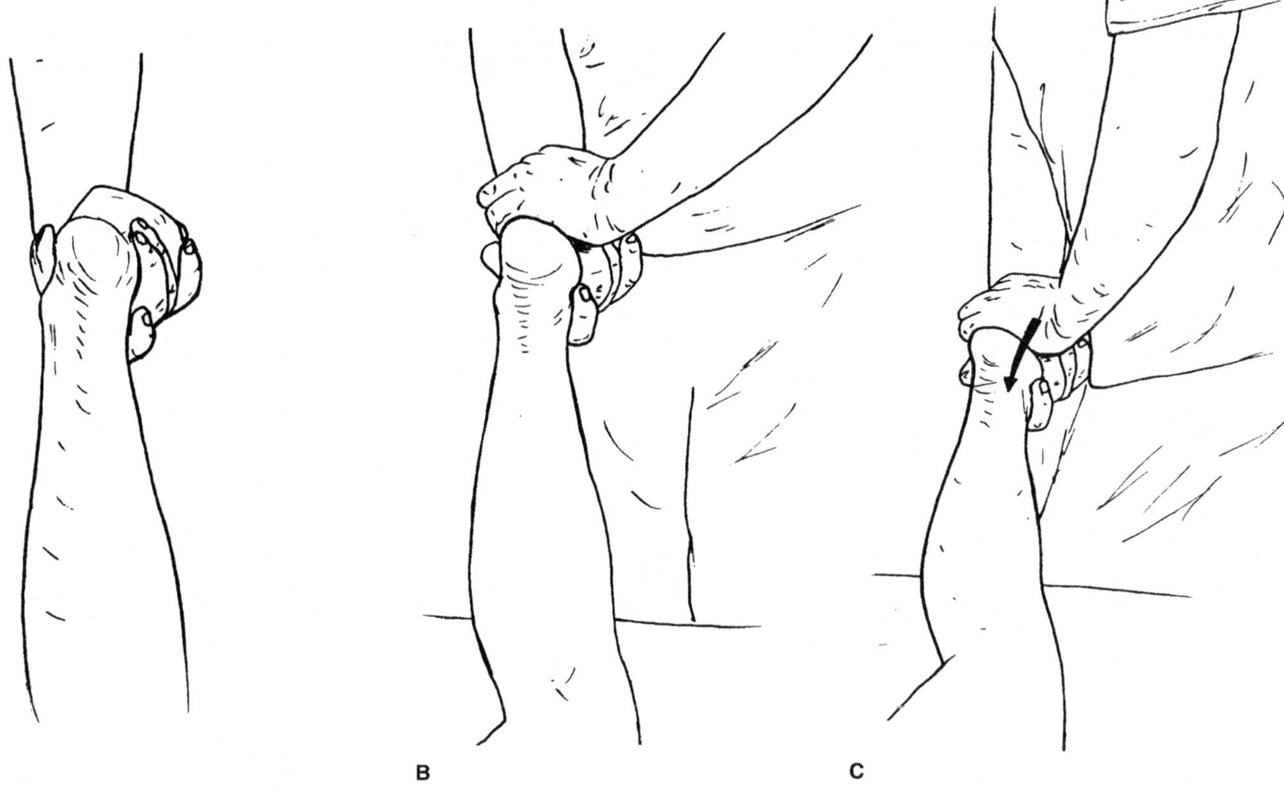

A   B   C

Fig. 6–48 **(A)** Plantar surface contact for plantar fixation of the first metatarsal on the first cuneiform. **(B)** Thrusting hand contact. **(C)** Thrust.

arch and for the patient's comfort during the thrust. The thrust is made with the inside hand; it is sharp, quick, and shallow while the outside hand restrains the foot (Fig. 6–48C).

Fixations of the Tarsals and Phalanges

Plantar Fixations of the Tarsals

Prone. With the patient prone, contact the plantarly fixed bone with the thumb of the outside hand. Reinforce the contact with the thumb of the inside hand. The thrust is executed in a fashion sometimes referred to as whip move: Allow the foot to drop toward the table and make a quick thrust with the thumbs (Fig. 6–49).

Standing. With the patient standing, the same whip technique may be applied but with much greater accuracy (Fig. 6–50A). Standing makes it possible to move the foot forward rapidly rather than plantar flexing the ankle, as in the preceding technique (Fig. 6–50B).

Alternative prone technique. The same technique as in Figure 6–50 may be applied by having the patient move to the side of the table with the leg off the table. This position allows the limb to move freely, enabling the technique to be applied.

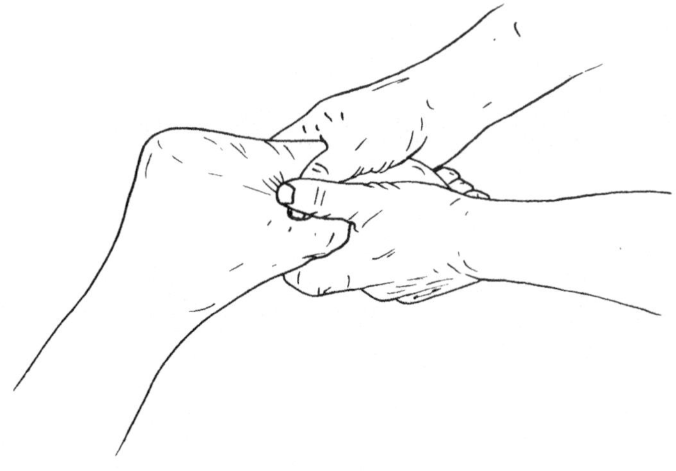

Fig. 6–49 Double thumb contact for plantar fixation of the tarsals.

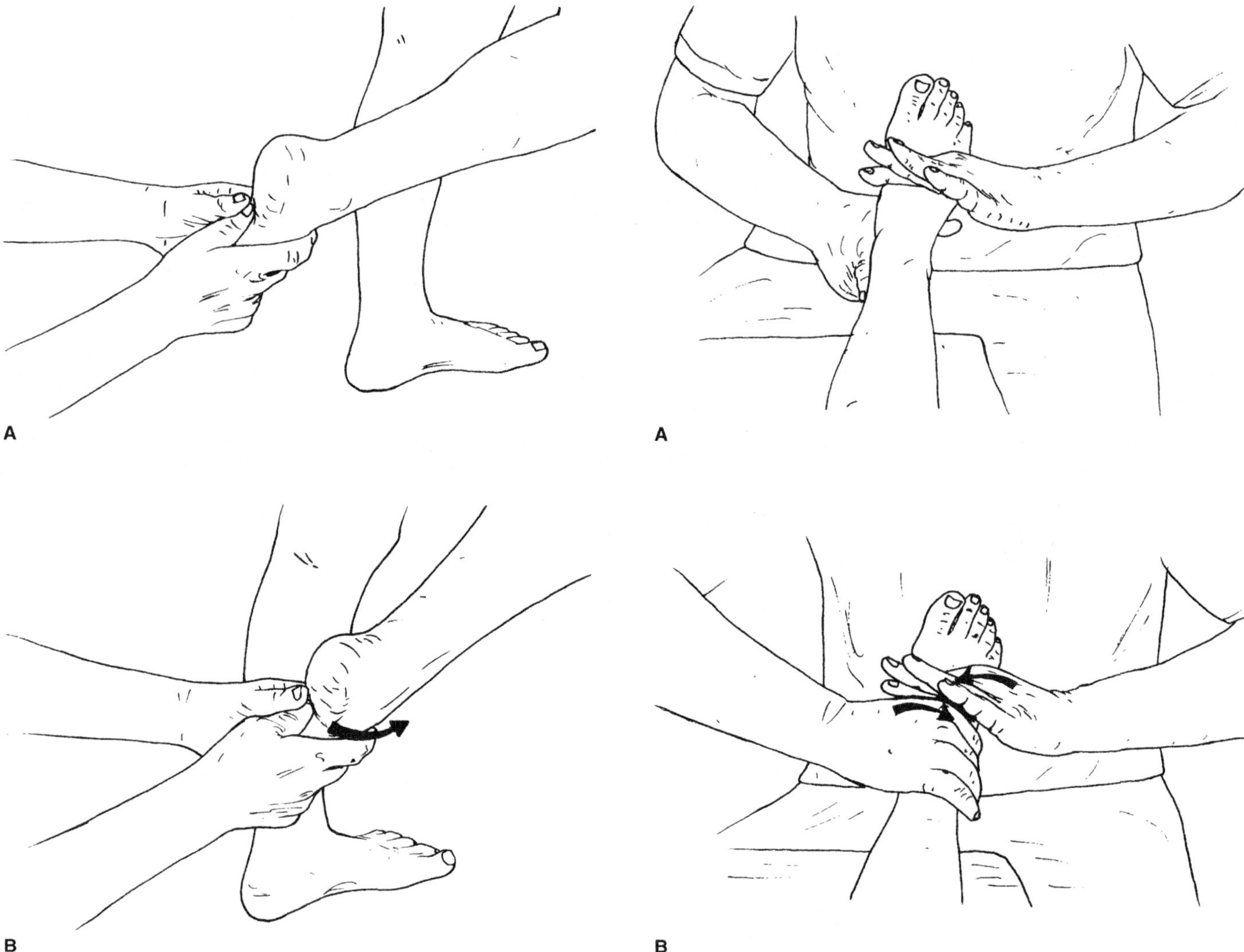

Fig. 6–50 (A) Standing contacts for plantar fixation of the tarsals. **(B)** Thrust.

Fig. 6–51 (A) Contacts for laterally rotated first metatarsal head. **(B)** Thrust.

Lateral Rotation of the First Metatarsal Head

With the patient supine, grasp the medial surface of the foot with the thumb web, securing the first cuneiform. With the outside hand, use an index contact on the lateral side of the first metatarsal head (Fig. 6–51A). The thrust is made in equal and opposite directions using a short lever technique (Fig. 6–51B).

Loosening of the Metatarsotarsal Articulations

Place the sides of the metatarsals against the open palms. Move the hands in opposite directions gently at first and then with increasing vigor and distance (Fig. 6–52).

Loosening of the Tarsals and the Tarsometatarsal Articulations

This general loosening technique may take care of many small undetected fixations and will allow greater flexibility of the foot. With the patient prone, take a firm grip of the tibia and hindfoot using the thumb web over the talar head (Fig. 6–53). With the footward hand, grasp the medial arch, securing the navicular. With these contacts, use a rotating, twisting, wrenching movement to loosen the talonavicular articulations (Fig. 6–54). By moving the hands progressively distally, each of the articulations may be loosened.

The two loosening techniques shown above do much more than correct minute fixations. Stimulation of the feet has a

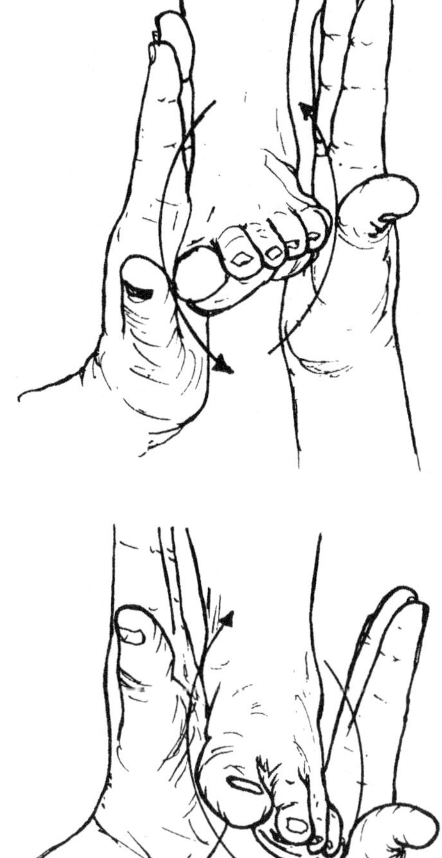

A

B

Fig. 6–52 (**A** and **B**) Loosening of the metatarsotarsal articulations.

definite relaxing effect on the majority of patients. Even if nothing specific is found in the lower extremities, the application of these techniques will often send the patient away feeling light of foot.

Plantar Fixation of the Distal Phalanx of the Great Toe

With the patient supine, grasp the distal phalanx using the proximal pad of the index finger underneath and the distal thumb pad over the toenail (Fig. 6–55A). Grip the phalanx lightly, and maintain the finger-thumb relationship. The adjustment is made by lifting up rapidly using wrist action (Fig. 6–55B).

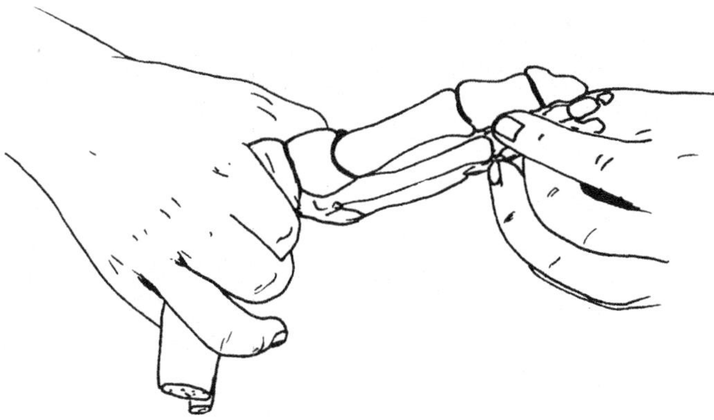

Fig. 6–53 First contact for loosening of the tarsals and tarsometatarsal articulations.

Adjustment of the Proximal Phalanx of the Great Toe with the First Metatarsal

Contact the first phalanx using the first (proximal) pad of the index finger and the first pad of the thumb. Maintain a light grip. The most common fixation is a lack of dorsal movement. The thrust is the same as in the distal phalanx: a quick upward flick of the wrist with a slight medial rotation (Fig. 6–56). Any rotational fixation can be adjusted by applying appropriate rotation in the thrust.

Plantar Fixation of the Second through Fifth Proximal Metatarsophalangeal Articulations

With the patient supine, place the thumb pad under the articulation. Place the index or middle finger on the dorsum of

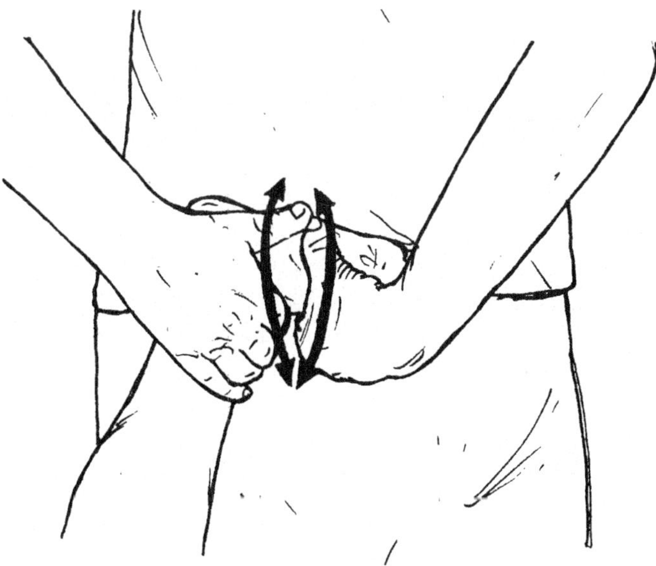

Fig. 6–54 Loosening technique.

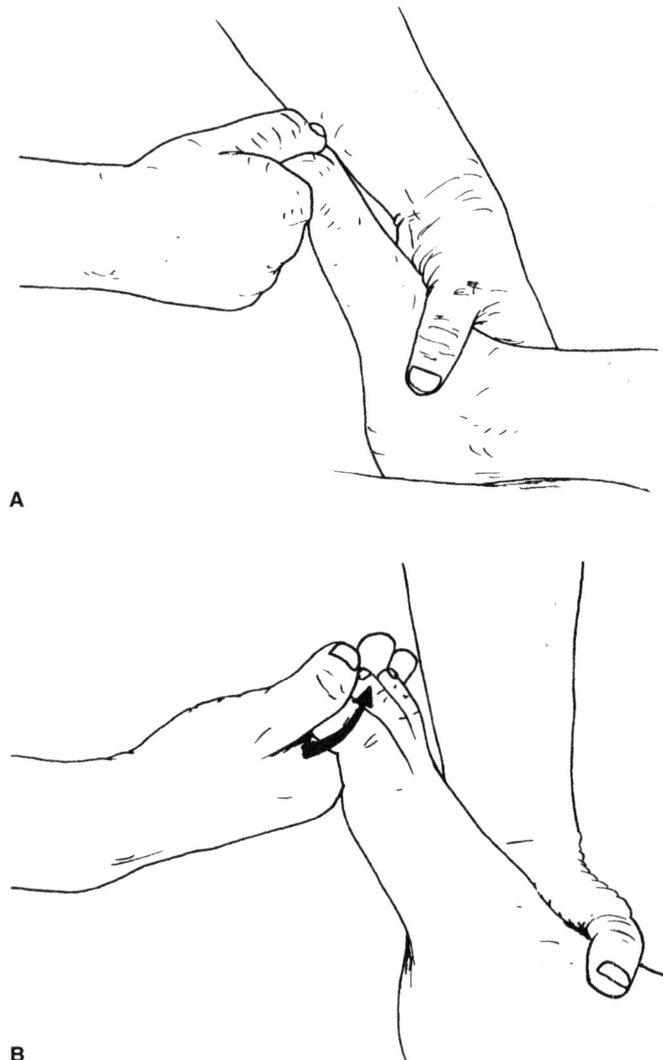

A

B

Fig. 6–55 (A) Contacts for plantar fixation of the distal phalanx of the great toe. **(B)** Thrust.

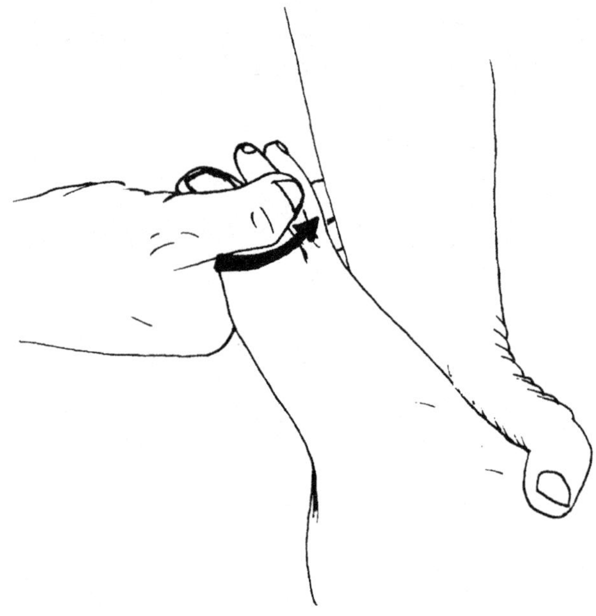

Fig. 6–56 Adjustment of plantar fixation of the proximal phalanx of the great toe.

---

the digit. Use a light grip; do not squeeze. The thrust is with the thumb in a dorsal direction while the finger simply maintains the digit position (Fig. 6–57). The same principle is applied in the prone position (Fig. 6–58).

It is important that the patient be instructed to relax. If the thrust is made quickly without a hard grip and is delivered at the point of tension, the technique should not be painful. A common error in both supine and prone techniques is attempting to do all the digits in one move. This is not only nonspecific but also usually painful to the patient.

Extension of the Articulations of the Second through Fifth Digits

Grasp the last phalanx with the index finger and thumb pad of the outside hand (Fig. 6–59A). Maintain a firm contact, but

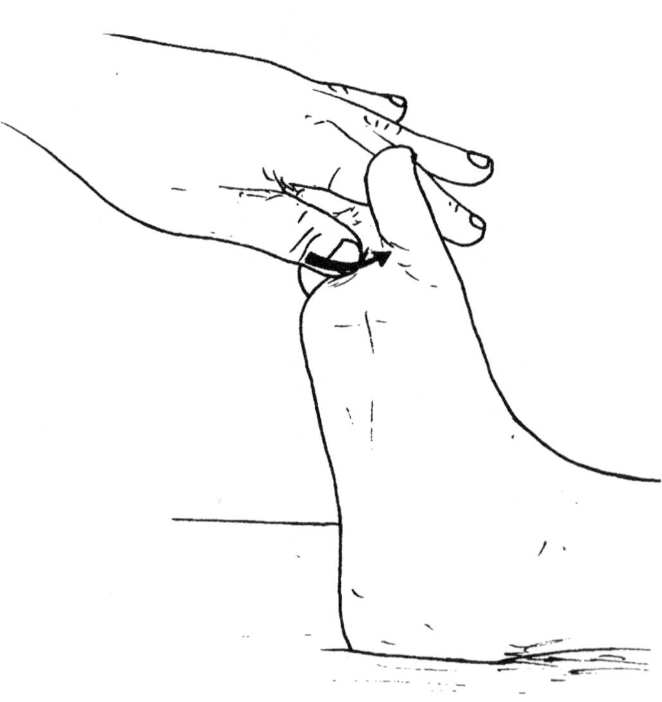

Fig. 6–57 Contact and thrust for plantar fixation of the proximal metatarsophalangeal articulation.

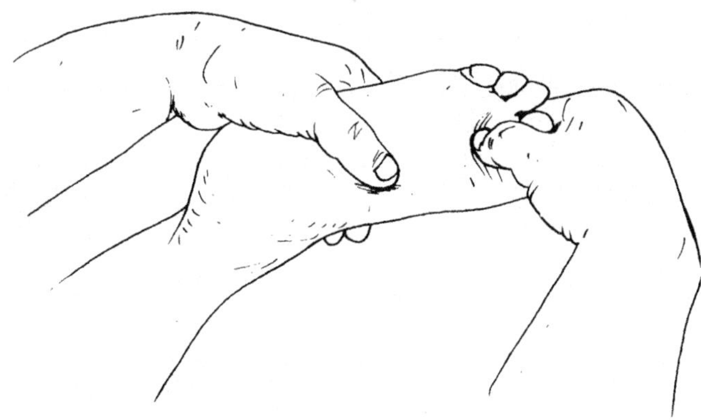

Fig. 6–58 Contact and thrust for plantar fixation of the proximal metatarsophalangeal articulation, prone technique.

---

do not squeeze. With the inside hand, take a pisiform or heel contact with the thumb. All the thrust is made with the inside hand using a rather shallow but quick thrust into extension (Fig. 6–59B).

USE OF AN ELEVATED CHAIR

One method of adjusting was developed by Hiss,[2] who worked in a pit with an elevated chair for the patient. His clinic was primarily for feet, so that a table was not necessary for other therapies. Most of the techniques described in this chapter may be adapted to this position. Alternatively, the patient may stand facing away from the adjuster while holding onto the chair, allowing examination and treatment of the plantar surface of the foot.

USE OF AN IMPACT TOOL

A dental impact chisel was adapted as an impact tool by using a small, hard, rubber insert rather than the chisel head (Fig. 6–60). The instrument has been improved and is now marketed under the name of Activator. This is not an endorsement of the techniques taught under the name Activator. I have found a use for the instrument under certain circumstances.

An impact tool may be used instead of the short lever technique. It is especially useful for a practitioner who has small or weak hands. A patient with large, almost immobile feet becomes a challenge even for practitioners with strong hands, however. I prefer the short or long lever techniques. Use of the Activator as shown (Fig. 6–61) helps break up fixations but does not improve the range of motion, as the other techniques will.

With the use of the Activator, apply thumb pressure to the dorsal surface of the affected bone structure and the tool to the plantar surface. It is usually necessary to impact several times for results.

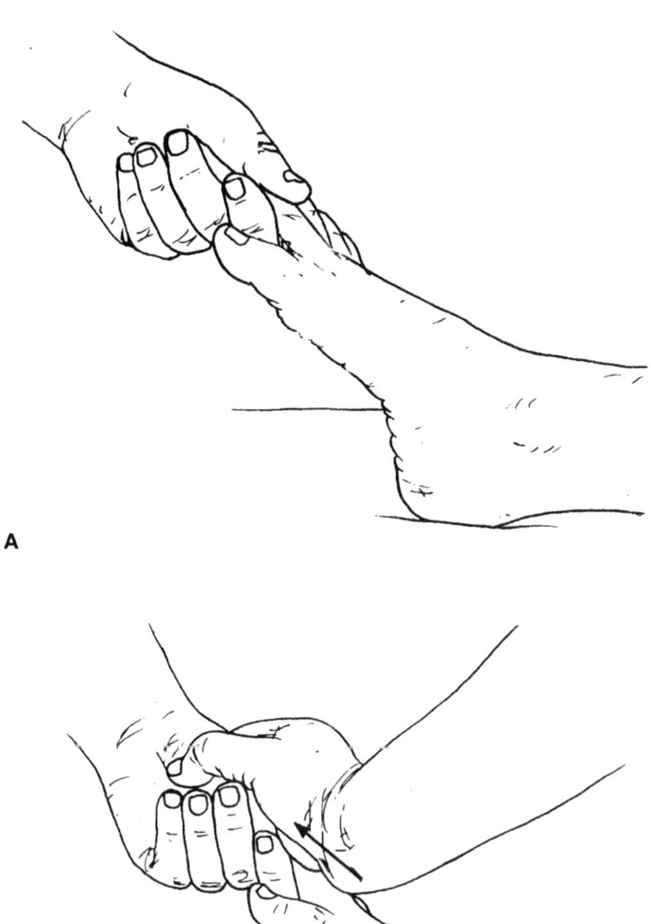

Fig. 6–59 **(A)** Contact for extension of the articulations of the second through fifth digits. **(B)** Thrust.

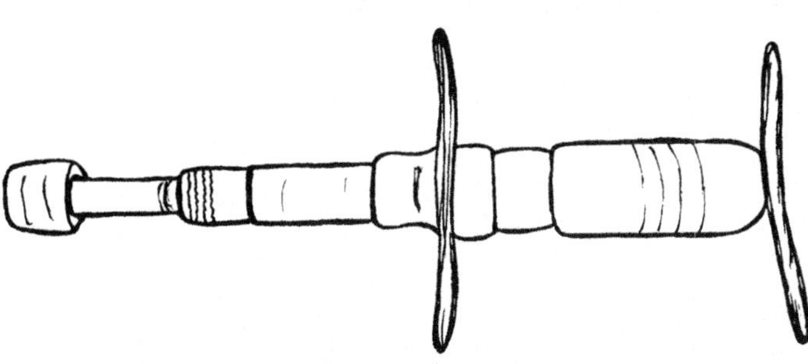

Fig. 6–60 Activator impact tool.

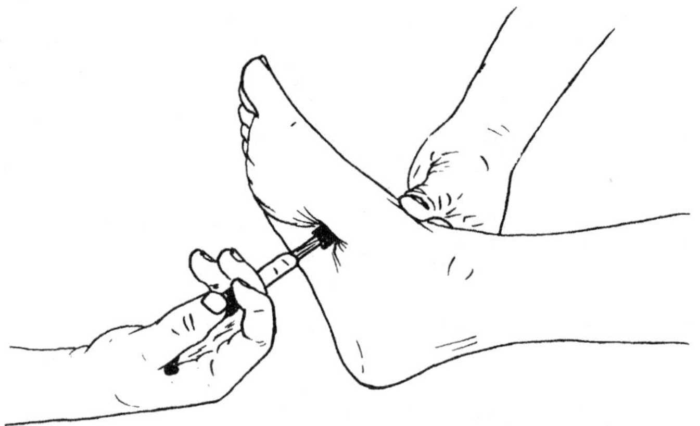

Fig. 6–61 Use of the Activator for short lever technique.

CONCLUDING REMARKS

No matter which technique is preferred, one caution must always apply: When any technique is used on a nonpliable, nonadaptable foot, the foot does not have to move on the first attempt. When movement has been restricted for some time, it is better to attempt the technique, give the patient some loosening-up exercises to do, and then follow up again at a later appointment.

REFERENCES

1. Broome RT. *The Foot and Ankle* [videotape]. Bournemouth, England: Anglo-European College of Chiropractic; 1987.

2. Hiss JM. *Functional Foot Disorders.* New York, NY: Oxford University Press; 1949.

Chapter 7

Conditions and Their Treatment

THE UNPLIABLE, UNADAPTABLE FOOT

One of the most common conditions found in practice is the foot that fails to move through its normal range of motion. In failing to do so, the foot is unable to adapt to variations in terrain while walking and is unable to support the rest of the body. When restrictions occur in one part of the body, another part often becomes hypermobile to make up for it. An example found in practice is a restricted forefoot accompanied by excessive range of motion of the talonavicular articulation.

Causes

Hiss[1] states that there are three main disturbances that are intrinsic causes of most foot symptoms: mechanical arthritis, muscle strain, and limited foot motion.

Mechanical Arthritis

With any displacement of a bone due to injury or misalignment, all slack that might exist in the joint is taken up. Joint surfaces become opposed with greater pressure, and the range of motion is limited. Greater pressure on the cartilaginous surfaces can cause inflammation and result in pain and dysfunction. Clinically, when this occurs it may be confused with systemic arthritis.

Muscle Strain

Muscle strain may be due to an injury, or muscles can be strained by abnormal postural stress. A fixation in a joint may cause a muscle to strain by interfering with normal antagonistic muscle action.

Limited Mobility

When the bone structures of the foot become locked into an abnormal position for whatever reason, the normal motion of the foot becomes limited. This may lead to alterations in posture, alterations in body movement, and/or alterations in other parts of the foot. When normal motion is limited, other articulations involved in the movement must become either hypermobile or restricted themselves.

Restricted mobility is usually accompanied by congestion. Venous and lymphatic flow depends on movement, especially in the lower extremity. Consider the person who wears tight-fitting shoes every day to work, sitting behind a desk and wearing the shoes for up to 16 hours per day. Without exercise, massage, or other activity, the entire lower extremity may become congested.

A demonstration may be made to show what congestion does to the foot. If palpation of the plantar surface of the foot reveals soreness and congestion along the plantar ligament, have the patient lie supine with one hip and knee flexed and the foot elevated. For approximately 1 to 2 minutes, have the patient wiggle the toes and move the foot around. Circulation may be increased with mild massage, but this is usually not necessary. If both feet responded to palpation with soreness and congestion to start with, the one that was mobilized will have the soreness either gone or greatly diminished.

Patients with limited mobility of the feet will respond favorably to mobilization and stimulation that increases circulation. On several occasions I have had to examine a patient, including checking for range of motion and fixations, without treating that day only to have the patient return the next day and report that the condition was greatly improved just from the mobilization.

Treatment

Correction of the unpliable, unadaptable foot should include correction of all postural faults that may affect the foot. To loosen the foot and begin the process toward normalcy, two methods have proved to be successful in practice.

Begin treatment by placing the foot between your open palms, and at the start gently mobilize the forefoot, rolling it back and forth between your hands. Within patient tolerance, increase the range and vigor of motion to establish mobility and to increase circulation (Fig. 7–1). In the other method, the patient is prone. Take a firm grip of the tibia and hindfoot with the thumb web over the talar head (Fig. 7–2). With the

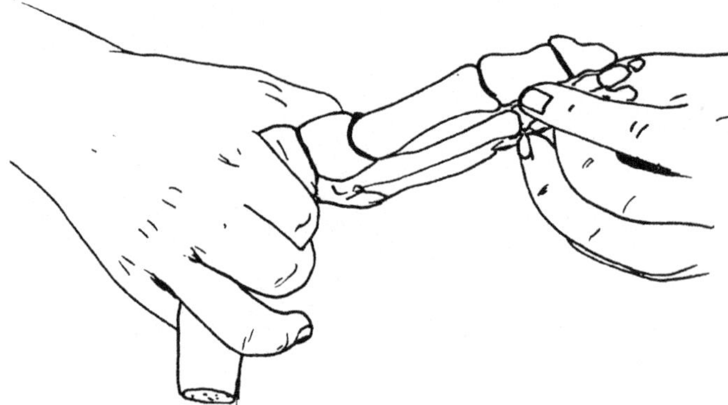

Fig. 7–2 First contact for loosening of the tarsals and tarsometatarsal articulations.

footward hand, grasp the medial arch, securing the navicular. With these contacts, use a rotating, twisting, wrenching movement to loosen the talonavicular articulations (Fig. 7–3). By moving the hands progressively distal, each of the articulations may be loosened.

The two loosening techniques described above do much more than correct minute fixations. Stimulation of the feet has a definite relaxing effect on the majority of patients. Even if nothing specific is found in the lower extremities, the application of these techniques will often send the patient off feeling light of foot.

The adjuster should explain thoroughly to the patient why mobility of the foot is important and should enlist the patient's energies to bring it about. The patient should understand that an unpliable foot does not develop overnight and that consistent effort on his or her part will be necessary to reestablish

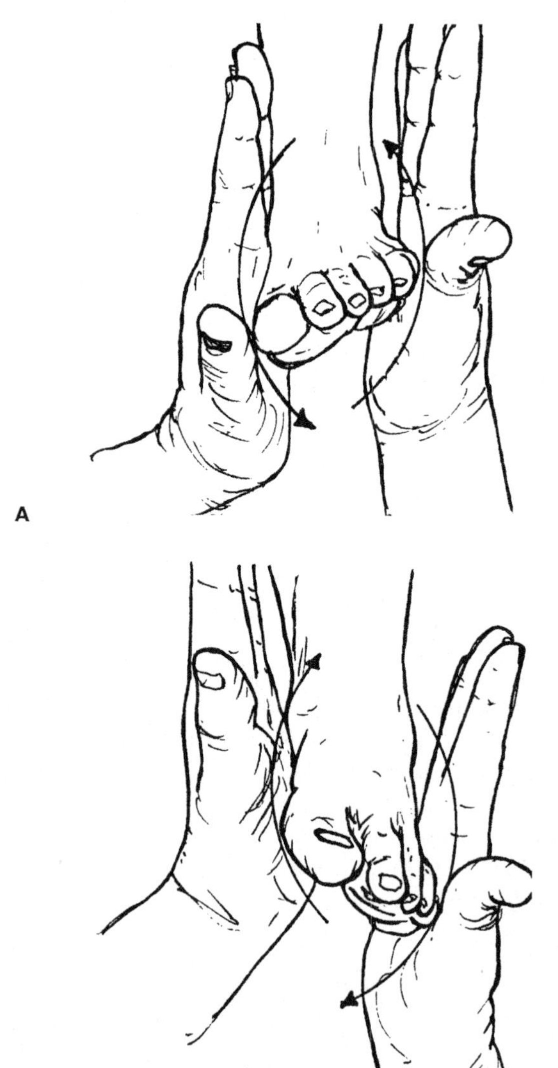

Fig. 7–1 (**A** and **B**) Loosening of the metatarsotarsal articulations.

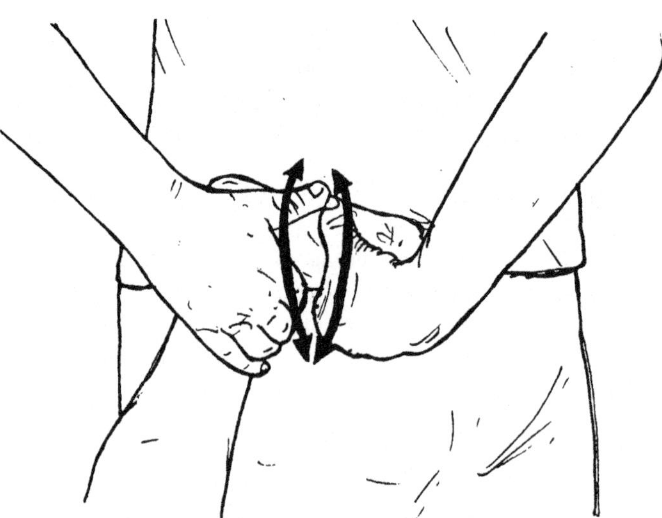

Fig. 7–3 Loosening technique.

mobility. Include the above manipulations each time the patient is seen in the office, and provide the following exercises for the patient to do at home.

With the leg resting on a stool, place a belt around the foot at the tarsal level. Pull on the belt to invert and evert the tarsals (Fig. 7–4). Begin gently, increasing the range of motion and the vigor of movement to tolerance. After 8 to 10 vigorous repetitions, move the belt to the metatarsal arch and repeat the exercise.

To establish movement and pliability, the above exercises should be performed several times per day. Improvement in symptoms may occur in a short time, but increased range of motion and pliability come only with time and effort. Muscles

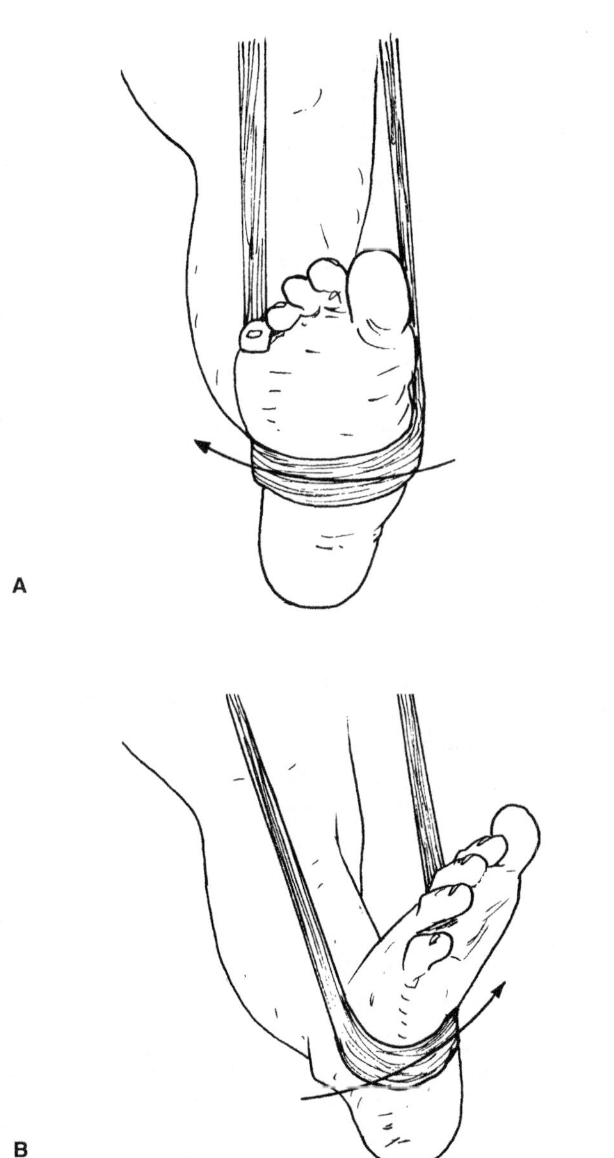

Fig. 7–4 Use of a belt to evert (**A**) and invert (**B**) the foot.

have to elongate, fascia must change, and the habit patterns of use must change.

The patient must be encouraged to participate in activities that increase the range of motion. Where possible, walking barefoot in sand or deep grass is a great help in increasing pliability and helps in improving adaptability of the foot.

Restricted mobility of the foot is usually accompanied by restricted dorsiflexion of the ankle, which must be addressed at the same time.

SHORTENED TRICEPS SURAE

Although a shortened triceps surae is referred to by Shands and Raney,[2] Calliet,[3] and Mennell[4] as a shortened Achilles tendon, I am of the opinion that the tendon itself is not at fault but the muscle is. Therefore, surgical intervention to lengthen the tendon seems rather drastic. This condition is present in some spastic conditions, especially in childhood, and may require bracing[5] to prevent the contracture from occurring. Mennell[4] states that metatarsal head pain may be a result of an Achilles insufficiency. Shortening may also be a result of excessive plantar flexion due to the wearing of high-heeled shoes.[2,3] I have found that a shortened triceps surae usually accompanies a foot that is restricted in its pliability. Whether it is the cause, the result, or just a part of the condition is unknown.

Another cause is often overexercising the plantar flexor muscles. Runners who do hard, long-distance running with a flatfoot gait, striding on the sole of the foot rather than on the heel, tend to have restricted dorsiflexion. Triathletes who participate in running, bicycling, and swimming have the same tendencies. Bicycling requires vigorous plantar flexion with less demand for dorsiflexion. Ankle movement during swimming begins in plantar flexion.

A shortened triceps surae should not be confused with Achilles tendinitis. Palpation along the tendon and its insertion into the calcaneus is necessary to differentiate the two.

In walking, as the body weight moves forward of neutral, dorsiflexion must occur to allow the full range of mobility and function of the foot (Fig. 7–5). Without the full range of dorsiflexion, a full stride is not possible without interference with the function of the foot (Fig. 7–6). Failure of full dorsiflexion results in the force from heel strike moving directly to the metatarsal arch. This places great strain on the plantar fascia and its attachments.

The foot provides stability and strength during standing and with all other demands. Its pliability and adaptability allow all these things to occur smoothly without strain to the foot or the body above. I have successfully treated patients with various symptoms, such as chronic midthoracic pain, low back pain, headache, knee pain, and pain in various areas of the foot, in whom the causal factors were traced back to a shortened triceps surae.

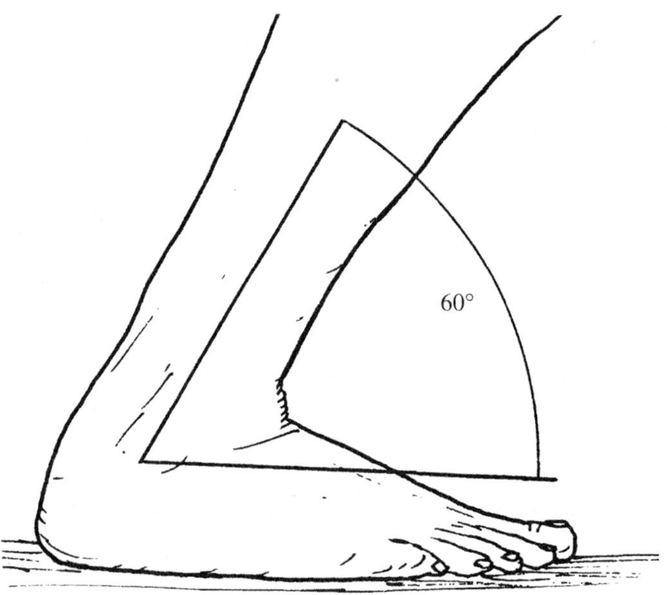

Fig. 7–5 Normal dorsiflexion of the ankle during a long stride.

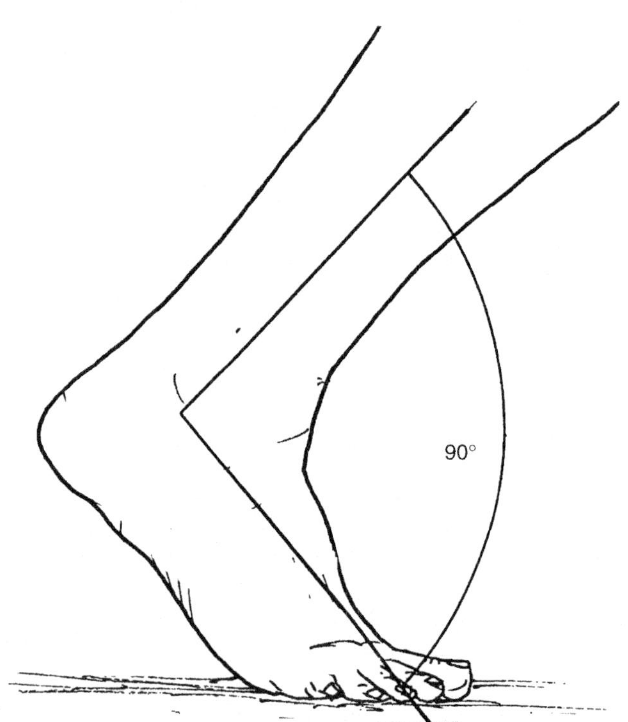

Fig. 7–6 Lack of dorsiflexion of the ankle during a long stride.

Consideration must be given to the premise that the short-ened triceps surae may be the result of other conditions as well. It may have occurred as a result of forefoot pain restrict-ing pressure on the forefoot, altering the habit pattern and minimizing dorsiflexion. Shortening can result from a low

back condition that prevents a shifting of body weight forward with resulting alteration of the use of the triceps surae. It may occur with the constant wearing of high heels without proper stretching exercises. Most often, I have found shortening to be the result of a lack of exercise coupled with sitting for long periods of time. It may also occur as a result of dorsiflexor muscle weakness if maintained over time. It is important to determine the cause of the shortening ultimately to correct the condition.

There are numerous methods that have been suggested to correct a shortened triceps surae:

- gradually altering the heel height to stretch the triceps surae[1,2,6]
- building up the heel to ease the tension on the Achilles tendon[1,2]
- using a brace for children[7]
- various stretching exercises

Stretching of the triceps surae is necessary to restore normal mobility to the ankle and, thus, the foot. Many methods have been used over the years, including standing with the forefoot on the edge of a stair. In my opinion, this method does tempo-rarily stretch the triceps but also increases the use of the muscles, defeating its purpose and failing to alter the habit pat-tern. Another method is to take a long stride forward and apply pressure down on the posterior heel to keep it on the surface.

I have found that the most effective way to stretch the tri-ceps is by using a slant board (Fig. 7–7). I use a slant board of 13×13 in, rising from the floor to $5\frac{1}{2}$ in at the front, to demon-strate to the patient the restriction and to show a part of the solution. With restricted dorsiflexion, standing in this position may not be possible. If it is possible, the stance is extremely distorted and/or is felt severely in the calf. The solution is to stretch the triceps surae.

At home the patient may stand on the board 10 to 15 times per day. Each time the patient should spend only 1 to 2 min-utes, attempting to stand up as straight as possible. This allows a gradual elongation of the muscles. Usually, 10 to 14 days of home stretching on the slant board will restore full range of motion in most patients. Stretching may remove all the symp-toms caused by the shortness. It is important to educate the patient in eliminating the causes at the same time to prevent a return of the problem.

The normal triceps surae allows the long stride to occur with the body well beyond the foot before it is necessary to elevate the foot from the ground (Fig. 7–6). When the triceps surae is shortened, not allowing dorsiflexion past 90° (Fig. 7–5), as the body weight approaches the midpoint directly over the foot the triceps surae must react. Either the knee must bend, giving the patient a shuffling gait, or the heel must im-mediately elevate from the ground (or both). With the heel-off occurring too soon, the entire normal process of the foot is interrupted, causing great strain.

tient remove the body weight from the foot, and apply pressure with two fingers just above the beginning of the Achilles tendon (Fig. 7–8). Ask the patient again to apply weight to the foot to reproduce the pain.

If a hypertonic portion of the musculature is causing the problem, a significant amount of the symptom will be gone. It may be corrected by a simple procedure. Fold adhesive tape into a 1-in square ⅛ in or more thick. Apply it over the same location at which finger pressure reduced the symptoms (Fig. 7–9). Secure the tape to the location with more adhesive tape. Wrap two to three times around, only tight enough to secure the square and to prevent greater expansion of the calf muscles. Do not constrict muscle function. Wearing of the tape for 36 to 48 hours usually removes the cause and allows normal function.

Pressure over the triceps surae at this location also applies pressure to the posterior tibialis muscle. It is possible that the pressure from the tape pad assists by affecting the posterior tibialis muscle as well.

Treatment of pain associated with a hypertonic triceps surae must include a careful analysis of the foot (see Chapter 5). As pliability returns, adjusting the individual articulations accelerates the process of restoring the foot to normal.

HEEL PAIN

Pain may occur in the heel from many causes, including postural disturbances, trauma, bursitis, tenosynovitis, and fasciitis. It can also be referred.

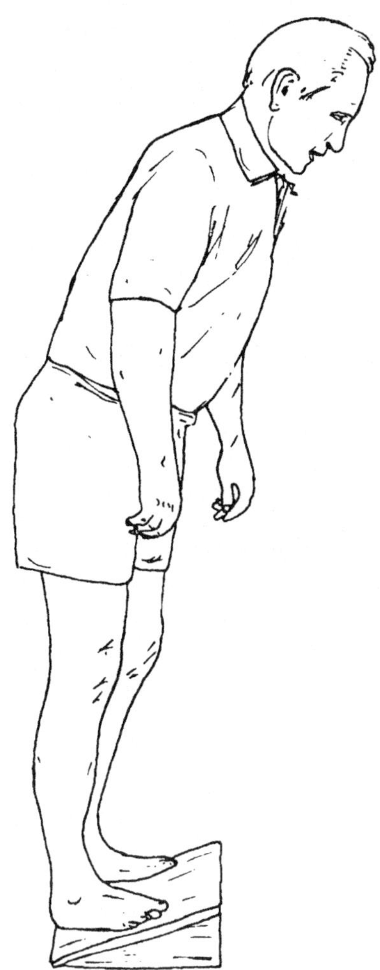

Fig. 7–7 Usual posture on the slant board with restricted dorsiflexion.

Restriction to 0° of dorsiflexion is not uncommon. Patients may have some degree of dorsiflexion, yet it is reasonable to assume that the degree of stress and strain on the foot is directly related to the degree of restricted dorsiflexion. Often, patients may present with symptoms of leg pain along the medial border of the posterior calf (soleus muscle) and low back symptoms. It is not unusual for symptoms in the midthoracics to clear up after stretching of the triceps surae.

Metatarsal pain may be the result of malfunction during the stride with restricted dorsiflexion. As the body weight passes the midpoint, instead of the pliable foot allowing normal movement, all the weight is thrust upon the metatarsal arch. The additional stress reduces the ligamental and muscular security of the metatarsal arch, resulting in pain.

A simple strain, resulting in a hypertonic portion of the triceps surae, may cause pain in the midfoot or the forefoot. A simple test to determine whether a strain exists is to have the patient stand on the limb to reproduce the pain. Have the pa-

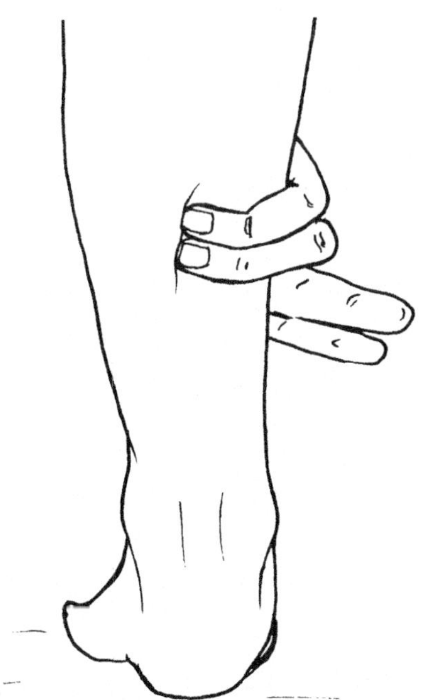

Fig. 7–8 Testing for hypertonicity of the triceps surae.

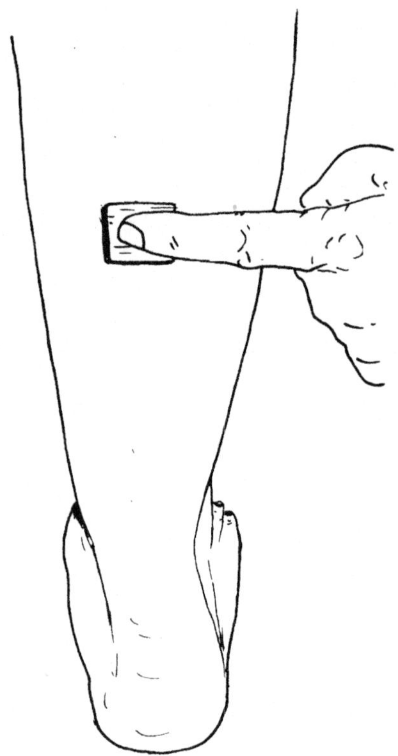

Fig. 7–9 Application of a 1 × 1 × ⅛ in square of adhesive tape.

Postural Disturbances

Postural disturbances allow the body weight to be borne on the posterior foot. In the erect posture, anteroposterior balance is maintained by many muscles. The dominant muscles are the psoas, projecting the weight forward, and the gluteus maximus, projecting the weight to the rear. Any disturbance in the body producing an imbalance, such as a weakened psoas muscle, may produce additional stress on the posterior foot. When the opposite occurs, a shortened psoas and a relatively weak gluteus maximus, a lordotic lumbar syndrome is the result. At first the weight is shifted to the forefoot. If the condition remains for some time, compensation may extend the upper lumbar and lower thoracic spine sufficiently to cause a sway back, and the weight then shifts to the hindfoot.

When either of the above conditions alters the weight balance on the foot, no amount of treatment to the foot itself will have any lasting effect. Only treatment of to cause of the stress and then treatment of the local symptoms will be of help.

Heel Pain after Trauma

Fracture must be suspected with heel pain after trauma. Proper examination, including the use of radiographs to eliminate the possibility, should be performed.

When gross signs of fracture are present, passive motion palpation will reveal even subtle interference with joint function. Examination of the heel after trauma should include the heel squeeze test (Fig. 7–10). The squeeze test will detect possible line fractures of the calcaneus. If positive and a line fracture is suspected, further imaging studies should be performed.

Achilles Tenosynovitis

This condition is referred to by most writers as tenosynovitis. Calliet[3] refers to this condition as paratendinitis because no synovial membrane exists with the Achilles tendon.

The sheath around the tendon is tender and may palpate slightly distended. Palpation of the tendon and the surrounding tissue during muscle activity produces pain and sometimes crepitus (Fig. 7–11). Trauma and stress of the tendon are believed to be the main causes.

Treatment of a mild case may only require cessation of activities that aggravate the condition, such as sports. Treatment of the more severe case should include complete rest, ice to reduce the edema, and manual stretching of the triceps surae muscles.

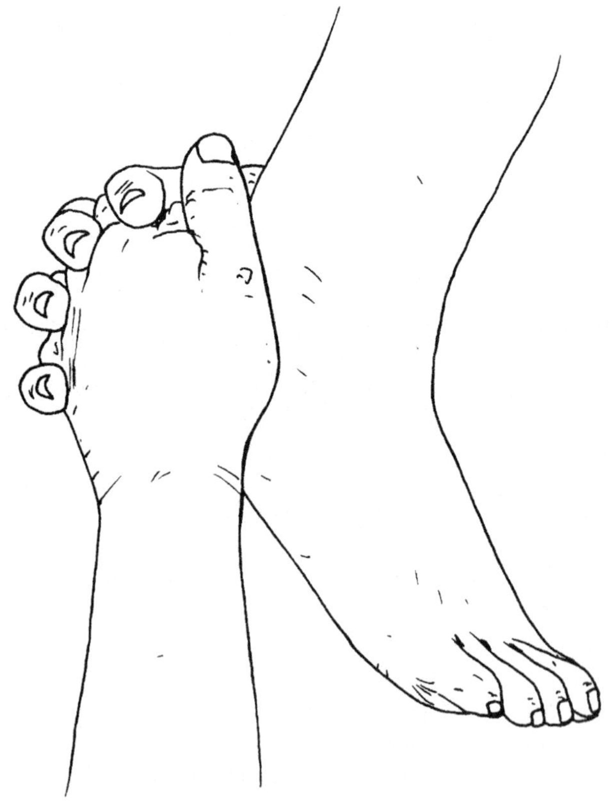

Fig. 7–10 Heel squeeze test.

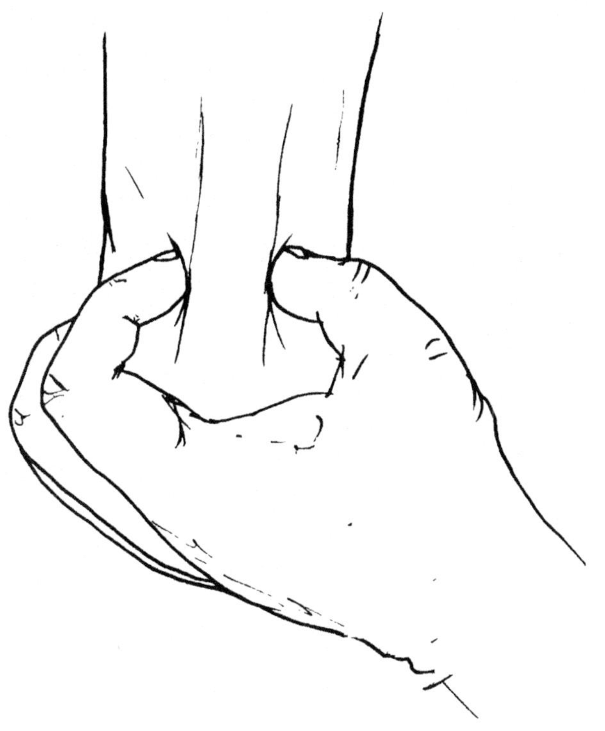

Fig. 7–11 Palpation of the Achilles tendon.

Inflammation and pain are usually accompanied by muscle reaction. With the application of ice to reduce edema, again the muscles may react. If the reaction is allowed to remain, the cycle of tension, inflammation, and lack of circulation will continue. Mild stretching of the musculature after the application of ice is necessary to break the cycle and allow healing to occur.

With the patient prone, stand at the foot of the table. Place the patient's foot on your thigh and apply pressure to dorsiflex the ankle. Using both thumbs, apply traction to the gastrocnemius and soleus muscles.

If the inflammation is on only one side of the Achilles tendon, it must be remembered that the tendon turns 180° during its descent. The lateral side becomes the medial side at the calcaneus attachment. An inflammation on one side only usually means that the gastrocnemius and soleus are affected on the opposite side and may be under greater tension.

Bursitis

There are a number of bursae that can become inflamed in the foot (Figs. 7–12 and 7–13).

Tendo Achilles Bursitis (Subcutaneous)

Inflammation of the subcutaneous bursa may be seen just above the calcaneus insertion of the Achilles tendon as an en-largement just below the skin (Figs. 7–12 and 7–13). Palpation of the tendon and the skin overlying it will reveal extreme tenderness (Fig. 7–14). Do not confuse palpation of this area with deeper Achilles bursitis under the tendon.

Subcutaneous bursitis is believed to be caused by pressure and friction of the shoe counter over the area and is found more often in women than in men. Treatment must start with the elimination of the cause of friction. A change to properly fitting shoes with a lower counter may be all that is necessary. Ice applied to the area to reduce edema followed by mild stretching of the triceps surae and rest may be needed, however.

Achilles Bursitis (Subtendinous)

The bursa between the Achilles tendon and the calcaneus, just above the insertion (Figs. 7–12 and 7–13), may become inflamed. Some of the causes, as in the subcutaneous bursa, are ill-fitting shoes, friction, and infection. If caused by an infection, it is usually severe with great edema and pain. Other systemic symptoms are usually present.[5] Palpate the bursa just above the insertion, between the tendon and the calcaneus (Fig. 7–15).

Treatment is of course the same as for subcutaneous bursitis: removal of the cause (ill-fitting shoes and friction). Again, the use of ice followed by mild stretching of the triceps surae may be necessary. If an infection is suspected, the patient should be referred to a medical doctor or podiatrist for consultation.

Other Bursae

Other bursae that may be affected include the subcutaneous bursae of the medial and lateral malleoli (Figs. 7–12 and 7–13) and bursae at the first and fifth metatarsophalangeal joints.

Referred Pain

Pain may be referred to the heel from two sources. It may be referred from an arthritic subtalar joint.[4] Arthritis that has developed after an old fracture may cause referred pain to the heel. It may also be referred from a fixation of the subtalar-calcaneus or cuboid-calcaneus articulation.

Painful Heel Pad

The elastic adipose tissue covering the plantar surface of the calcaneus provides a cushion that springs back after impact. As aging occurs, degeneration can cause a loss of the spring action. With a sudden, severe impact, some of the fibers may become ruptured, resulting in the spilling of fat cells.[5] Clinically, the patient presents with localized heel pain upon standing. It is relieved with rest.

Treatment not only must include rest but also must address

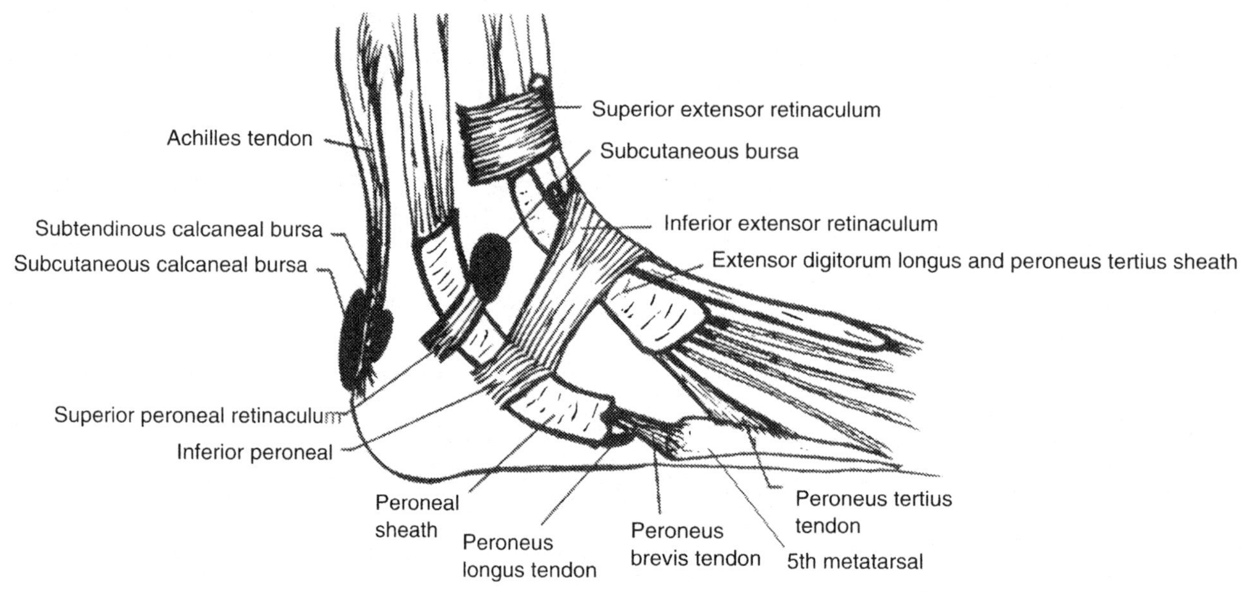

Fig. 7–12 Right foot, lateral aspect showing bursae.

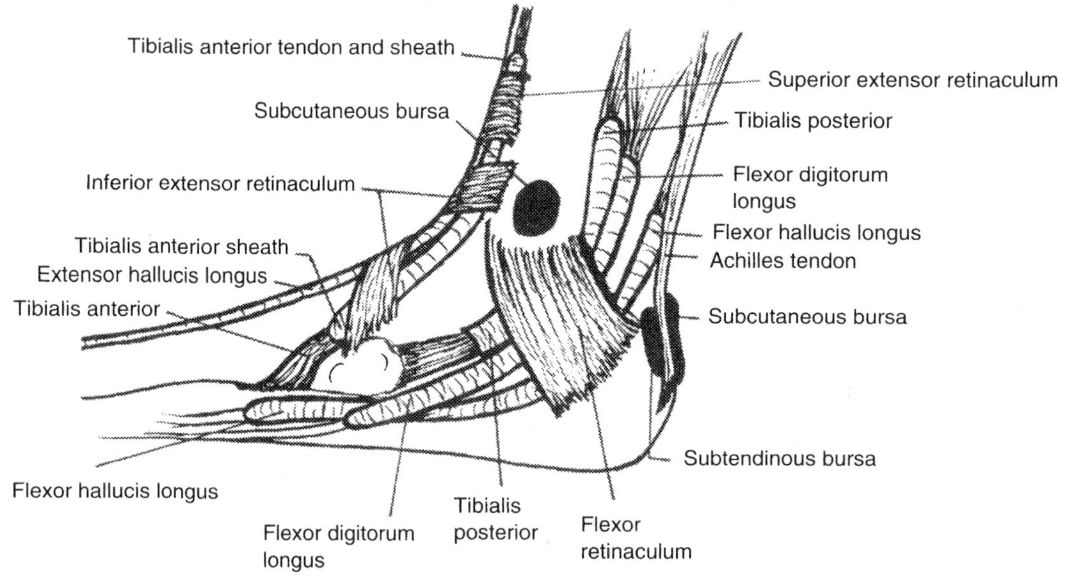

Fig. 7–13 Right foot, medial aspect showing bursae.

the possibility of postural stress on the heel, as discussed at the beginning of this chapter.

Plantar Fasciitis

Plantar fasciitis is a common condition found in adults and is believed to be caused by excessive strain to the plantar fascia. It may result from bursitis, traumatic periostitis, tearing of some of the fibers' attachments to the bone, or focal sepsis causing localized inflammation. Palpation of the plantar surface will reveal pain in the area of the origin of the plantar fascia at the calcaneus (Fig. 7–16).

Plantar Calcaneal Spurs

Spurring may occur along the origin of the plantar fascia (Fig. 7–17). The spurring is believed to be caused by traction

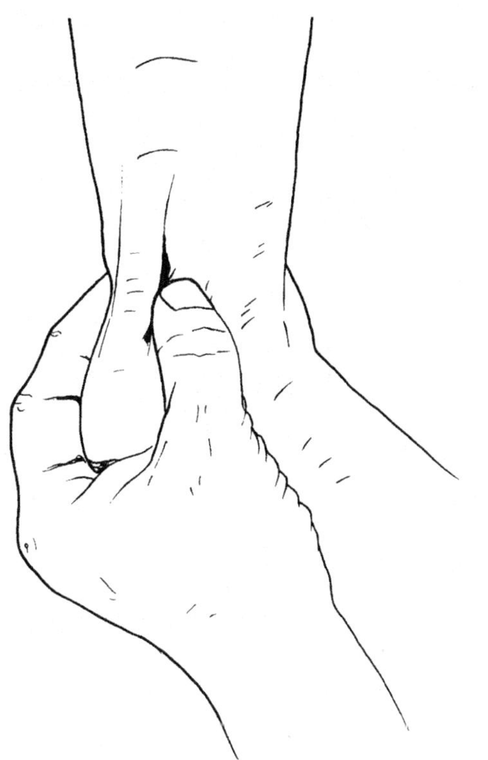

Fig. 7–14 Palpation of the subcutaneous bursa.

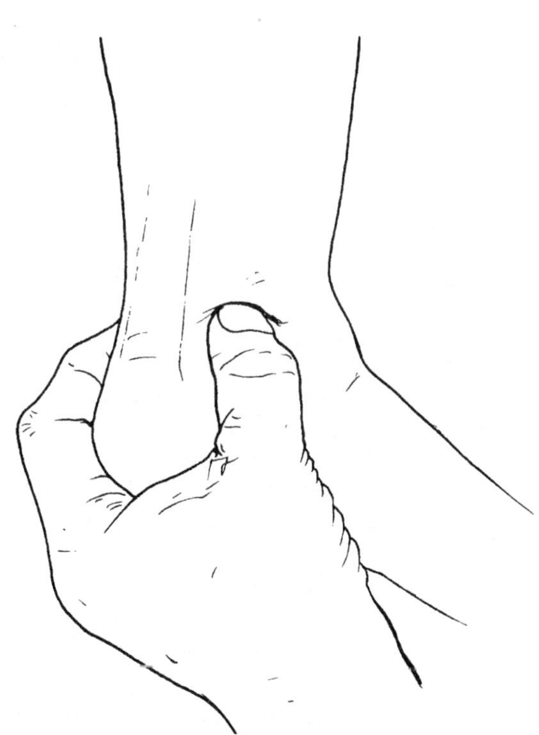

Fig. 7–15 Palpation of the subtendinous bursa.

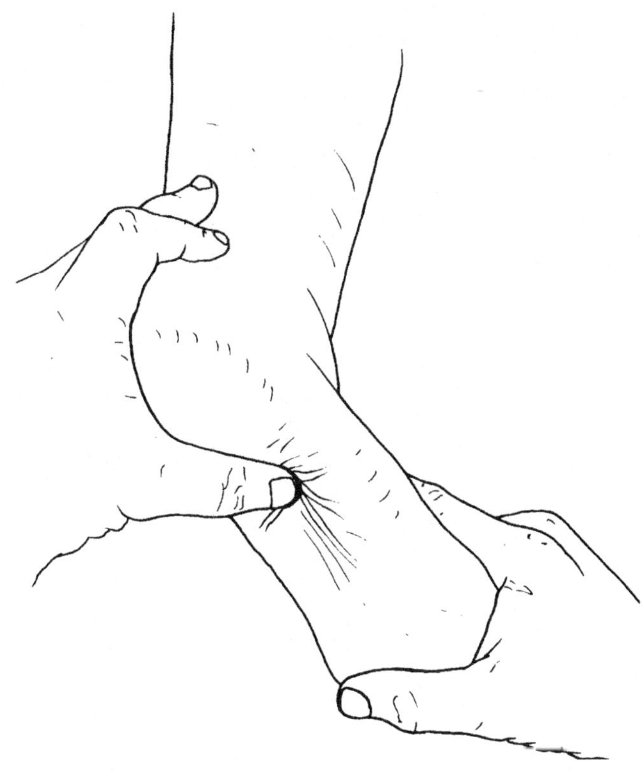

Fig. 7–16 Palpation of the plantar fascia.

on the periosteum, resulting in subperiosteal ossification. Cailliet[3] states that spurs are found more often in men than in women, being commonly found in a pronated foot that has a flattened longitudinal arch. He further states that spurring occurs frequently after a period of bed rest or in occupations requiring excessive walking and standing, especially if the patient is unaccustomed to the activity.

Hiss[1] states that fasciitis and spurs occur more often in the everted foot. He further states that the great majority of patients with heel pain in this area do not have heel spurs.

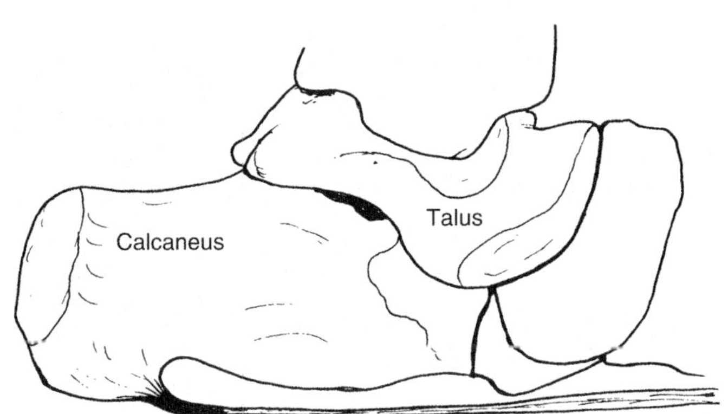

Fig. 7–17 Plantar calcaneal spur.

Spurs are present frequently in asymptomatic feet. The spur is a result of the cause of fasciitis, not the cause of symptoms. In cases where continued activity occurs, however, trauma to the area of spurring, especially if a great deal of elongation is present, may produce its own inflammation.

Treatment should be directed toward relieving tension on the plantar fascia. Turek[8] states that rest, hot soaks, the use of local anesthetic and hydrocortisone, and the wearing of a rubber heel pad constitute conservative treatment. Surgical intervention to remove the spur is a last resort and is seldom successful. Without correction of the cause, the spur soon returns. In the rare case where spurs occur pointing inferiorly rather than forward along the fascia, surgical removal may be necessary. Hiss[1] states that manipulation to correct the eversion and/or the fixed foot is the treatment of choice with good results.

I have found plantar fasciitis with and without spurs associated with several conditions:

- the unpliable, unadaptable foot
- the foot with a fixed tarsal arch of long standing
- the so-called short Achilles tendon
- postural distortions placing strain on the foot

Treatment should be directed toward the following:

- restoration of normal mobility to the entire foot
- correction of postural distortions that place stress on the foot
- changing to properly fitting shoes, if necessary
- use of a cushion for the heel as a temporary measure
- rest

INJURIES TO THE ANKLE

Injuries to the ankle include strains, sprains, and many types of fractures and dislocations. In this text, fracture and dislocation are not discussed except as they relate to peripheral strains and sprains. There are many texts covering the wide variety of fractures and their treatment.

Strains

As defined in *Dorland's*,[9] straining is overexercising or using to an extreme and harmful degree or overstretching or overexerting some part of the musculature. Cailliet defines strain as "the physical force imposed upon the ligamentous tissues possibly exceeding normal stress but not causing deformation or damage to the tissues. Physiological recovery is expected."[3(p62)] For the purposes of this text, strain refers to injuries to musculature only with no injury to the ligamental structures and may be classified as follows:

- *mild*—stress or injury to the musculature that would interfere with normal function with little or no fiber damage.

- *moderate*—injury to the musculature sufficient to prevent muscle function without pain. There are palpable areas of pain and/or edema within the muscle, its origin, or its insertion. Some fibers are damaged, yet the muscle may function in spite of the pain.
- *severe*—tearing of a major portion of muscle fibers, preventing use of the muscle.

Mild strain may constitute minor injury to the muscle sufficient to cause a reaction, overpowering some muscle fibers and interfering with normal function. It may not produce edema or blood loss into the tissue, however. Upon examination, some of the signs may be the following:

- Posture and gait may be altered as a result of muscle malfunction. A mild strain may produce a hypertonic reaction (eg, a knuckle blow to the deltoid). A muscle may not function up to par (eg, the popliteus muscle may be stretched after sitting with the legs suspended with the feet on a stool, allowing hyperextension and resulting in poor function).
- Testing of the muscle may cause cheating by the patient (ie, shifting to allow recruitment of other muscles to respond to the command).
- Testing of the muscle may be nearly normal, yet the muscle may shake during the test.

Palpation of the muscles is important. Areas of hypertonic muscle fibers or the lack of muscle tone may be detected only by palpation. Without careful palpation, many strains may be overlooked simply because the muscle tested nearly normal. If the areas are left untreated, altered patterns of function could lead to more problems in the future.

In the study of muscles and their function, the tendency often is to assume that if the muscle tests nearly normal no damage has occurred. Many of the larger muscles of the body that originate or insert over a large area may test 100%, with the bulk of the muscle providing the resistance. A smaller portion of the muscle may be functioning at only 50%, however. A good example of this is the gluteus maximus muscle, with origins on the ilium, sacrum, and coccyx and insertion into a long area on the posterolateral femur. It may test normal even though the coccygeal fibers are strained because the bulk of the muscle is normal. Palpation therefore is the key to detecting portions of muscles that are reactive or lacking in muscle tone.

If severe damage to the ankle structures has been eliminated and only a strain has occurred, treatment should be directed toward the following:

- Elimination of fixations of all the affected joint structures to ensure normal function.
- Stretching of the hypertonic muscle or portion thereof.
- Stimulation of the fibers that are lacking in tone. If dur-

ing palpation most of the muscle seems normal and a portion is relatively flaccid, it would indicate the portion of the muscle that received minor damage. Goading (digital stimulation with the contact stationary on the skin and deep enough to stimulate the origin of the muscle) often is all that is necessary, other than rest, to restore circulation and normal muscle tone.

- Application of moist heat. Apply for 2 minutes and follow with passive or mild active mobilization within patient tolerance. Repeat five to six times, alternating heat and exercise. The application of moist heat increases arterial blood flow and relaxes the musculature to allow circulation. Mild exercise produces movement, and the stretching and contracting of the muscle activate the venous and lymphatic system, carrying off the by-products of tissue damage.
- Rest.
- Correction of causal factors where possible.

Moderate strain includes greater muscle fiber damage, not only overpowering the fibers but causing a degree of tearing. With tearing, not only is function interrupted but so is the normal blood, venous, and lymphatic flow, with loss of fluid into the tissue.

During the examination, again palpation is the key. In the moderate strain, palpation will probably reveal areas of edema, pain, and lack of tone. Palpation of fiber tearing is usually not possible because of the edema.

The examiner must keep in mind that when a moderate strain occurs the continued use of the joint structure may cause the uninjured portions of the same muscle to react and become hypertonic. If other support muscles of the same function are involved, they too may be reactive and may require treatment. The only benefit to stretching the hypertonic reactive muscle at the beginning of treatment would be to relieve pain and to increase circulation. The results of stretching are usually only temporary. The reactive muscles will malfunction with the first activity.

Treatment of a moderate strain is more aggressive and includes the following:

- Ice to reduce the edema. Ebrall et al[10] found that ice 10 minutes on and 10 minutes off followed by a second 10 minutes of wet ice provides a temperature of less than 15°C for 33 minutes and less than 20°C for at least 63 minutes. They concluded that this produces a lower temperature for twice the length of time compared with 20 minutes of continuous application.
- Gentle, passive mobilization of the joint structure involved to produce movement, not contraction.
- Total rest.
- Correction of all fixations of the joint structures affected by the muscle or that may affect the muscle.

- After sufficient time (varying with the severity), application of moist heat. Apply for 2 minutes and follow with passive or mild active mobilization within patient tolerance. Repeat five to six times, alternating heat and exercise. The time to change to this technique is a matter of judgment on the part of the practitioner, and caution must be used on the first application of heat. If sufficient healing has taken place, the application of heat will not increase or cause edema. If edema occurs with the first application, cease the heat treatment, and return to the first line of therapy: ice. After sufficient time, a return to heat and exercise may occur.
- Taping if the limb must be in use. Taping should be directed toward preventing the necessity of use of the affected muscle.
- Exercise to restore normal function and strength. If necessary, gait evaluation may be needed to restore normal habit patterns.

A severe strain is the tearing of a major portion of a muscle, the tendon, or the periosteal attachment. Pain is immediate, and ambulation is not possible. Furthermore, pain is excruciating with forced stretching of the muscle. Careful palpation reveals a depression in the muscle accompanied by massive edema.

Treatment is directed toward immobilization by splint with the joint in a position to relieve any tension on the affected muscle. The use of antiinflammatory agents may be necessary, requiring medical consultation. If the tear is extensive enough to require surgery, the patient should be referred to a competent surgeon who will cooperate for the patient's benefit and allow rehabilitation under chiropractic care. Surgery, if necessary, is not possible at the early stage and, if performed, would probably fail.

A review of the literature reveals a wide variety of methods for treatment of ankle sprains. Each study seems to reach a conclusion as to a method, yet there is no consensus on the best method.

Scotece and Guthrie,[11] in their research study, listed numerous methods and their advocates. Some of these include:

- non–weight-bearing for 3 weeks and no athletic activity for 5 weeks
- ice, compression, crutches, strapping, and gel cast or plaster cast
- muscle reeducation and proprioceptive training
- heel cord stretching (recall that the triceps surae will be hypertonic)

Their study included the following three methods of treatment; each used 650 mg of CAMA, an OTC pain reliever, four times a day for 5 days on entrance to the study:

1. strapping with athletic tape for 3 days

2. application of a gel cast for 3 days
3. daily strapping for 3 days

Each group, on the day of treatment, had three repetitions of an ice bath for 5 minutes followed by walking until sensation returned. The subjects used a balance board with as much weight as possible. Achilles tendon/soleus muscle stretching and resistive ankle exercises using rubber tubing were also used. The study's conclusion was that group 3 returned to 60% of full duty in 3 days or less.

Again, many therapies were involved. In my opinion, it seems difficult to determine what therapy was best. Stretching of the gastrocnemius/soleus would be called for only if examination demonstrated the need. With recognition of which muscles or ligaments are involved, strapping should be done accordingly to reinforce the structures that are injured, not just general strapping.

Inversion Strain

Most texts concentrate on the ankle sprain because the symptoms are more severe. Mild strains can also occur, however, leaving a susceptibility to further injury, including a sprain. If recognized and corrected, the more severe damage may be prevented.

Inversion strain (little or no ligamental damage) may occur with the ankle in any position, but the ankle is most susceptible during plantar flexion. The muscles involved are the peroneus longus, peroneus brevis, peroneus tertius, and extensor digitorum longus.

A major part of the treatment and rehabilitation of the strain and sprain patient must be a consideration of the muscle involvement. When an injury is sufficient to do ligamental damage, the musculature has been overpowered and must be involved.

Figure 7–18 reveals that the major origin of each of the muscles involved in an inversion strain (or sprain) is the fibula. These muscles, individually and as a group, affect not only the foot but also the relationship of the fibula to the tibia and thus affect many other structures.

Recall from Chapter 5 the movements of the proximal and distal fibula on passive motion palpation:

- *anteroinferior*—by actions of the peroneus longus, peroneus tertius, extensor hallucis longus, and extensor digitorum longus muscles

- *superior*—by action of the biceps femoris with the knee extended

- *superoposterior*—by action of the biceps, depending on the degree of flexion (past 90° the movement is posterior)

- *inferior*—by action of the flexor hallucis longus, peroneus brevis, and extensor digitorum longus muscles

Movement at both the ankle and the knee may be altered as a result of muscle spasms or weakness. If the fibula is fixed su-

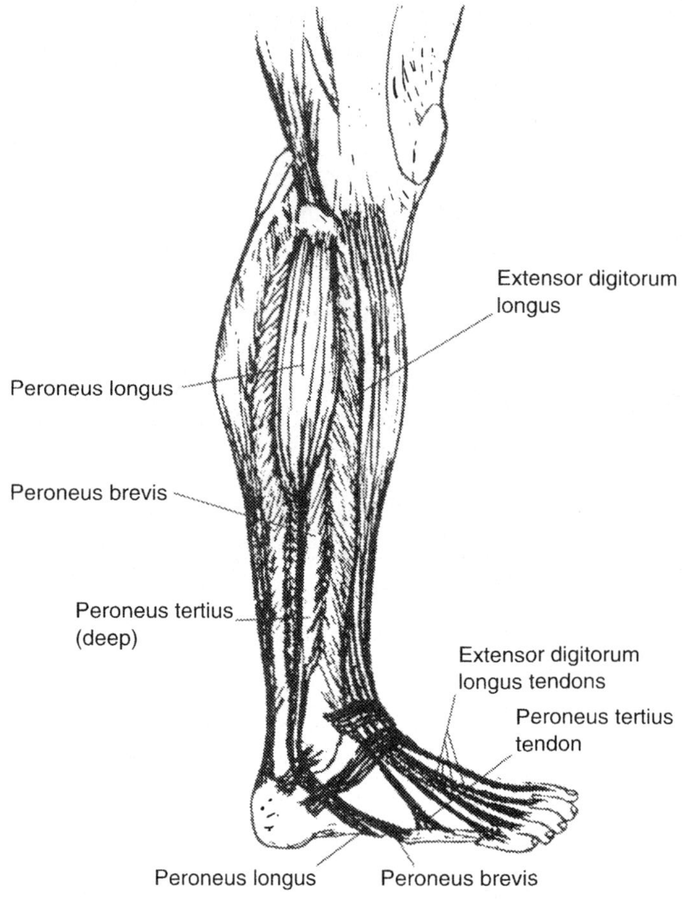

Fig. 7–18 Right leg, lateral view showing muscles and tendons involved in inversion sprain.

periorly as a result of contracted biceps and a weakness of the everter and dorsiflexors of the foot (originating on the fibula), no movement will be felt on motion palpation.

Motion palpate the distal fibulotibial articulation during dorsiflexion of the ankle (Fig. 7–19). Beginning with the ankle in slight plantar flexion, move the ankle into dorsiflexion while palpating the anterior fibular and tibial surfaces. With dorsiflexion, the anterior fibula should separate slightly from the tibia, rotate laterally, and glide proximally. Repeat dorsiflexion, and palpate the proximal end of the fibula at the knee (Fig. 7–20). Movement should correspond with the movement felt distally.

Movement of the fibula on the tibia is governed by the former's location on the posterolateral surface of the tibia as the condyle begins to narrow and by its muscle attachments. An injury sufficient to interfere with the function of the muscles involved in the inversion strain will undoubtedly interfere with the actions of the other muscles involved in fibular function. With an injury producing weakness, the opposite muscles and the support muscles tend to compensate and be-

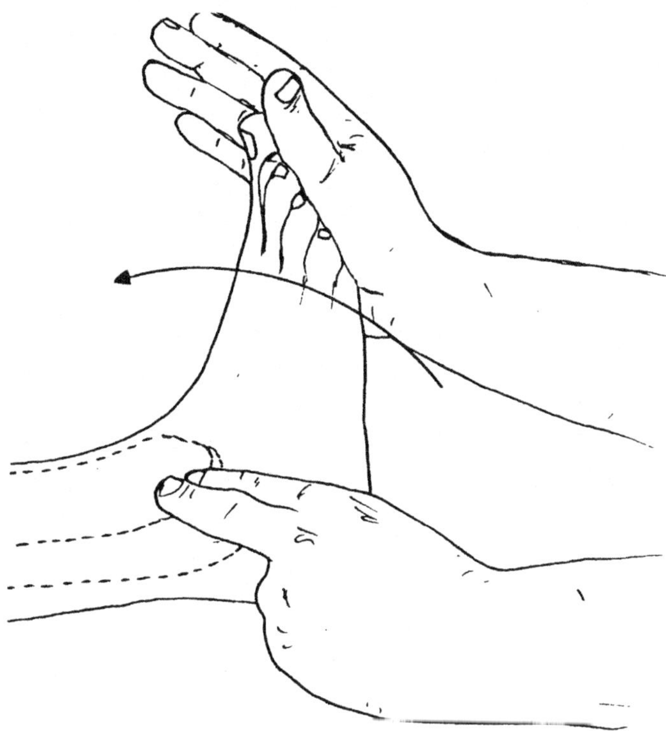

Fig. 7–19 Palpation of fibular movement during dorsiflexion of the ankle.

come hypertonic. If the extensor and flexor hallucis longus muscles are affected, they interfere not only with the motions of gait but also with the inversion-eversion action of the calcaneus as it assists the posterior tibialis muscle with inversion.

Any injury interfering with action that pulls the fibula distally must affect biceps function. Therefore it is reasonable to assume that, through its sacrotuberous ligament attachment, pelvic and thus spinal function is affected.

Inversion strains that occur with the ankle in dorsiflexion to neutral would involve primarily the peroneus longus and brevis muscles. The tendons of the peroneus longus and brevis may be palpated as they traverse the fibula posteriorly and as they pass behind the lateral malleolus below the peroneal retinaculum. Each tendon may be distinguished by alternatively plantarflexing-everting and everting without plantar flexing.

The peroneus longus muscle produces plantar flexion and eversion through its passage under the cuboid and its attachment to the first cuneiform and first metatarsal (Fig. 7–21). Its pull on the two bone structures laterally and proximally assists in the support of the longitudinal arch and opposes some of the function of the anterior tibialis.

The tendon of the peroneus brevis passes under the peroneal retinaculum, crossing over the longus tendon, and inserts into the tubercle on the base of the fifth metatarsal (Fig. 7–22). The direction of pull and the attachment to the tubercle of the fifth metatarsal make the peroneus brevis especially susceptible to strain. Strain of the brevis will allow excessive lateral rotation of the fifth metatarsal during the stride and eliminates some of the necessary kick-off as the weight passes through the lateral arch. The attachment should be palpated carefully. Avulsion fracture of the fifth metatarsal is not uncommon.

Inversion strains that occur with the ankle in neutral or plantar flexion show greater involvement of the peroneus tertius and the extensor digitorum longus muscles. The bellies of both muscles may be palpated on the anterolateral aspect of the leg one-half to two-thirds of the way from the knee to the ankle. They become apparent with extension of the lesser digits (Fig. 7–23).

The peroneus tertius tendon can be considered the fifth tendon of the extensor digitorum longus. The tendons of both muscles pass under the anterior retinaculum at the ankle. The peroneus tertius portion separates below the ankle and inserts

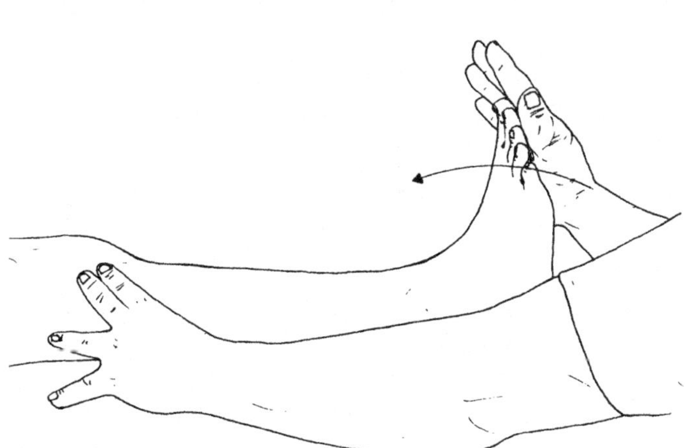

Fig. 7–20 Palpation of the fibular head during dorsiflexion.

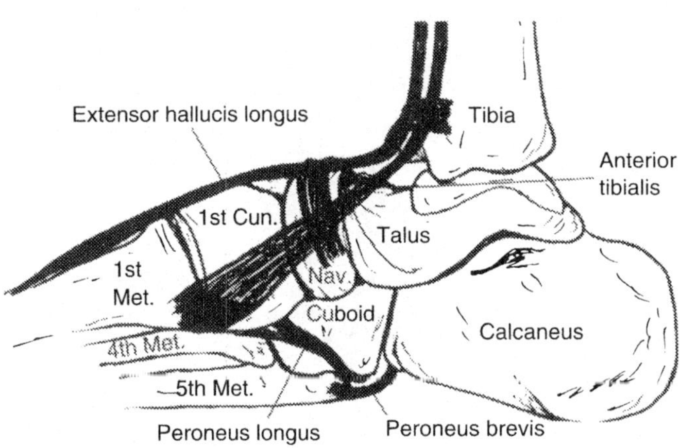

Fig. 7–21 Right ankle and foot, medial-plantar view showing tendons.

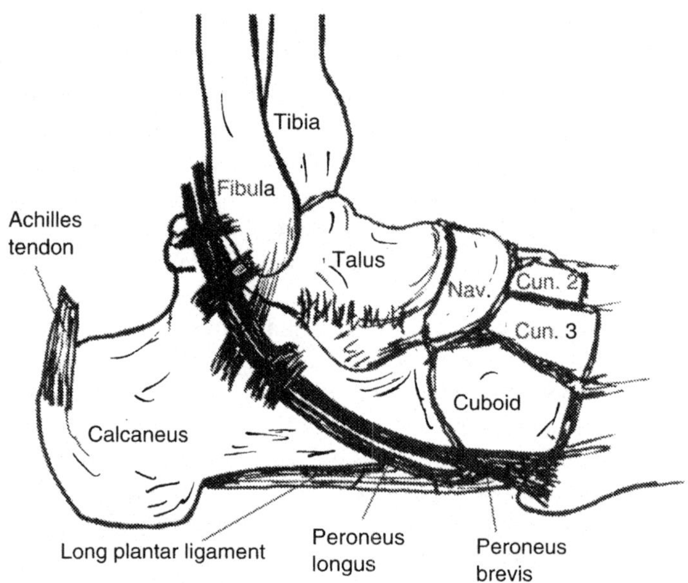

Fig. 7–22 Right foot, lateral view showing peroneal tendons.

into the dorsal surface of the base and shaft of the fifth metatarsal.

Eversion Strain

Eversion strains as well as sprains are a result of excessive medial force with the ankle in external rotation and abduction. The muscles involved with this type of injury are the posterior tibialis and the flexor hallucis longus (Fig. 7–24).

The posterior tibialis, with its insertions on the sustentaculum tali, the tubercle of the navicular, and the other tarsals (Fig. 7–25), is the primary force that brings the foot into medial rotation and inversion. When the braking action of the posterior tibialis fails, eversion sprain may take place.

Assisting the posterior tibialis is the flexor hallucis longus. Its passage inferior to the sustentaculum tali, on its way to the great toe, provides part of the leverage preventing excessive eversion of the calcaneus (Fig. 7–25).

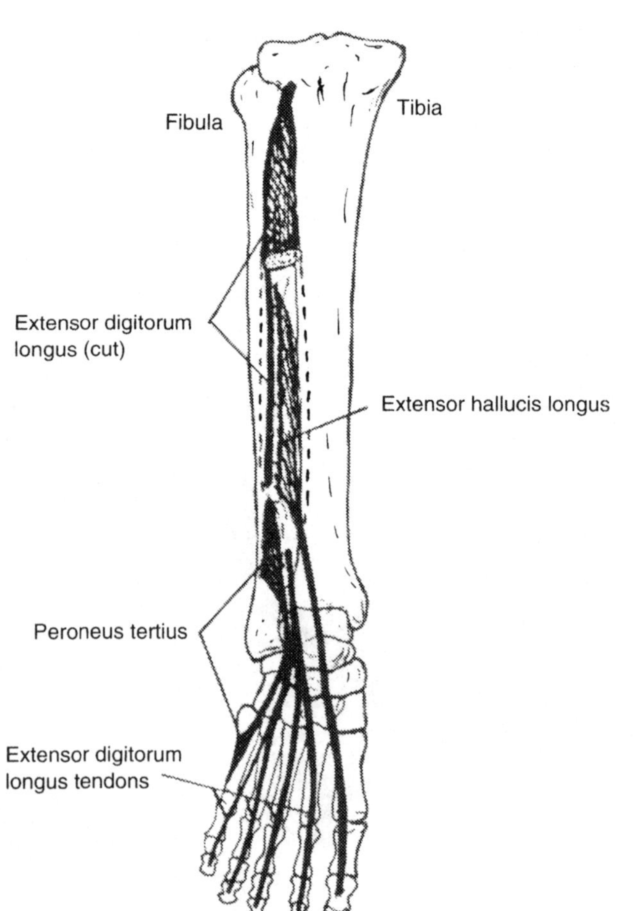

Fig. 7–23 Right leg and foot showing extensor muscles.

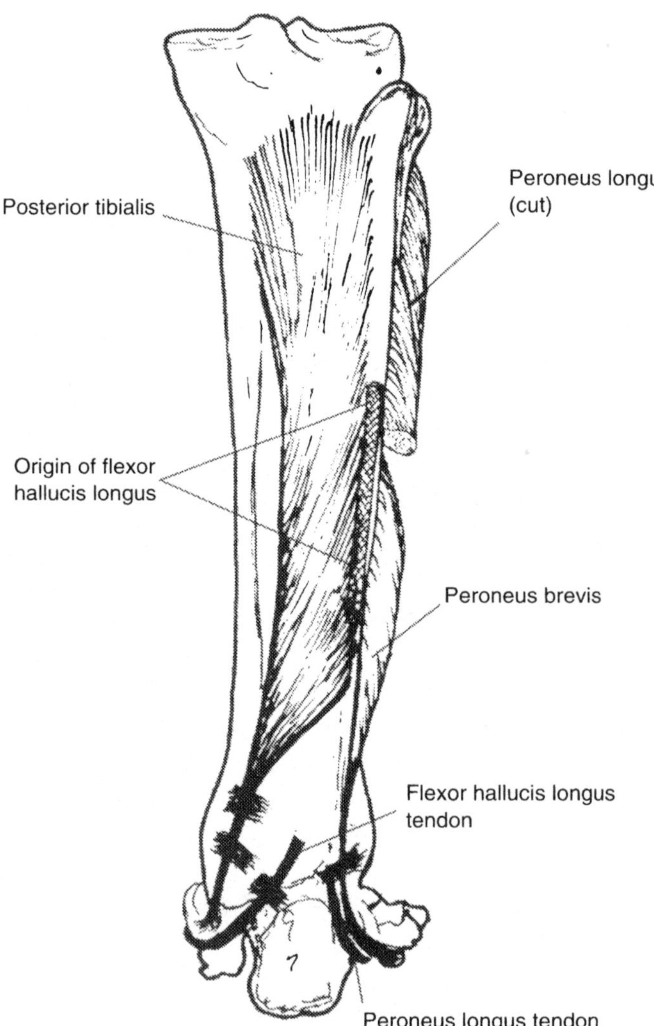

Fig. 7–24 Right leg, ankle, and foot, posterior view.

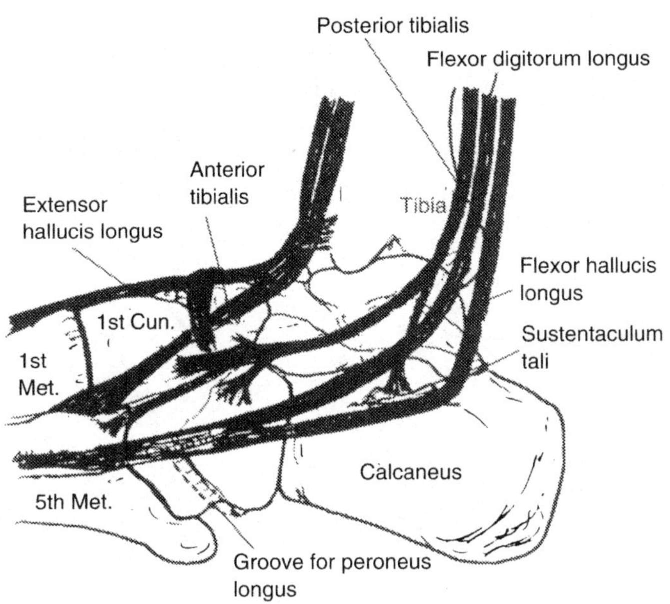

Fig. 7–25 Right ankle and foot, plantar-medial view showing tendons.

Treatment of Strains

Once the determination is made that no ligamental damage exists, treatment may include the following:

- Correction of all fixations of the low back, pelvis, hip, and knee to ensure normal circulation and nerve integrity. Fixations in the foot may be adjusted by using the short lever techniques described in Chapter 6 or the Activator instrument.
- Taping, if necessary, to support the muscle until an exercise program restores the muscle to normal strength.
- Exercise, which should be designed to include all four muscles. The patient should be instructed to emphasize the one with the most damage (see Chapter 8).
- Ice therapy, which is useful before and after exercise.
- Neuromuscular reeducation, retraining the foot and ankle to function normally. With injury to the muscles, only a few days of walking in an abnormal manner will change the habit pattern.

I use the following method:

1. Have the patient deliberately and slowly step off on the unaffected foot while you watch the entire process.
2. Follow by repeating on the affected ankle and foot, making sure that the same procedure is repeated. If not, a correction in habit must be made.
3. Repeat 40 to 50 times slowly down a hallway and back. Repeat 3 times per day for 3 to 4 days, and the normal habit pattern should be restored.

Sprains

A sprain may be defined as a partial or complete rupture of the fibers of a ligament. This may include injuries all the way from minimal tears to complete rupture of the ligament and may also include avulsion of the periosteum at the bony attachment. Sprains may be graded as mild (grade 1), moderate (grade 2), or severe (grade 3).[12]

A mild sprain may be associated with limited swelling, no discoloration, a small amount of pain, and no loss in range of motion. Some fibers of the ligaments involved may be torn, yet their integrity is maintained. A moderate sprain diagnosis may be considered with greater swelling, discoloration, greater pain, and sufficient fibers torn to allow some excess range of motion. A severe sprain represents complete severance of a ligament.

Inversion Sprain

Inversion (or lateral) sprain (Fig. 7–26) may involve any of the ligaments on the lateral ankle, depending on the position of the ankle when the excess stress occurs. Jahss[13] states that the anterior talofibular ligament (Fig. 7–27) is the only ligament preventing anterior slipping of the talus. Palpation of the talofibular ligament is possible over the sinus tarsi (lateral surface of the talocalcaneal articulation).

To test for anterior talofibular ligament integrity, the drawer test is performed by holding the fibula and tibia posteriorly while pulling the calcaneus (and with it the talus) anteriorly (Fig. 7–28). An end feel at the limit of normal motion, rather than movement, should be felt.

Jahss[13] further states that both the anterior talofibular ligament and the calcaneofibular ligament must be torn for instability. To test the calcaneofibular ligament, invert the calcaneus while holding the fibula. Again, end feel is all that should be felt (Fig. 7–29).

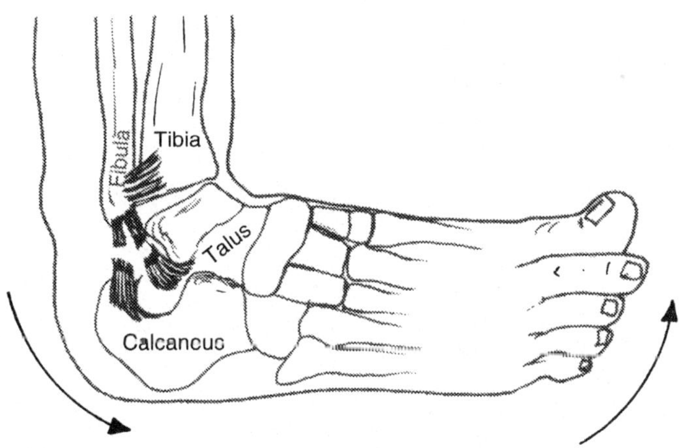

Fig. 7–26 Inversion sprain.

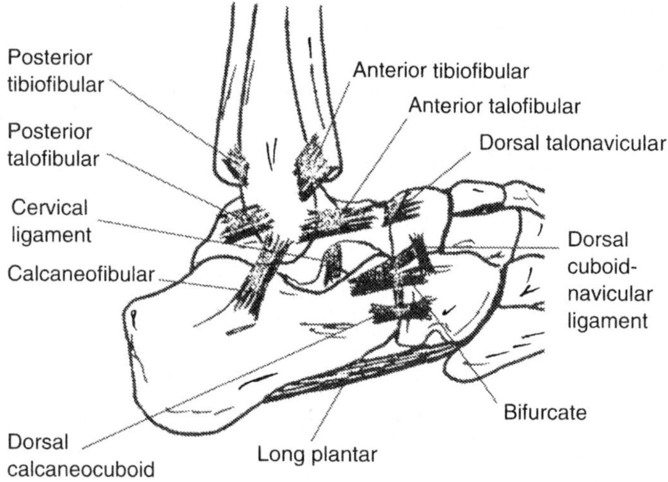

Fig. 7–27 Right ankle, lateral view showing ligaments.

Colville et al[14] state that the anterior talofibular ligament is most likely to tear if the ankle is inverted in plantar flexion and internally rotated. They further state that the calcaneofibular ligament tears primarily in inversion. If the ankle is dorsiflexed, the anterior tibiofibular ligament tears when dorsiflexion is combined with external rotation. The posterior tibiofibular ligament tears with extreme dorsiflexion (Fig. 7–27).

Eversion Sprain

Eversion (or medial) sprain involves the deltoid ligament (medial collateral ligament) with its four segments (Fig. 7–30).

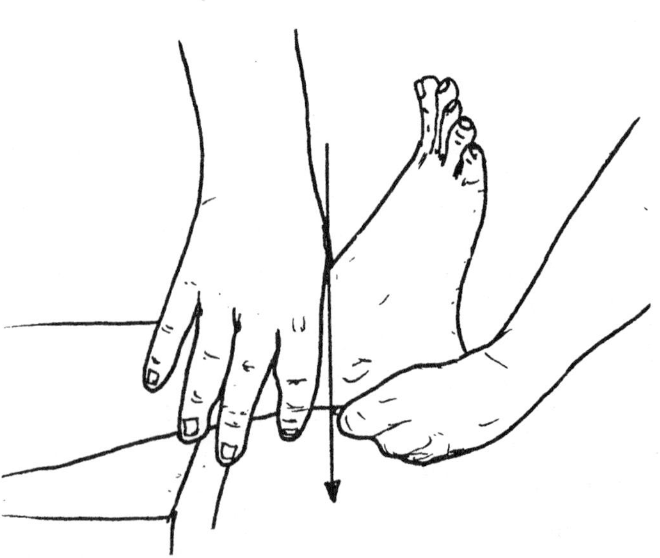

Fig. 7–28 Drawer test.

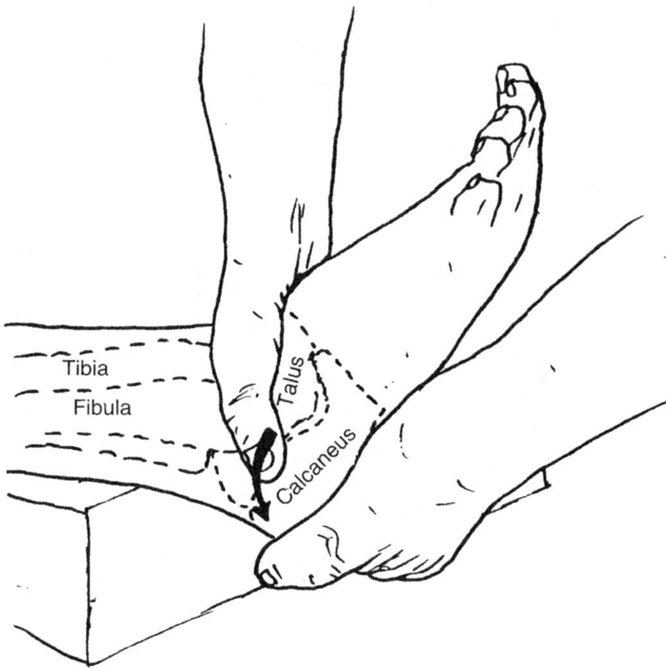

Fig. 7–29 Posterolateral ligament test.

The ligaments run from the medial malleolus to (anterior to posterior) the navicular, talus, and calcaneus.

The medial ankle is less susceptible to sprain because of the greater number and size of the ligaments (Fig. 7–31). The integrity of the medial ankle is most susceptible when in external rotation and abduction.[12]

Abduction Sprain

An abduction sprain of the ankle (Fig. 7–32) will involve the anterior tibiofibular ligament. To test for possible anterior tibiofibular ligament damage, support the tibia and fibula with the inside hand (Fig. 7–33A). With the outside hand, hook the thumb over the talonavicular articulation and the index finger along the lateral surface of the calcaneus. Apply pressure to produce abduction of the foot on the tibia (Fig. 7–33B). Only minimal separation should be felt, if any. With ligamental tearing, movement would of course be greater and accompanied by pain.

Treatment

Roycroft and Mantgani[15] concluded that active management of grade 1 and 2 sprains, when initiated within the first 24 hours, achieves results in a shorter time. Treatment consists of ice packs, strapping, and weight bearing followed by therapeutic ultrasound and mobilization. Cote et al,[16] in a comparison study of cold immersions, hot immersions, and hot-cold contrast, found that cold therapy produced the least amount of

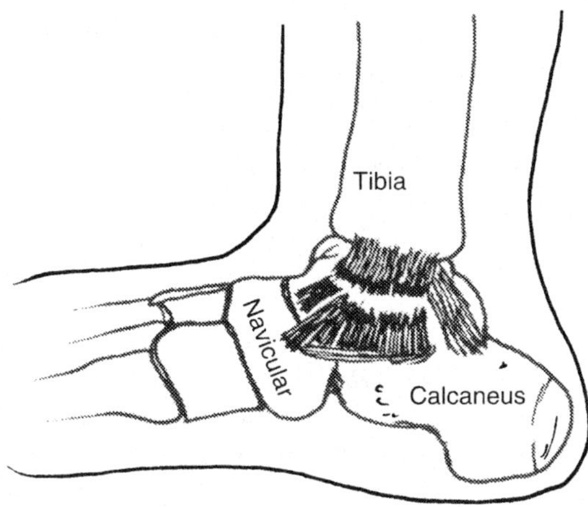

Fig. 7–30 Eversion sprain.

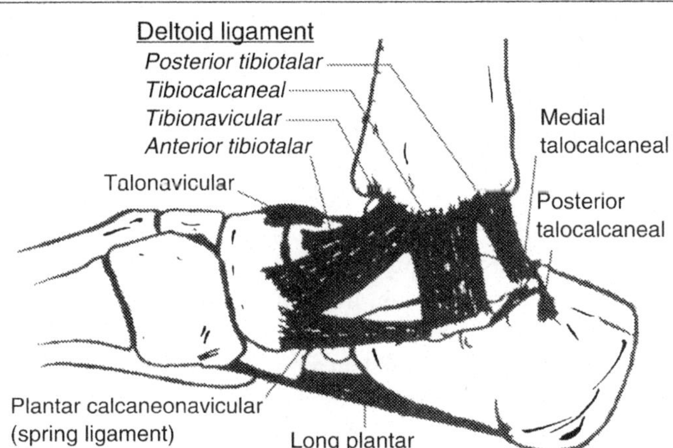

Fig. 7–31 Right ankle and foot, medial view showing ligaments.

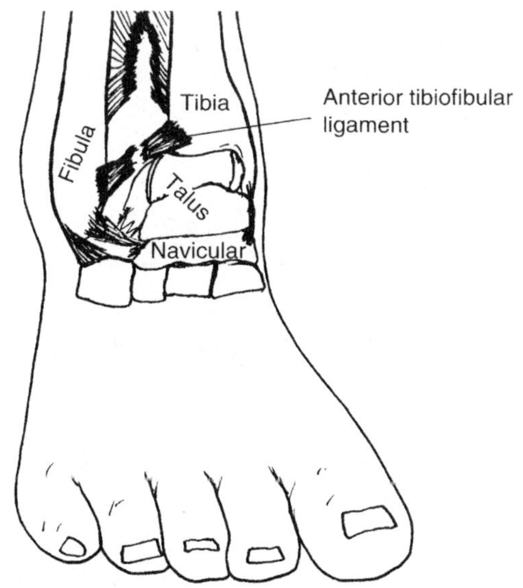

Fig. 7–32 Abduction sprain.

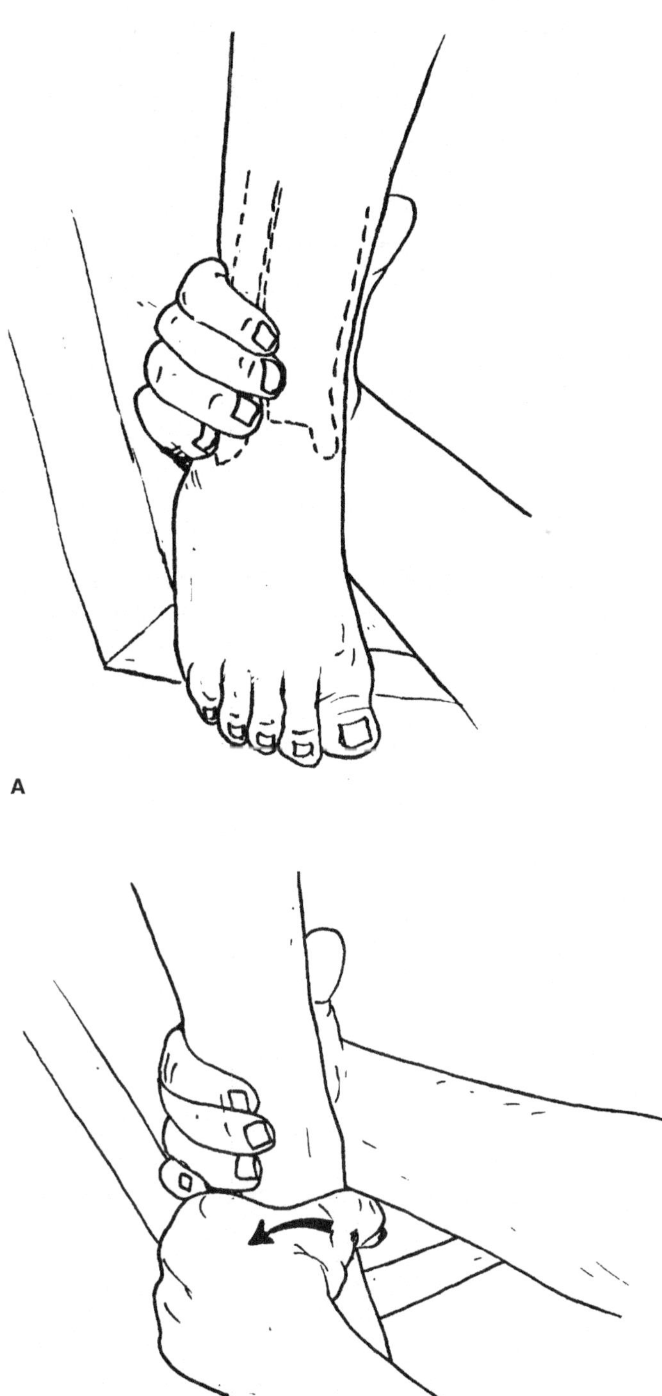

Fig. 7–33 **(A)** Support contact for tibiofibular ligament test. **(B)** Test for tibiofibular ligament damage.

edema. Briner et al[17] state that with the anteroinferior tibiofibular sprain the most effective treatment program is ice, elevation, compression, and avoidance of weight bearing for 1 to 3 days. With more severe sprains, cast immobilization and medication for pain are necessary.

Treatment of a grade 3 sprain is not without controversy. Athletes and patients with occupations that require great stress to the ankle may benefit from surgery. Other patients may have good results with conservative care. I recommend the following treatment course:

1. Adjust all fixations of the low back, pelvis, hip, and knee to ensure circulation and nerve integrity to the ankle.

2. Apply wrapping to retard edema.

3. Elevate the foot.

4. Apply ice. In the initial, acute stage, any available ice will do. For use at home, my recommendation is to fold two or more towels into 12×12 in squares, wet them slightly, and freeze them. With the ankle wrapped and elevated, the towels may be applied to the ankle with one posterior and one anterior. No ice burn will occur on any bare area as a result of the immediate thawing of the first layer of the towel upon contact.

5. When the edema is reduced, adjust fixations of the foot using the short lever techniques or the Activator instrument (see Chapter 6).

6. Apply tape after the swelling is reduced. The tape should be applied to reinforce the injured structures, not just for general support. A knowledge of the origin and insertion of the ligament involved allows the practitioner to tape accordingly.

7. When it appears that the edema is reduced and stays reduced for 2 to 3 days, wet two towels as described above except heat them in a microwave oven. Apply moist heat to the ankle for 2 minutes and follow with mobilization of the ankle within its normal range of motion. Repeat five to six times. *Caution:* If edema returns afterward, cease and return to ice therapy for another 2 to 3 days before attempting heat therapy. The application of moist heat therapy coupled with mobilization not only brings circulation to the ankle but helps in movement of fluids from the area through lymphatics.

8. Begin mobilization exercises as soon as the severe edema is reduced.

9. Use mobilization exercises with elastic tubing for the affected muscles before any weight bearing is allowed. Icing before and after exercise is helpful. As progress is made, ambulation with crutches to start may be added.

10. Introduce neuromuscular reeducation, retraining the foot and ankle to function normally. With injury to the

muscles, only a few days of walking in an abnormal manner changes the habit pattern. Use the same procedure described in the treatment of strains.

TARSAL TUNNEL SYNDROME (SINUS TARSI SYNDROME)

The tarsal sinus is the cavity running lateral to medial between the anterosuperior surface of the calcaneus and the inferior aspect of the neck of the talus (Fig. 7–34). Within the cavity is the cervical ligament with its two portions: the anterior portion of the subtalar joint capsule and synovium, and the posterior portion of the talocalcaneonavicular joint capsule and synovium and the three roots of the inferior extensor retinaculum. The inferior extensor retinaculum crosses the proximal portion of the dorsum of the foot. The lateral strap is anchored to the talus and calcaneus. As it progresses medially, it bifurcates and encases the tendons of the peroneus tertius, extensor digitorum longus, extensor hallucis longus, and tibialis anterior muscles.

Bernstein et al[18] stated that 70% of 220 reported cases of sinus tarsi syndrome were thought to be caused by complications from inversion ankle sprains. Other causes thought to be responsible are pes cavus, hypermobile pes planus, and chronic subtalar joint instability. Byank et al[19] state that the causes may be numerous, including dilated varicosities, fibrous bands, neural tumors, and trauma (including injury from calcaneal fractures), but that most commonly tarsal tunnel syndrome is considered idiopathic. Obviously, malfunction of the subtalar joint leads to problems involving the structures within. Instability after injury is believed to be the most common cause.

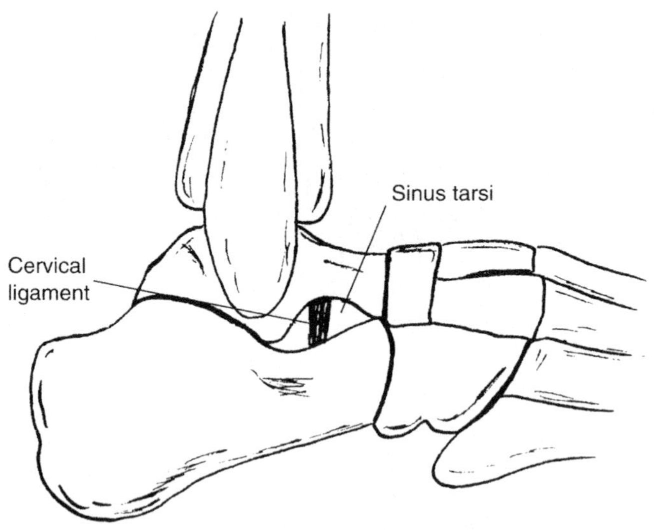

Fig. 7–34 Right ankle and foot showing the sinus tarsi and cervical ligament.

Symptoms of burning and paresthesias on the sole of the foot are common, but heel pain and sensory loss are occasionally seen as well. Patients usually localize the painful area by placing two or three fingers over the anteroinferior border of the fibular malleolus. They may complain of a sense of instability of the hindfoot when walking.

The best course of treatment is prevention. Proper management of the lateral ankle strain or sprain to will stabilize the subtalar joint, minimizing the possibility of tarsal tunnel syndrome. If conservative care fails, surgery may be necessary.

PRONATION (PES PLANUS)

D'Ambrosia[20] states that pes planus is the normal appearance of feet seen in many cultures of the world. On weight bearing, the pes planus foot assumes a position of heel valgus and a dropped arch. The deformity often disappears or becomes mild when the weight is removed.

Hiss[1] states that true flatfoot can be diagnosed by the fact that the inner spring arch is absolutely flat. There is no curved contour or external appearance of an archlike structure in the sole of the foot. It lacks all the elements of an arch from both an architectural and an anatomic standpoint. Hiss further states that this cannot come under the definition of a broken arch. It is his opinion, and many writers on this subject agree, that the foot is flat in infancy and that the arch develops as the child begins to stand and walk. Hiss states that children who are overweight, walk late, or are malnourished during this formative period do not develop enough intrinsic strength in the foot to cope, so that their arches remain flat with the ligaments and muscles accommodating. He emphasizes that comfort varies directly with function and that practitioners in his clinic, after seeing thousands of patients, seldom saw patients with flat feet who suffered much unless the function was disturbed. The flatfoot is subject to injury the same as the normal foot.

Lawrence[21] states that pes planus may be acquired as a result of osseous fracture, disease, ligamentous tears, muscular imbalance, or degenerative joint disease but that the most common cause is postural problems.

From the beginning, I was taught that the entire body has to be considered in all problems, and I have been treating feet, or at least examining feet, for more than 37 years. Some of my observations include the following:

- Patients who appear to have true flatfoot are often of a stocky build, would make a good lineman on a football team, and, when planted, would be difficult to move. This type of patient is seldom able to run as fast or jump as far as the patient with a normal arch.
- Patients presenting with symptoms elsewhere who have flat feet seldom have any more fixations in the foot than patients with similar complaints and with a normal arch.
- Patients with foot symptoms who have flat feet usually respond to treatment at the same rate as patients with normal arches.

- Foot symptom patients with what appear to be a normal arch in non–weight bearing and a flatfoot in weight bearing usually display a postural distortion or have experienced an injury to the feet.

The old adage "if it ain't broke, don't fix it" applies to the true flatfoot. Attempting to support the arch with an orthotic is a gross error in judgment and can only lead to problems.

The acquired flat foot may be unilateral or bilateral and should be treated locally if injured. If caused by postural distortion, the condition that has produced the stress should be treated and then local treatment should be applied. Some of the most common causes are anatomic short leg and lordotic lumbar syndrome. Distortions associated with an anatomic short leg usually produce a laterally rotated tibia in response to a rotated femur medially or, more often, laterally (in an attempt to elongate the leg). This forces the patient to walk in a Charlie Chaplin style. Lordotic lumbar syndrome is usually caused by obesity or lack of proper exercises after pregnancy. The associated anterior rotation of the pelvis and weak gluteus maximus and piriformis muscles produce a valgus knee, forcing the tibia to rotate laterally.

If the patient with a true flatfoot is complaining of pain or has an excessive amount of fixations, treatment should be the same as with the normal arch. The true flatfoot should not be supported unless there has been trauma. Treatment of an acquired flatfoot should be addressed to the postural cause, where applicable.

Locally, support may be used as a temporary aid while therapeutic exercises produce the necessary intrinsic support. Exercises (see Chapter 8) should include the following:

- the posterior tibialis muscle, which supports the entire arch posteriorly, medially rotates the foot on the ankle, and inverts the calcaneus
- the anterior tibialis, which provides the strength to invert the foot by elevating the key bones of the arch
- the peroneus longus muscle, which plantar flexes and everts the foot; it is one of the stabilizers of the arch along with the above muscles
- the flexor hallucis longus, which assists in the support of the arch as well as assists the posterior tibialis muscle in inverting the calcaneus

FOREFOOT STRAINS AND SPRAINS

One of the most common conditions found in practice is pain between the metatarsals, sometimes extending to the distal ends and the metatarsophalangeal joints.

The presence of a Morton neuroma should be considered when one is examining the forefoot with pain. D'Ambrosia[20] states that Morton's neuroma may produce symptoms that appear to be metatarsalgia and may produce a sensory deficit of the involved digital nerve. Tenderness may be more severe on the plantar surface of the web space rather than in the metatarsal heads and is found most often between the third and fourth metatarsals. Alexander[6] states that the term *neuroma* is a misnomer because the lesion is a fusiform swelling of the nerve rather than an abnormal overgrowth of nerve tissue. In advanced cases a small mass may be palpated between the fingers, and a definite click (Mulder's click) may be appreciated when the forefoot is squeezed.

When one is considering a diagnosis of neuroma, it is important to consider the cause of the patient's complaints and to ascertain an accurate history. It is my opinion that many doctors are too quick to make the diagnosis of neuroma. It should be realized that a simple strain can also cause fusiform swelling and pain between the metatarsals. The majority of intermetatarsal pain patients with suspected Morton's neuroma whom I have seen did not have one.

Examination should proceed as follows:

1. Squeeze the intermetatarsal spaces for pain or abnormal tissue (Fig. 7–35).
2. If pain is present, apply pressure on the first and fifth metatarsal toward the center of the foot (Fig. 7–36). Use about 3 to 4 lb of pressure only, and palpate the intermetatarsal area with the other hand. If a Morton neuroma is present, the pain will become more severe.
3. If the pain is present with the patient standing, have the patient remove the weight from the foot. Apply 3 to 4 lb of pressure as in Figure 7–36, and have the patient, while maintaining the pressure, replace the weight on the foot.
4. If the pain is relieved, nothing more than a splaying, or strain, of the metatarsal arch has occurred, and the patient should be treated accordingly. I have successfully treated numerous patients over the years who originally were scheduled for surgery.

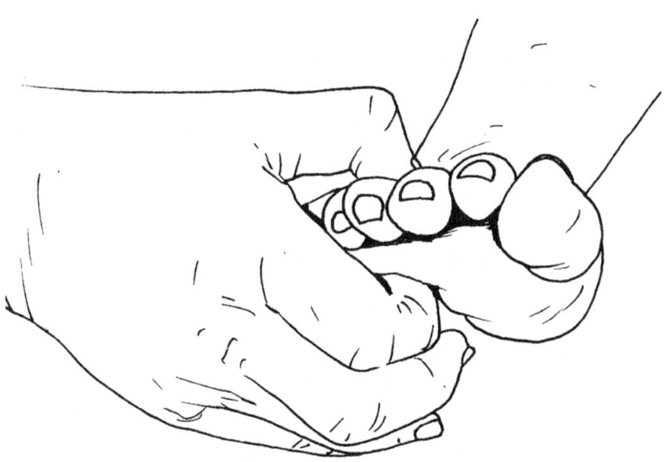

Fig. 7–35 Test for Morton's neuroma or unstable metatarsal arch.

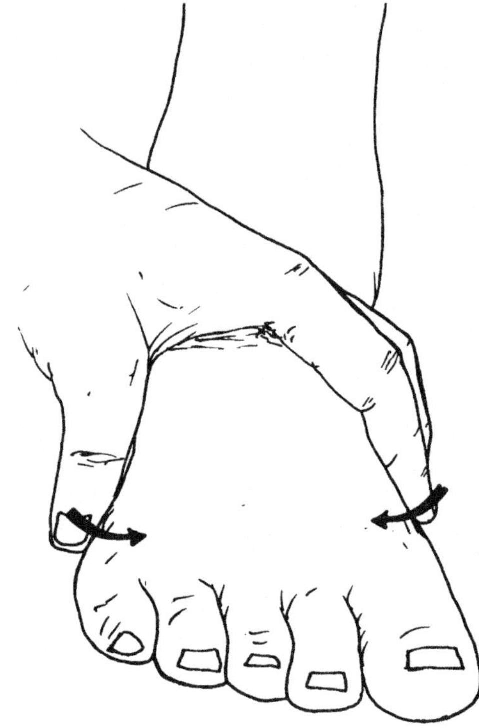

Fig. 7–36 Application of minimum pressure to relieve pain.

Causes

Patients used to wearing tight-fitting shoes and/or those with a sedentary occupation who suddenly become overactive in loose-fitting shoes or barefoot commonly experience forefoot strains. Running barefoot in the park or taking a long walk on the beach without shoes can cause problems.

The metatarsal arch is supported by ligaments yet is maintained by the dorsal interosseous muscles. The inactive patient who tries to act as a teenager one weekend can strain the metatarsal arch.

Abnormal conditions that produce unusual strain on the metatarsal arch also cause forefoot strains. A tight, hypertonic triceps surae with restricted dorsiflexion produces a lack of the fluid, rolling movement of the foot during the long stride with a more direct heel to metatarsal arch movement. Other causes are an acquired unpliable, unadaptable foot that prevents fluid movement and an anomalous condition, such as bridging of the calcaneus to the talus or navicular, that produces abnormal movement.

Treatment

Apply two to three turns of rigid adhesive tape around the distal metatarsal shafts (Fig. 7–37). Do not try to secure the arch with the tape. The application is meant only as a retainer to prevent the splaying; therefore, use only minimal tension, and wrap the tape while making sure that no wrinkles are on the plantar surface. This should relieve the pain, as did the digital pressure applied in the examination (Fig. 7–36). The tape should be worn for several days and thereafter whenever an unusually heavy activity is anticipated.

Exercises, with tubing for resistance, to move the metatarsal arch from dorsiflexion and eversion into plantar flexion and inversion and then the reverse should be performed to help in strengthening the interosseous muscles. (See the inverter and everter exercises in Chapter 8.)

HALLUX VALGUS

Hallux valgus, or lateral deviation of the great toe, is usually accompanied in the extreme case by medial deviation of the first metatarsal bone (bunion). The deviation gives the forefoot a deformed look (Fig. 7–38).

The plantar surface of the great toe has two sesamoid bones that articulate with the metatarsal head (Fig. 7–39). They articulate within their respective grooves. The medial sesamoid is contained within the tendon of the medial head of the flexor hallucis brevis and the abductor hallucis muscles. The lateral sesamoid is contained within the tendons of the adductor hallucis muscle and the lateral head of the flexor hallucis muscle.

As the great toe migrates laterally, the first metatarsal slides medially, and the majority of the body weight is borne by the medial sesamoid. As the migration continues, the medial sesa-

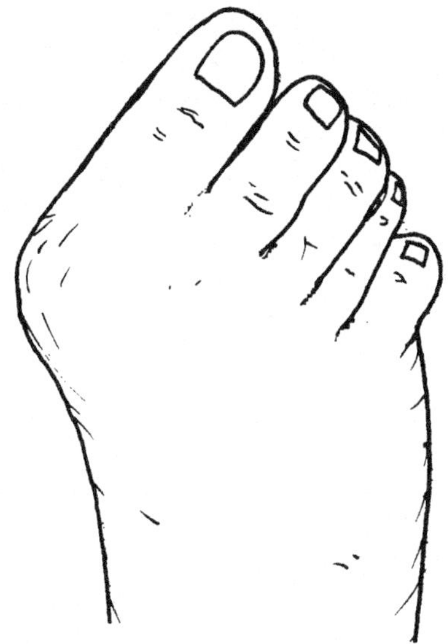

Fig. 7–38 Hallux valgus.

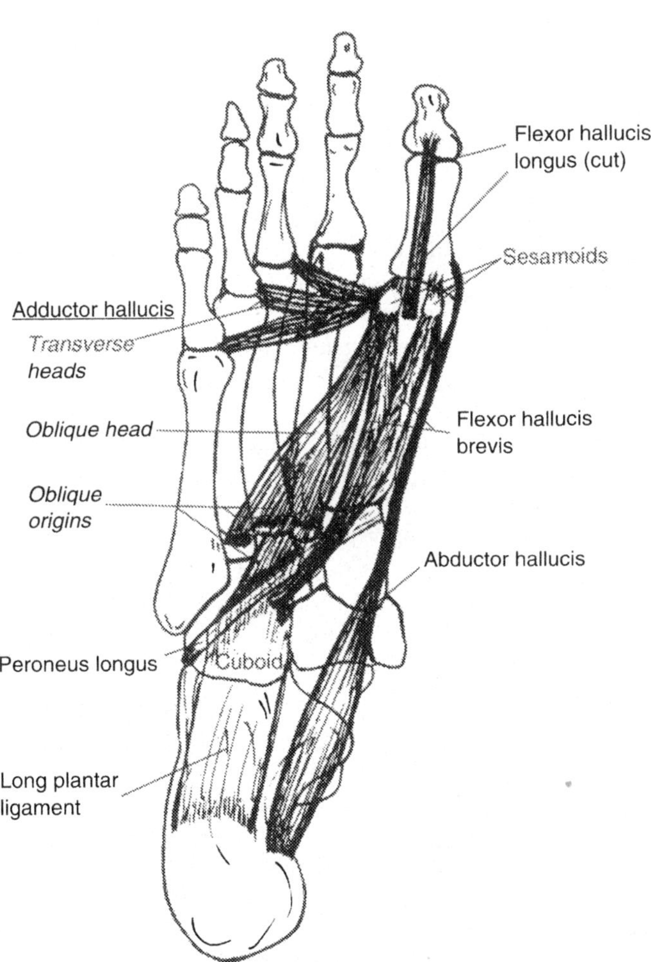

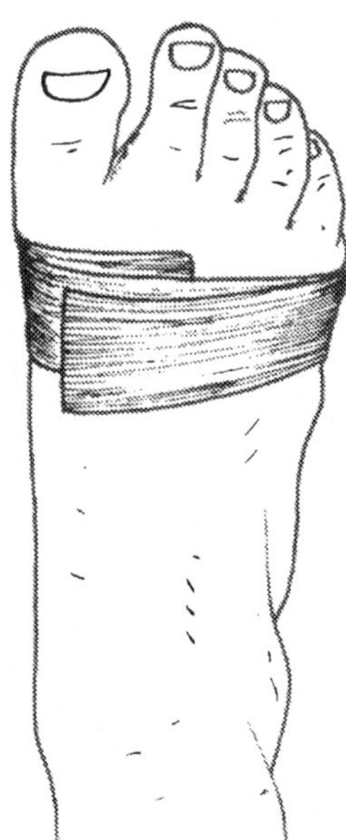

Fig. 7–37 Taping of the metatarsal arch.

Fig. 7–39 Right foot showing deep muscles of the plantar surface.

moid is now bearing the weight on the angulation of the bone rather than on the smooth articular surface. With this, the abductor hallucis muscle slides under the metatarsal and allows the joint to buckle further. The lateral head of the flexor hallucis muscle pulls the lateral sesamoid between the metatarsals. The result is friction and the formation of a bursa medially, further deforming the foot.

The cause of hallux valgus is believed to be hereditary, associated with tight, ill-fitting shoes, or related to pronation and eversion of the foot.[1]

In the early stages, conservative chiropractic care (correcting the cause of the pronation, relieving the fixations of the foot, and instituting appropriate exercises) is the treatment of choice. Once the sesamoids have migrated and the angulation reaches 30° to 35°, surgical intervention is necessary for correction. It is important to remember that rehabilitation after the surgery must be the same as in normal conservative care (ie, correction of the cause and restoration of normal function of the foot) to prevent the stresses from simply recurring.

TENDINITIS

Causes and Diagnosis

Overuse of a muscle can result in a straining injury. The same overuse may affect the tendon, resulting in an inflammatory process. Tendinitis can occur at the tenoperiosteal junction or elsewhere in the tendon. It can lead to scarring in the tendon, which can be chronically painful. In areas where the tendon runs through tendon sheaths, there can be inflammation. In this case, tenosynovitis may result in chronic thickening of the sheath. Careful palpation of the muscles and the tendons from their origins to their insertions is important in determining the tissues involved.

Palpation of the anterior retinaculum compartment (Fig. 7–40) for areas of pain allows the examiner to check for tearing of the fibrous tissue itself as well as of the tendons in the anterior compartment. Palpation of the anterior retinaculum, beginning from the medial surface of the tibia, first reveals the tendon of the anterior tibialis muscle followed by the extensor hallucis longus, extensor digitorum longus, and peroneus tertius muscles (Fig. 7–40).

The tendons of the posterior tibialis, flexor digitorum longus, and flexor hallucis longus may be palpated just posterior to the medial malleolus (Fig. 7–41).

The peroneus longus tendon may be palpated from its insertion on the lateral surface of the first metatarsal and first cuneiform as it passes under the cuboid (Fig. 7–42). The peroneus longus tendon may be palpated as it passes from the groove in the cuboid onto the lateral surface of the calcaneus, where it traverses alongside the peroneus brevis tendon (Fig. 7–43). The peroneus brevis tendon may be palpated at its insertion on the tubercle of the fifth metatarsal. While palpating along the

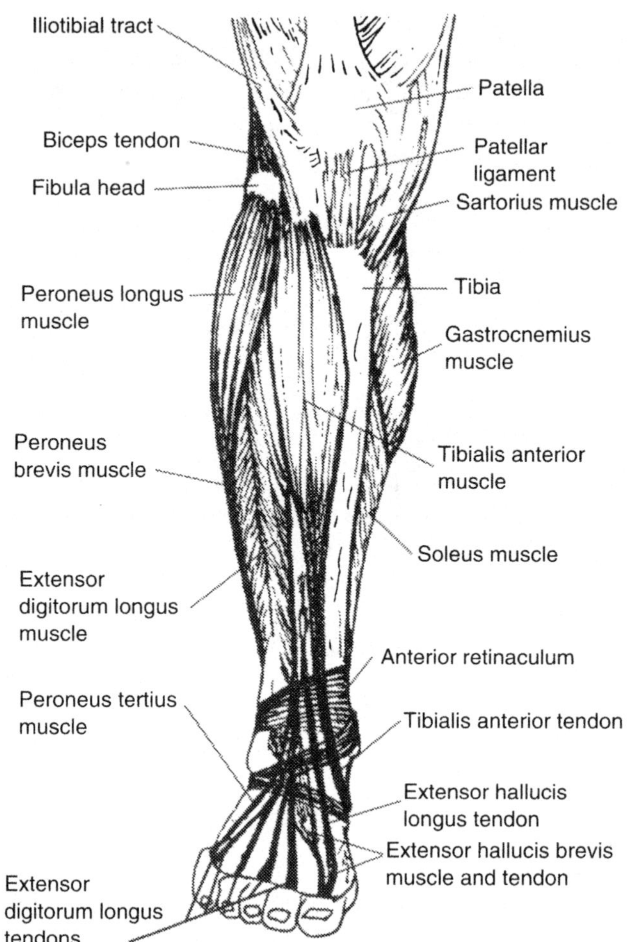

Fig. 7–40 Right leg, anterior view showing muscles and tendons.

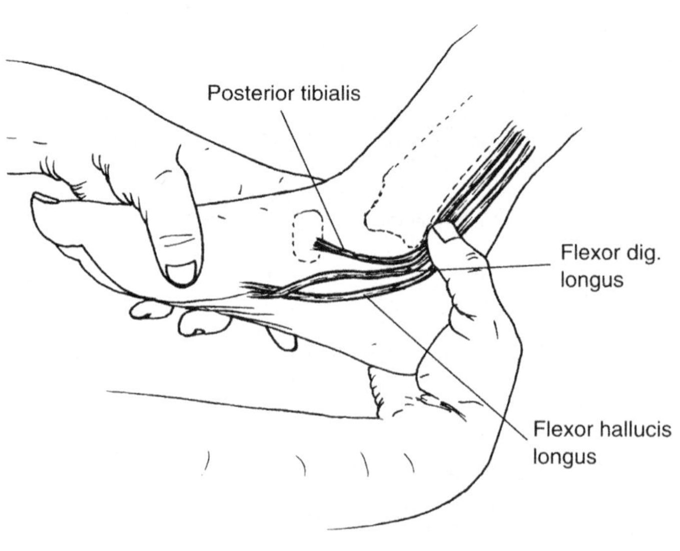

Fig. 7–41 Palpation of the tendons at the medial malleolus.

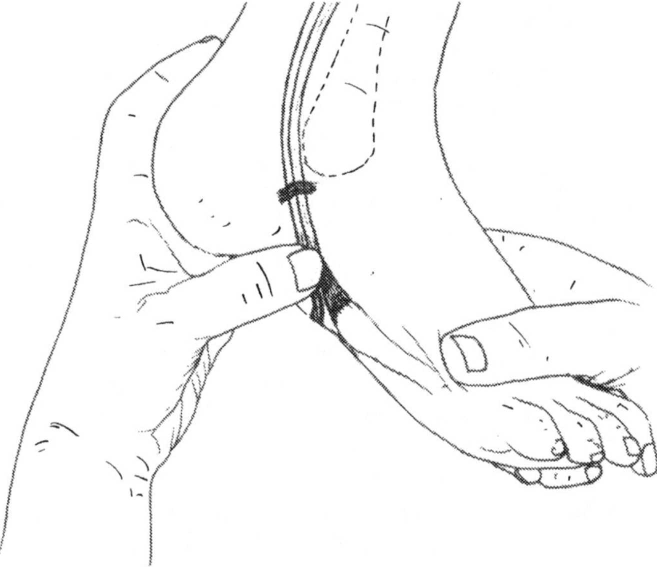

Fig. 7–43 Palpation of the peroneus longus tendon, lateral aspect.

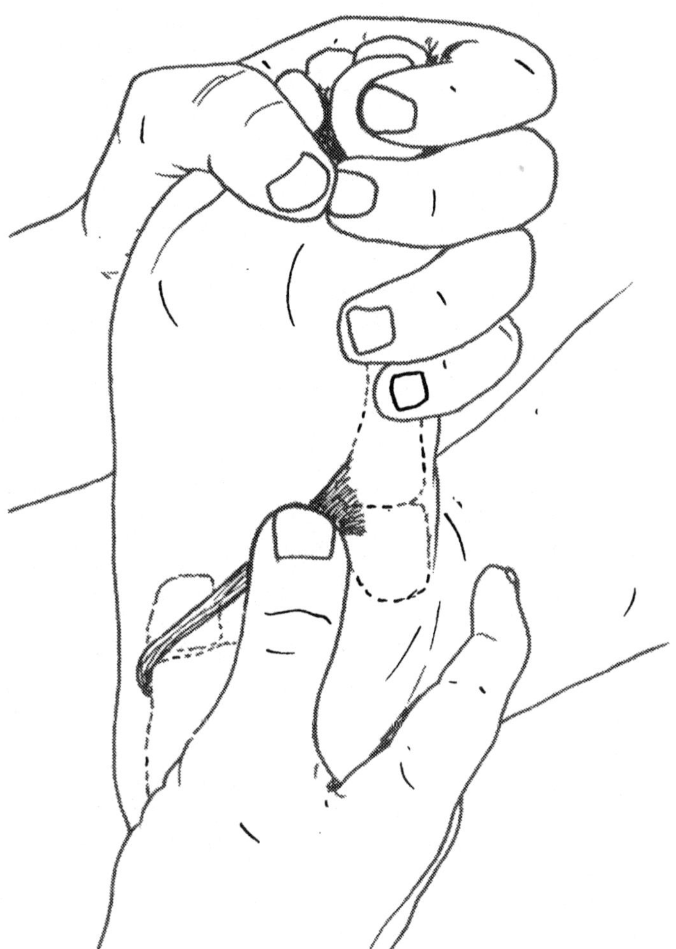

Fig. 7–42 Palpation of the peroneus longus tendon, plantar aspect.

course of the two tendons inferior to the lateral malleolus, note that they are retained by the peroneal retinaculum posterior to the fibula (Fig. 7–43).

The term *shin splints* describes an overuse irritation of the muscles in the leg that results in a strain on muscle and tendon and, in some cases, periostitis. Shin splints refers to an area of pain along the anteromedial or anterolateral portion of the distal two-thirds of the tibia. Brody[22] states that it usually develops in poorly trained athletes running on hard surfaces, wearing improper shoes, or running on a banked track or surface. He further states that the runner with a malalignment problem repeatedly pulls the posterior tibialis tendon. The repetitive pull stresses the interosseous membrane, resulting in pain in the anteromedial area of the tibia. Patients present with complaints of pain along the distal two-thirds of the shaft of the tibia. Some may complain of pain on the anterolateral surface, which usually indicates involvement of the anterior tibialis, or on the posteromedial surface, which may indicate involvement of the most medial origin of the soleus muscle.

Whether the patient presents with a complaint of shin splint or other pain suspected to be from overuse of a muscle, the examiner should palpate from the tendon insertion along its course to, and including, the muscle.

Treatment

Treatment for tendinitis includes rest and correction of any fixations that may affect the lower extremity. Correct the dysfunction that has caused the problem, where applicable.

If the patient is an athlete, taping may be necessary to support the structure. The runner or other athlete may listen to the practitioner's advice about rest, but as one athlete put it to me, "You tell me not to run, and I'll tell you that I will not run. However, when I return on Monday we'll start this discussion all over again, because I probably will run." Athletes who get a "high" out of their activity, compete with their peers, or are professionals are stubborn. If practitioners wish to continue working with such patients, then we must give assistance that allows them to participate and recover if possible. If the practitioner feels that this is not possible, then it is his or her turn to be just as stubborn and to insist that the patient cease the activity or seek help elsewhere.

Correction of the muscle dysfunction is essential. It is my opinion that the majority of the muscle pain syndromes found associated with the foot are from hypertonic musculature, whether from trauma or microtrauma (misuse syndrome). The problem may be from postural dysfunction, wearing the wrong shoes, or doing the wrong activity or from a muscle weakness that allows the dysfunction to take place. The pain is usually related to the hypertonic muscle, however.

Treatment should include the following:

- manual stretching of the affected muscle
- use of moist heat applications, 2 minutes on and 2 minutes off, with mild non–weight-bearing movement through the joint's range of motion and repeated five to six times per session; this should be repeated five to six times per day
- gradual return to activity after correction of the cause of the problem

The use of ice therapy on the affected musculature may relieve the symptoms temporarily, but in my opinion it may retard the progress.

To illustrate the effectiveness of this approach, I submit the following case history. A professional basketball player injured the second metatarsophalangeal joint just as the playoffs were starting. He had received three cortisone shots to the area and had been packed in ice from the knee down when I was asked to see him. He could not wear a regular shoe and was confined to using a postsurgical rigid shoe. A thorough examination revealed fixations throughout the tarsal arch, the knee, the sacroiliac joint on the same side as the injury, L4–5, and the atlas.

Treatment consisted of adjusting all the above except the foot followed by manual stretching of all the musculature of the leg, with an emphasis on the extensor digitorum longus, the flexor digitorum longus, and the interosseous muscles of the region. Stretching of all the musculature was necessary because of the restricted movement of the foot and the amount of ice therapy the patient had received. After the stretching, each of the fixations of the foot were adjusted. The above was followed by applications of moist heat, 2 minutes on and 2 minutes off, with non–weight-bearing range of motion exercises during the time off. When treatment was ended, the athlete immediately was able to walk barefoot with minimal discomfort. The trainer was instructed to continue the therapy five to six times per day.

Treatment was initiated on a Saturday. Sunday, on national television, the player sat at courtside watching his fellow players, wearing the shoes he would normally wear. On Tuesday night, again on national television, he played the entire game without even a trace of a limp.

Needless to say, not all patients respond that well. Even so, I have found remarkable success by adhering to this procedure.

COMPARTMENT SYNDROMES

An important diagnostic consideration in evaluating a patient with apparent straining injury to the muscles and tendons of the leg and foot is differentiating among strains, tendinitis, simple shin splints, and compartment syndromes. The compartment syndromes can be a serious medical emergency. Failure to recognize the difference can result in avascular necrosis of the muscles and nerves in the leg.

The patient who presents with aching pain in one or both legs with a history of unaccustomed heavy exercise 10 to 12 hours before onset is possibly experiencing a compartment syndrome and should be evaluated carefully. The pain and swelling can be palpated along the distal two-thirds of the tibia anteromedially, anterolaterally, or laterally.

The mechanism of injury is a swelling of overworked muscles and a loosening of muscular fascia from the periosteum of the tibia and/or fibula, resulting in excessive intercompartmental pressure. This can cause compression of the blood vessels and may lead to necrosis. The pain is usually intense, swelling is often evident, and the skin may be taut, glossy, warm, and red. Active and passive movement of the foot is painful, and muscle weakness is often evident, with foot drop being the most evident sign.

There are three compartments that can be involved (Fig. 7–44).[8] The anterior compartment is the most common, involving the anterior tibialis and extensor hallucis longus. The peroneal compartment is much less commonly involved and affects the peroneal muscles and the common peroneal and/or superficial peroneal nerves. The deep posterior compartment contains the flexor digitorum longus, flexor hallucis longus, and posterior tibialis muscles and the posterior tibial nerve and artery. This compartment is affected in fractures of the tibia and fibula and, less often, in soft tissue injuries.

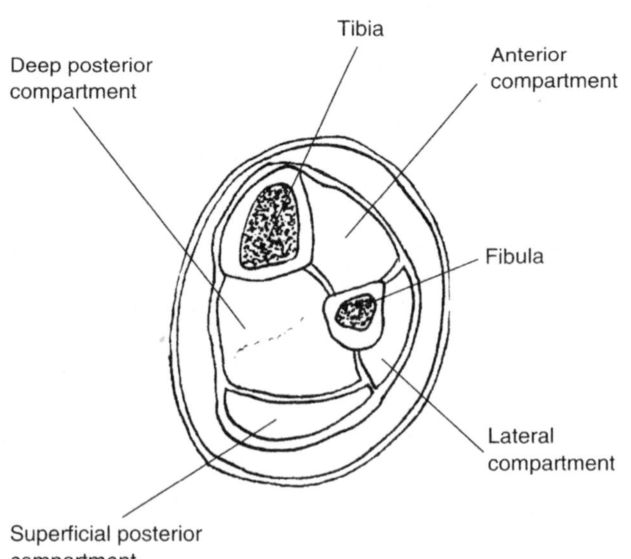

Fig. 7–44 Distal two thirds of the right leg, cross-section showing compartments.

REFERENCES

1. Hiss J. *Functional Foot Disorders*. New York, NY: Oxford University Press; 1949.

2. Shands AR, Raney RB. *Handbook of Orthopaedic Surgery*. St. Louis, Mo: Mosby; 1967.

3. Cailliet R. *Knee Pain and Disability*. Philadelphia, Pa: Davis; 1976.

4. Mennell R. *Foot Pain*. Boston, Mass: Little, Brown; 1969.

5. Scholl W. *The Human Foot*. Chicago, Ill: Foot Specialists; 1920.

6. Alexander U. *The Foot: Examination and Diagnosis*. New York, NY: Churchill Livingstone; 1990.

7. Hoppenfeld S. *Physical Examination of the Spine and Extremities*. New York, NY: Appleton-Century-Crofts; 1976.

8. Turek S. *Orthopaedics Principles and their Application*. Philadelphia, Pa: Lippincott; 1967.

9. *Dorland's Illustrated Medical Dictionary* (25th ed). Philadelphia, Pa: Saunders; 1974.

10. Ebrall PS, Bales GL, Frost BR. An improved clinical protocal for ankle cryotherapy. *J Man Med*. 1992;6:161–165.

11. Scotece G, Guthrie M. Comparison of three treatment approaches for grade I and II ankle sprains in active duty soldiers. *J Orthop Sports Phys Ther*. 1992;15:19–22.

12. Birrer R. Ankle trauma, looking beyond the sprain. *Diagnosis*. 1984;6:32–36.

13. Jahss M. *Disorders of the Foot*. Philadelphia, Pa: Saunders; 1982.

14. Colville M, Marder R, Boyle J, Zarlins B. Strain measurement in lateral ankle ligaments. *Am J Sports Med*. 1990;18:196–200.

15. Roycroft S, Mantgani A. Early active management: ankle sprain. *Physiother*. 1990;69:355–356.

16. Cote D, Prentice W, Hooker D, Shields E. Comparison of three treatment procedures for minimizing ankle sprain swelling. *Phys Ther*. 1988;68:101–118.

17. Briner W, Carr D, Lavery K. Anterioinferior tibiofibular ligament injury. *J Phys Sports Med*. 1989;17:63–69.

18. Bernstein R, Bartolomei F, McCarthy D. Sinus tarsi syndrome: anatomical, clinical and surgical considerations. *J Am Podiatr Med Assoc*. 1985;9:475–480.

19. Byank R, Clarke H, Bleecker M. Standardized neurometric evaluation in tarsal tunnel syndrome. *Adv Orthop Surg*. 1989;12:249–253.

20. D'Ambrosia R. *Musculoskeletal Disorders*. Philadelphia, Pa: Lippincott; 1986.

21. Lawrence D. Pes planus: a review of etiology, diagnosis and chiropractic management. *J Manip Phys Ther*. 1983;6:185–188.

22. Brody D. Running injuries. *Ciba Clin Symp*. 1980;32:15–19.

Chapter 8

Exercises

Exercise is important in prevention of problems, recovery from trauma, and rehabilitation to preinjury status and beyond. Trauma or symptoms make it necessary for patients to present themselves for treatment, with success being measured by the cessation of symptoms and the return to normal. Normal, of course, may not be what is correct.

If examination reveals abnormal posture or poor habit patterns, the practitioner should make sure that the patient is fully informed of the problem, and a treatment program should be provided. The patient with a chronic postural fault must not merely be introduced to corrective exercises. The practitioner must look further into the habit patterns of activities during work or recreation and advise the patient in altering the activity.

Patients who have experienced trauma should be given exercises to restore muscle function as soon as practical. In the severe stage, where edema and pain are present, exercises may be harmful, but as soon as the edema is reduced exercises may be introduced within the normal range of motion and within the patient's tolerance.

If ligamental damage has occurred that does not require surgery, taping to reinforce the joint structure is a necessity before introducing an exercise. Always start with mild exercises, increasing as symptoms will allow for the muscles that produce the movement, which will reduce the strain on the injured ligamental structure.

Two types of exercise may be used: isometric, involving no joint movement (contraction of the musculature only), and isotonic, involving active movement against resistance. Isotonic exercise may be performed with weights or an apparatus providing the resistance. Exercising in a gym is convenient for the patient who belongs to one, but it does have its drawbacks. The average person will not go to the spa more than three to five times per week. It requires driving to and from and changing in and out of clothes and in general occupies a lot of time without the benefits necessary for rehabilitation. I prefer the use of stretchable tubing. Most supply houses now provide several sizes of tubing with various strengths. Before stretchable tubing I used bicycle inner tubing, and this is still preferred for one of the exercises for the foot.

Getting a patient to perform exercises at home is, at best, difficult. Getting a patient to do the correct exercises at home is even more difficult. It is easy and simple to hand out a set of standard exercises for a patient to perform, but this method is fraught with problems:

- Unless designed specifically for the problem this patient is experiencing, some of the exercises may be harmful.

- Without actually going through an exercise, the patient usually has difficulty in figuring out exactly how to perform the exercise.

- If the patient performs the exercise incorrectly or does the wrong exercise, the condition may deteriorate, with the patient getting discouraged and not returning. If and when the patient does return, it is still necessary to review the exercises, so that it is more efficient to rehearse the patient to start with.

Patients with work-related injuries, and for that matter most patients who work, are interested in returning to work as soon as possible. Therefore, if necessary the patient should be brought into the office to perform the exercise for 1 to 3 days to ensure that the exercises are being performed as instructed.

It has been my experience that to ensure that exercises are performed correctly the following must be done:

1. Give a careful description in lay terms of exactly what the problem is.
2. Test the muscle and demonstrate to the patient how weak it is and why exercise is necessary.
3. Demonstrate the exercise.
4. Have the patient perform the exercise, making sure that cheating (recruitment of other muscles) does not occur.
5. Provide, where possible, a drawing of the exercise to be used as a reminder.
6. Make available exercise tubing if it is to be used. Do not rely on the patient to purchase one somewhere else.
7. If a spouse is available, recruit him or her to assist in reminding the patient to do the exercises and to observe to see whether they are being done correctly.
8. Explain exactly how many repetitions at each session and how many sessions per day are expected.
9. On the following visit, not only review the results but have the patient repeat the exercise to ensure that it is being performed correctly.

Stretchable tubing allows a patient to perform exercises at home, at work, or while traveling. A length of about 5 ft will allow most exercises to be performed. If a bicycle tube is used, cut out the stem. With either, tie a knot in each end, and the exercises may begin.

Why tubing? Why not just send the patient to a gym or fitness center for exercises? There are several reasons:

- Some patients cannot afford to join.
- Some of the acute patients could not go.
- Some patients have no transportation.
- Most would not go more than once per day. Most would perform the exercises three to four times per week.
- By having tubing and proper instructions, patients may do the exercises as many times per day as needed.

Active participation of the patient in the treatment process is essential. Patient attitude all too often is one of placing all the responsibility on the practitioner's shoulders. After the initial diagnosis and treatment of the acute stage, patient participation is a must if complete rehabilitation is to be accomplished.

LORDOTIC LUMBAR SYNDROME EXERCISES

The lordotic lumbar syndrome (Fig. 8–1) is one of the most common postural distortions found in practice. One of the reasons is the conveniences of our modern society. Sitting down is a way of life; often the work force drives an auto for 1 to 2 hours per day and then sits at a desk or in front of a computer

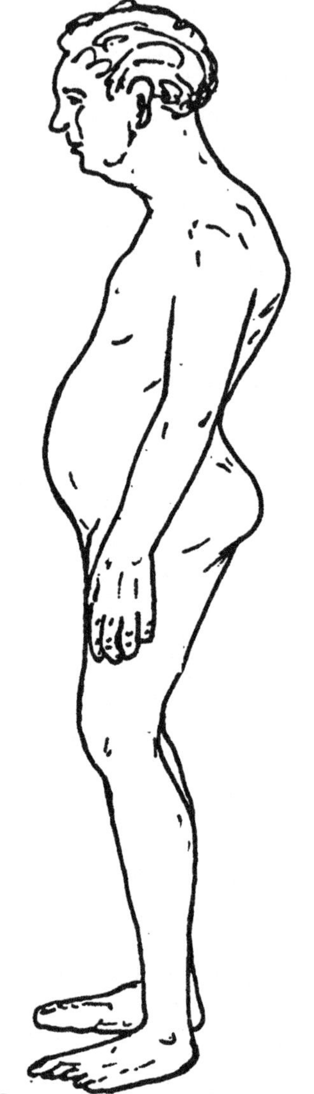

Fig. 8–1 Lumbar lordosis and resulting posture.

for 8 hours. Without the proper exercises to make up for the deficit in activity, the lordotic lumbar syndrome can be the result.

As if the above was not enough, add abdominal surgery, pregnancy, and obesity, and we have the middle-aged female patient who has had problems since her first child. She now has not only back problems but valgus knees with their associated laterally rotated tibias, and she is forced to walk with the foot turned out. Thus she complains of foot pains (Fig. 8–2). The anterior rotation of the pelvis and increased lordosis of the lumbar spine must be reduced before exercises for the lateral rotators of the hip will be effective. As long as they exist, the Q or valgus angle of the knee will remain increased as a result of the medial rotation of the femur. Female patients who have

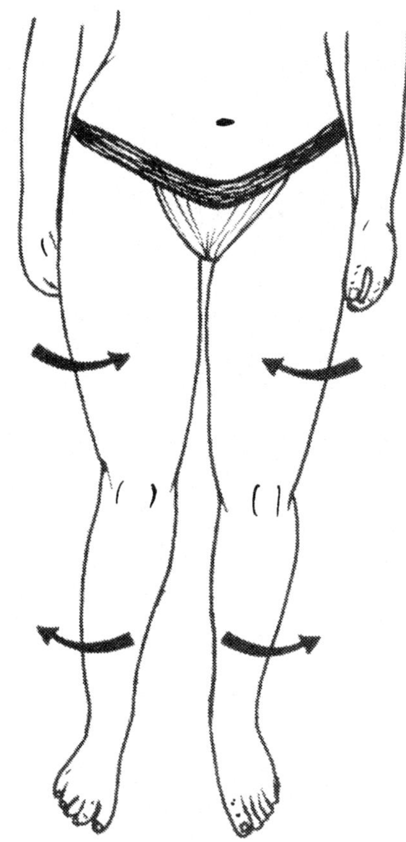

Fig. 8–2 Distortions common to the lordotic lumbar syndrome.

had children must be screened for abdominal muscles that not only may be weak but may have ceased functioning during the later stages of pregnancy, breaking the normal habit pattern. The habit pattern must be reestablished for the rest of the lordotic lumbar exercises to be effective.

To accomplish this, have the patient perform a bilateral straight leg raise (Fig. 8–3). Observe the pelvis at the start of the effort. As the hip flexors begin to contract, the abdominal muscles should contract, securing the pelvis to provide a fulcrum for the function. If the habit pattern is broken or the abdominals are weak, the pelvis will rotate anteriorly before the legs leave the table. To prove the necessity of doing this exercise, place your hand on the lower abdominal area and help abdominal function by stabilizing the pelvis (Fig. 8–4). The legs will rise more easily.

Reestablishing a normal habit pattern takes effort and patience on the part of the patient and physician. With the patient supine, place one hand underneath the patient on the sacrum. With the other hand, contact the lower abdomen and physically rotate or rock the pelvis posteriorly for the patient several times to show what is expected. Then have the patient start helping in the movement and then doing it unassisted. Stop,

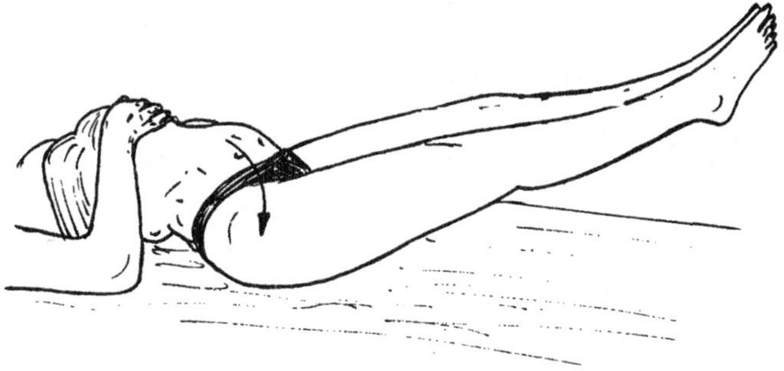

Fig. 8–3 Abdominal weakness on bilateral straight leg raise.

remove your hands, and ask the patient to perform the pelvic rock again. Most of the time she cannot: Everything may move but the pelvis. Assistance should be provided again and the process repeated. The patient may think that she is performing the movement when in fact the pelvis does not move. Have the patient place her hand on the pubic area so that she can feel the lack of movement during the attempt.

Instruct the patient to attempt the pelvic rock at home 10 times per session for three sessions per day and to return in 2 days. Some patients may return and be able to rotate the pelvis. Most require at least one more session in the office with assistance before the habit pattern is reestablished. Once this has been accomplished, the patient is ready to perform the rest of the exercises.

The following illustrations and directions are for exercises that I have used successfully for many years.

LORDOSIS EXERCISE

Instruct the patient to lie on the floor, couch, or bed and to place 5 to 10 lb of weight on the abdomen below the umbilicus. (The weight is determined by the patient's size and basic build.) Have the patient bend one knee as shown in Figure 8–5 and, using that leg only, raise the buttocks off the surface while rotating the pelvis posteriorly (ie, move the pubic bone

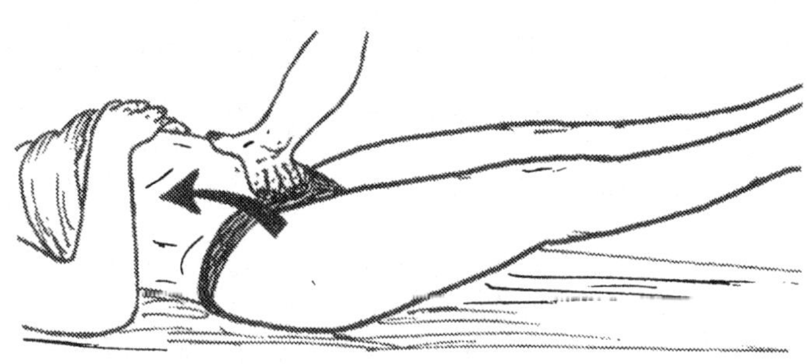

Fig. 8–4 Manual assistance to the abdominals to help in the bilateral straight leg raise.

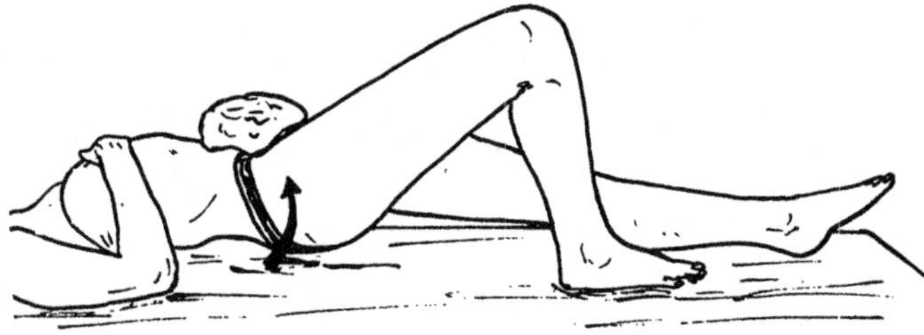

Fig. 8–5 Lordosis exercise.

toward the chin). Hold for 5 to 6 seconds, and then return to the table slowly. Repeat six to eight times, and then repeat on the opposite side. Compare one side with the other, and if one side takes more effort the patient should repeat the exercise on that side six to eight more times. Having the patient compare one side with the other for the amount of effort to perform the exercise is a simple way of achieving balance of the muscles.

The above constitutes one session. The patient should perform at last one to five sessions per day (as determined by the patient's condition).

The weight on the abdomen is an important part of the exercise. When asked to do the exercise without weight, the patient usually will increase the lumbar curve. Patients who are obese or who cannot raise the buttocks off the table many times may do so if the operator applies hand pressure of 5 to 10 lb on the abdomen. The weight seems to trigger a reflex to rotate the pelvis posteriorly and to allow raising to occur.

Some general exercises for the low back include raising the buttocks using both legs. If done, this exercise increases the lordosis of the lumbar spine.

SIT-UPS

Have the patient lie on the floor with the legs in a chair. Make sure that the hip is flexed to 90°. With arms outstretched, the patient should try to rise up and touch an imaginary point to his or her extreme right (position 1, Fig. 8–6A), hold, and then slowly return to the floor. Repeat progressively across to position 6 (Fig. 8–6B). Rest, and then repeat back from position 6 to position 1. After all 12 sit-ups have been performed, compare position 1 with position 6. If one takes more effort than the other, repeat it an additional three to four times. Then compare positions 2 and 5, then positions 3 and 4, and repeat each one that takes more effort an additional three to four times.

The above constitutes one session. The patient should perform one to three sessions per day.

By having the patient flex the hips to 90°, most of the function of the psoas muscle is removed from participation. (The psoas is usually hypertonic and/or shortened.) Using six positions exercises all the abdominal muscles, with the extreme outside ones exercising the transverse abdominals.

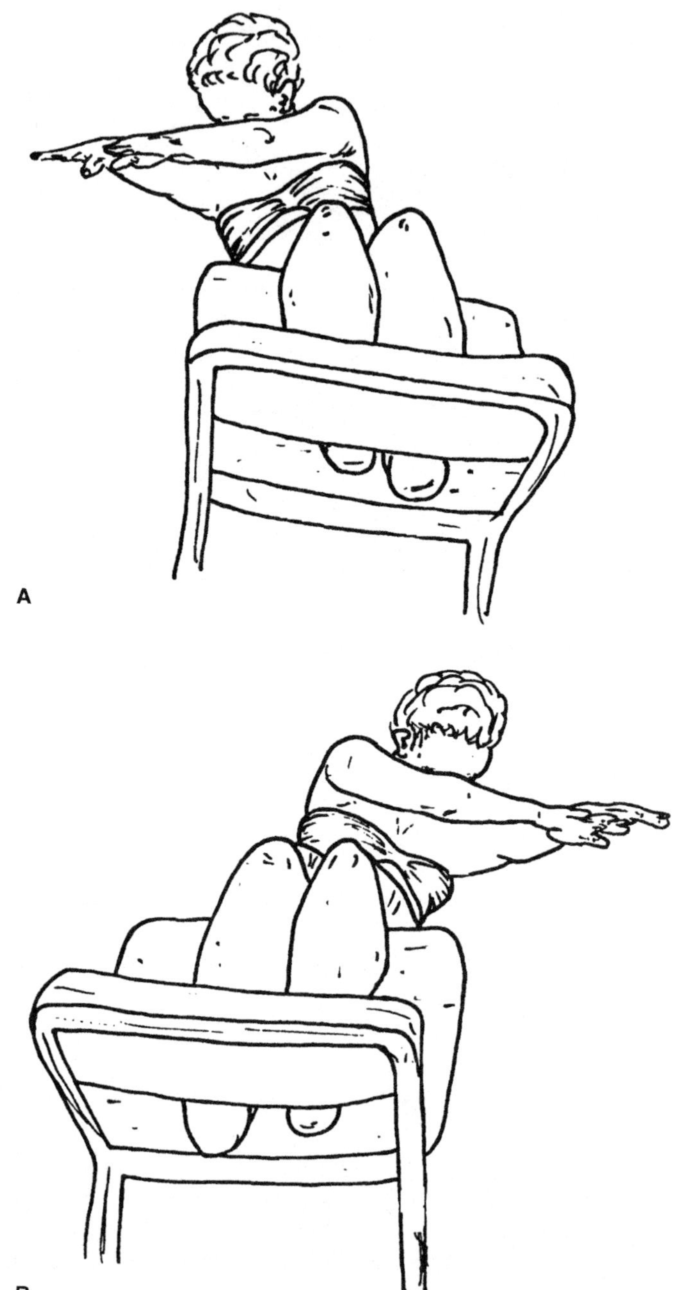

Fig. 8–6 **(A)** Sit-up position 1. **(B)** Sit-up position 6.

OTHER POSTURAL FAULTS

An anatomic short leg is another postural fault that produces changes resembling a lordotic lumbar syndrome. At first glance, in the upright position the anteriorly rotated pelvis may have the appearance of a lordotic lumbar syndrome. With an anatomic short leg the anteriorly rotated pelvis is part of the attempt to stand erect, and exercising for it would be a mistake.

On the short leg side, most of the time the patient will laterally rotate the femur in an attempt to make the leg longer, thus laterally rotating the foot (Fig. 8–7). The proper treatment and correction for the problem should be done before exercising for the foot itself; otherwise, as soon as the patient takes a few steps the problem starts all over again.

Sitting on the foot is another habit pattern that places undue stress on the lateral ankle and foot. Women with short legs who sit on a regular chair soon get the circulation cut off because their feet never touch the floor. To make up for that, they will sit on one foot and then the other (Fig. 8–8).

If it is determined that the foot problem is a result of another postural fault, not only should the postural fault be corrected but any poor habit patterns that started as a result should be corrected as well.

When examining the patient with a poor habit pattern observed during gait, I use the following method of correction. Have the patient look down at his or her feet during this exercise. Place the heel on the floor, then slowly and deliberately place the forefoot forward, not rotated. Slowly and deliberately move the body weight from the heel to the forefoot. Repeat on the opposite side. Have the patient repeat this 40 to 50 times down a hallway and back while looking down at the feet at all times. This should be repeated two to three times per day until the habit pattern is broken.

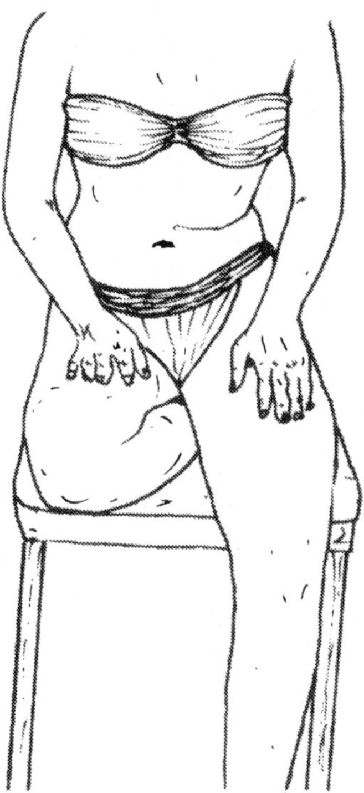

Fig. 8–8 Ankle strain from sitting on one foot.

SHORT TRICEPS SURAE

I use a slant board 13×13 in with a rise of $5\frac{1}{2}$ in in the front. Place the board at a convenient location, usually behind a chair. The patient should stand on the board for 1 to 2 minutes at a time for as many times per day as possible (Fig. 8–9). If the slant board is placed in the TV room, I suggest that every time the commercials come on the patient stand on it. Usually, with a patient who is consistent, 2 weeks is sufficient to stretch completely. If the patient is a woman who must wear high-heeled shoes at work and then is required to sit down, the problem is perpetuated. The board must be a way of life for that patient until she can be convinced to wear better shoes.

EVERTER EXERCISE

A bicycle inner tube works best for this exercise because of its flat, broad surface. Place the tubing around the leg of a heavy piece of furniture. Sit in a chair and, with the foot plantar flexed and inverted, hook the foot into the tubing. Against the resistance, pull into eversion and dorsiflexion (Fig. 8–10).

INVERTER EXERCISES

With the foot in plantar flexion and everted, hook the foot into the tubing. Against resistance, pull into inversion and dorsiflexion (Fig. 8–11).

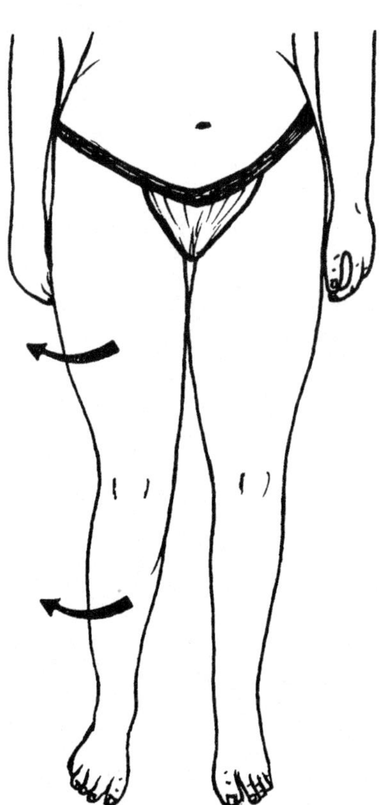

Fig. 8–7 Rotated limb associated with an anatomic short leg.

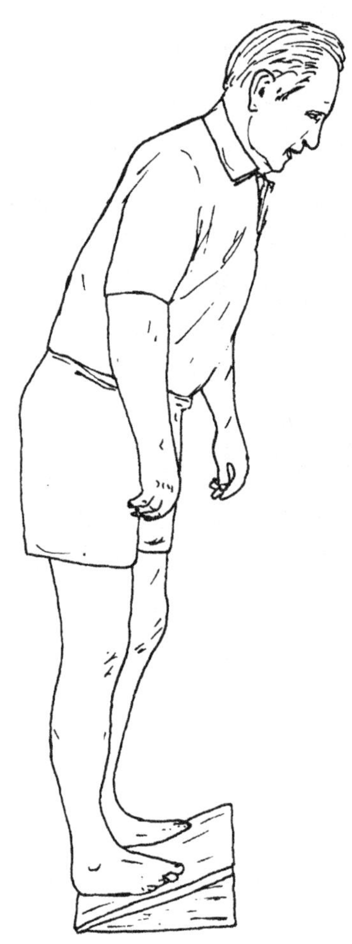

Fig. 8–9 Posture while standing on the slant board with restricted dorsiflexion.

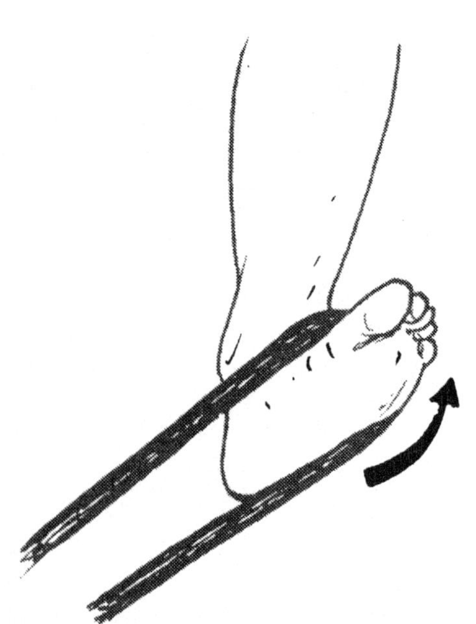

Fig. 8–10 Everter exercise.

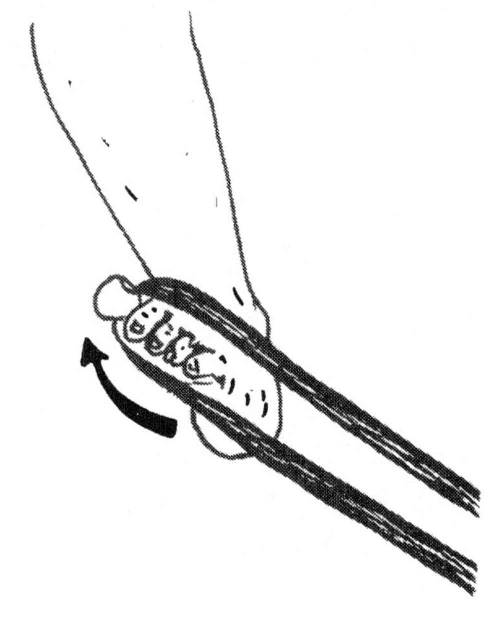

Fig. 8–11 Inverter exercise.

POSTERIOR TIBIALIS

The posterior tibialis produces plantar flexion, but much less than the triceps surae. It also has a role in medial rotation of the foot on the tibia. An effective method of isolating the posterior tibialis is as follows. Place the foot on a slanted surface, keeping the knee at 90° (Fig. 8–12). Secure the tubing to the lateral side of the foot, and take up the slack (Fig. 8–13).

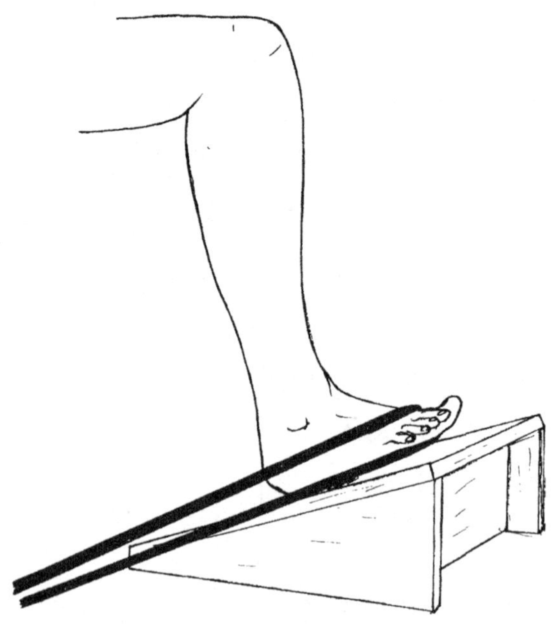

Fig. 8–12 Starting position for posterior tibialis exercise, side view.

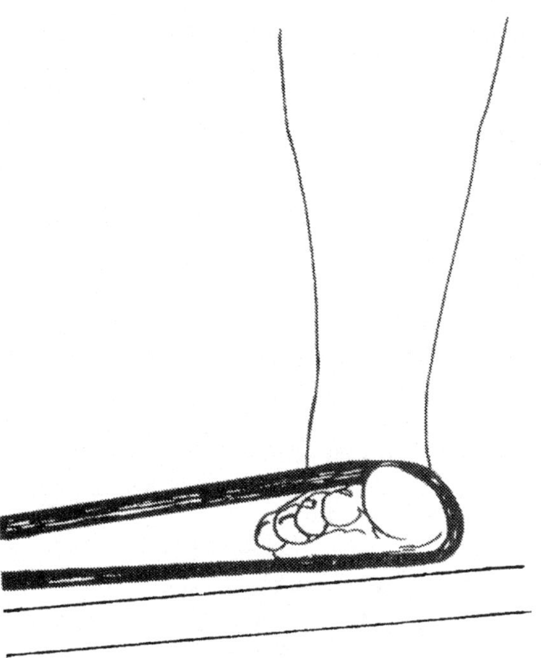

Fig. 8–13 Starting position for posterior tibialis exercise, front view.

Medially rotate the foot as far as possible (Fig. 8–14). Most of the movement is medial rotation of the tibia, with the popliteus and semitendinosis performing the work. The last 5° is rotation of the foot on the tibia, which is produced by the posterior tibialis.

ANKLE STABILITY

To stabilize the ankle and restore proprioception, several methods are used. For circumduction, use a round cut-out board (available in most home improvement stores). To this, attach half a 3-in round ball to the middle (Fig. 8–15).

For mediolateral and plantar-dorsal stability, use a board 12 × 18 in with a 2 × 2 in centerboard attached down the middle. Round the edges of the 2 × 2 in board (Fig. 8–16). With the centerboard down, place the feet with one on either side of and parallel to the centerboard. Tilt back and forth for strengthening the inverters and everters. By placing the feet directly above and across the centerboard, the plantar flexors and dorsiflexors can be worked.

I find the two preceding methods good for younger patients or athletes but not so good for 60-year-olds, who may not be so steady on their feet. My preference is the exercises described earlier using tubing.

If a steep hill is available, the following is a good exercise for the whole body as well as for helping stabilize the ankle and foot. Walk 10 paces straight up the hill, then turn and walk at 45° across the hill for the width of a street. Continue 10 paces up, and then recross at 45° in the other direction. Repeat this process five to six times (Fig. 8–17). This stabilizes the ankle, foot, and knee and causes many muscles to be activated throughout the body that otherwise may never get exercised.

One of the problems with runners, especially marathon runners, is that they run consistently over relatively smooth terrain. All the muscles that propel the body forward get exercised, and sometimes overexercised. I have had success with

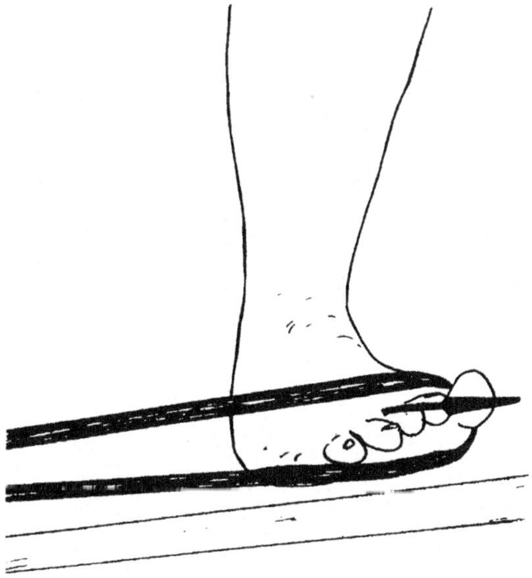

Fig. 8–14 Movement for posterior tibialis exercise.

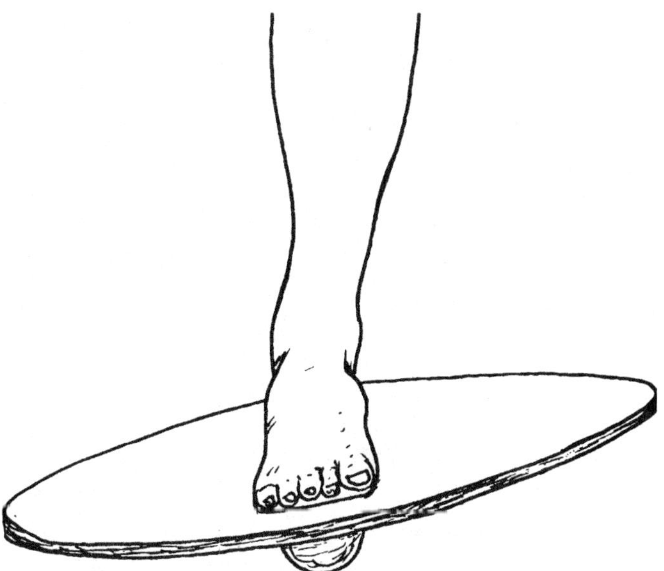

Fig. 8–15 Use of the circumduction board.

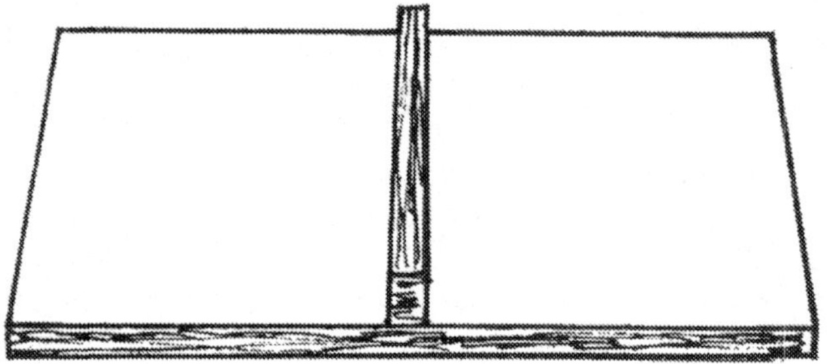

Fig. 8–16 Exercise board for mediolateral and dorsiflexion-plantar flexion (shown upside-down).

several marathon runners by having them do the following. Run in a zig-zag manner (similar to what football players do with auto tires). This is best done in sand because the feet tend to sink in and drag through the sand. Most runners are reluctant to participate because they do not get anywhere fast, which is what they want. By doing so, however, the medial to lateral stabilizers are exercised in the feet and ankles as well as in the knees. The runners who participated in this exercise had

improved marathon times, and, more important, their injury rates decreased dramatically.

EXERCISE FOR CIRCULATION

The prevalence of sedentary occupations, plus the type of shoes worn by many women, make exercises for circulation important to both male and female patients. The woman who is required (or chooses) to wear high-heeled shoes, keeping the ankle in plantar flexion, may travel to work in an auto. After arriving, she then sits down at the computer for 8 hours and then drives home. The arterial flow to the extremities is propelled by heart action. The venous return from the periphery has a more difficult time with the weight of the body on the chair. Lymphatic flow is dependent on muscular action.

Careful palpation of the plantar surface of the foot in this typical female patient will reveal rather congested, sensitive tissue. Gentle massage with the foot higher than the buttocks will remove most of the discomfort in a few minutes.

One of the most effective methods that I have found is a mobilization exercise using resistance tubing. A bicycle inner tube is the best equipment for this exercise. It will lie flat and will not slide, as does exercise tubing. Have the patient lie on his or her back with the tube looped over the forefoot (Fig. 8–18). Pull first on one side and then on the other, gradually in-

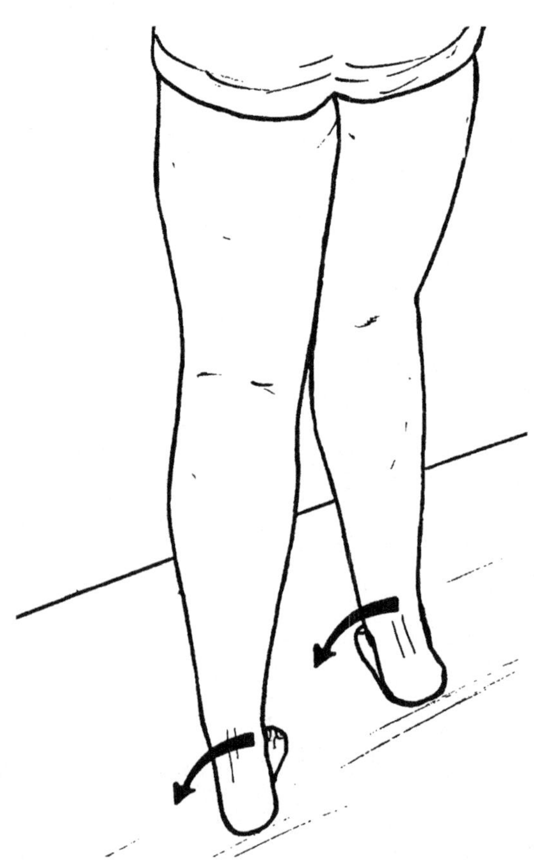

Fig. 8–17 Exercise on a steep hill for ankle stability.

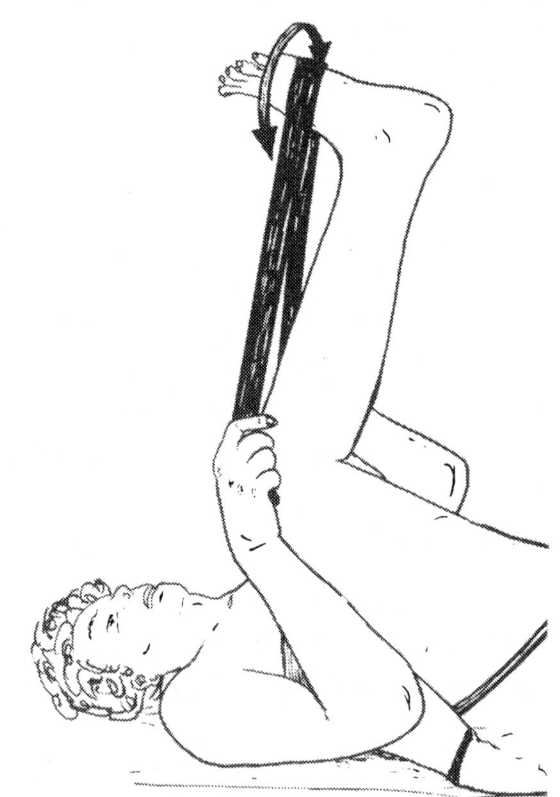

Fig. 8–18 Exercise to improve the circulation.

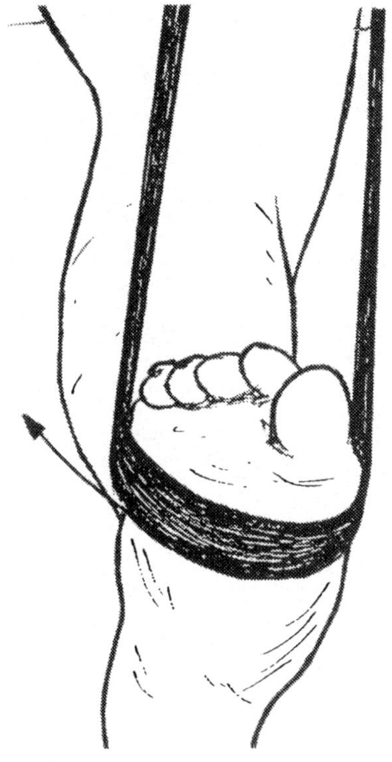

A

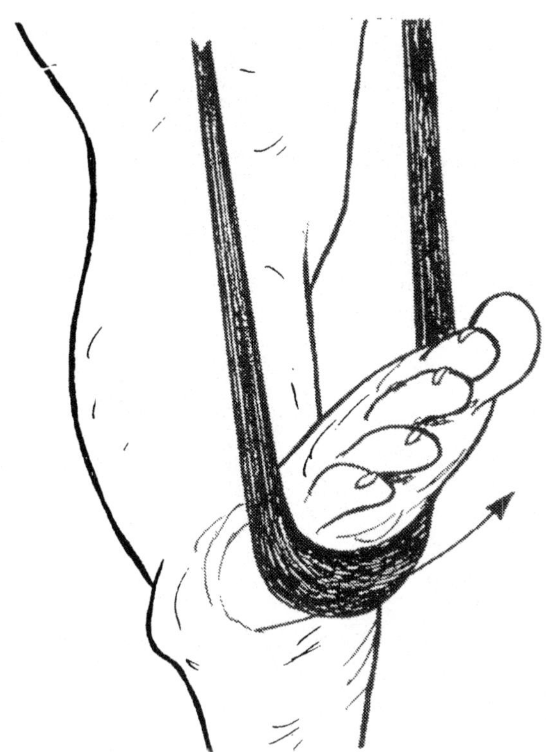

B

Fig. 8–19 (A) and (B) Mobilization exercise for the unpliable foot.

creasing to tolerance. If performed one to two times per day, much of the discomfort will be removed.

It goes without saying, however, that doing away with the high-heeled shoes and getting some regular exercise, even walking at lunch, would help. Many women now wear comfortable athletic shoes to and from work and wear their high-heeled shoes only when they must. I always encourage patients to do this.

LOOSENING THE UNPLIABLE, UNADAPTABLE FOOT

Several things are useful in loosening the rigid foot:

- daily walks and runs in dry sand, if available
- daily walks and runs over uneven, grassy terrain
- use of a foot roller (I used to recommend the old heavy Coca-Cola bottle; the newer ones are too fragile. A simple foot roller also can be made from a short piece of 1¼-in dowling.)
- use of a bicycle inner tube to continue the loosening process started in the office at home or at work

The mobilization exercise is a more complete work-out than the decongestion exercise described previously. A bicycle inner tube provides the best grip on the foot. With the leg extended, loop the tube over the forefoot just proximal to the distal metatarsal ends to start. Begin with gentle mobilization in a back-and-forth action, gradually increasing the pressure to tolerance (Fig. 8–19). Move the tube toward the heel and repeat the exercise in several positions, working the metatarsals and the metatarsotarsal and tarsal articulations.

Organic Problems and the Foot and Ankle

Organic problems may produce many signs and symptoms, which may include interference with the normal function of specific muscles. Muscle weakness in the foot and ankle area should warn the examiner of at least the possibility of an organic problem. Questioning the patient about other signs and symptoms makes it mandatory either to investigate further or to eliminate organic problems as a cause of or contributor to the foot problem.

Organ-muscle relationships are controversial. Therefore, before discussing the specific organ-muscle relationships of the foot I must relate my opinion of the history and theory as well as the methods I have used to prove or disprove it clinically.

The earliest recorded signs of organ-muscle relationships are found in drawings of Indian therapeutic yoga exercises. The positions used in therapeutic yoga apply pressure to or stretch specific muscles for each organic problem. The muscles being affected by the yoga exercises are strikingly similar to the organ-muscle relationships introduced by George Goodheart, DC in the 1960s.

With the introduction of muscle testing, goading of muscle origins and insertions, and then organ-muscle relationships, I set out to prove or disprove the organ-muscle theory clinically. To my knowledge, no studies have been done to prove or disprove the organ-muscle theory, the fixation-organ theory, or Bennett's neurovascular dynamics (NVD) theories. An explanation of my interpretation of each of the theories is necessary to convey fully the methods I used.

FIXATION-ORGAN THEORY

For many years, organic areas have been taught as areas of fixation found by doctors of chiropractic to accompany organic problems. Successful treatments of organic problems after adjustment of the related areas of fixation have been reported by various writers. D.D. Palmer reported that by adjusting he restored the hearing of a deaf person;[1] this was the first patient of chiropractic. Thus the relationship of an organ to an area started from the beginning of chiropractic in 1895.

Many technique proponents have related various areas of the spine as organic places. These include Biron, Welles, and Houser, whose *Chiropractic Principles and Technic* was published in 1939[2]; they refer to the centers and organic places in use by many chiropractors at that time. The most prominent chiropractic system to propose organic places has been the Meric system. The fixation levels for organs may vary from writer to writer but are usually no more than one vertebra apart. Variations in patient anatomy and methods of palpation used by the writers may account for the differences. The following are the levels of fixation and the organs related to them as I use them:

- T1–2, heart
- T-3, lung
- T4–5, gall bladder
- T6–8, liver
- T7–8, pancreas
- T7–11, small intestine
- T-9, adrenals
- T9–11, kidneys
- T12–L1, ileocecal valve and appendix
- L-5, uterus and prostate

Even though there are overlapping areas in the list above, persistent fixation in the area should alert the practitioner to investigate the possibility of organic problems associated with the area. Further investigation may be necessary to prove that the fixation is from organic causes and not a structural fault missed during the examination.

All methods of palpation are fraught with the variables of patient reaction and the examiner's experience and ability. I prefer palpation of the thoracic and lumbar spine in the supine, non–weight-bearing position for greater accuracy. The distortions and stresses of the prone position for static palpation and the weight-bearing problems in motion palpation interfere with accuracy.

NVD

Terrence Bennett, DC, established reflex areas that he believed related to each organ of the body, and he claimed success in some organic problems by using the reflexes as treatment points.[3]

On the front (Fig. A–1), the reflex points are either over the location of the organ or, as Bennett described them, reflexes from the organ (or valve). The reflex point on the back (Fig. A–2) is felt as a tight muscle and is usually sensitive to the patient when palpated. Some of the posterior points coincide with the fixation places. If nothing else had ever come from Bennett's work, the location of the reflex points alone is helpful in diagnosing possible organic problems.

Treatment consists of passive contacts of the two reflexes. With the patient supine, use the right hand and palpate the abdominal area (Fig. A–1) corresponding with the organ that is associated with the area of persistent fixation. With the left hand, contact the area related to the organ (Fig. A–2) along the area of the transverse processes and simply hold. In my opinion, this technique helps greatly in decongesting the organ or relaxing the sphincter. I have helped many patients with known organic problems with the use of NVD as an adjunct to adjustive procedures. When possible, all reflex techniques should be used only after an adjustment is made. Along with the organic place, NVD should be taught as an integral part of diagnosis.

ORGAN-MUSCLE RELATIONSHIPS

Chapman, an osteopath, found that patients with organic problems usually had sensitive areas related to them: one next to the spine and one on the anterior part of the body. (Generally these are different areas than the NVD areas.)[4] Chapman claimed success in treating organic problems by stimulation of the reflexes by goading.

George Goodheart, DC, introduced to the profession the importance of muscle balance and function as a part of diagnosis and treatment.[5] He found that patients with known organic problems also had specific muscles that tested weak. He also found that stimulation of the reflex areas located by Chapman for the same organ many times resulted in an increased re-

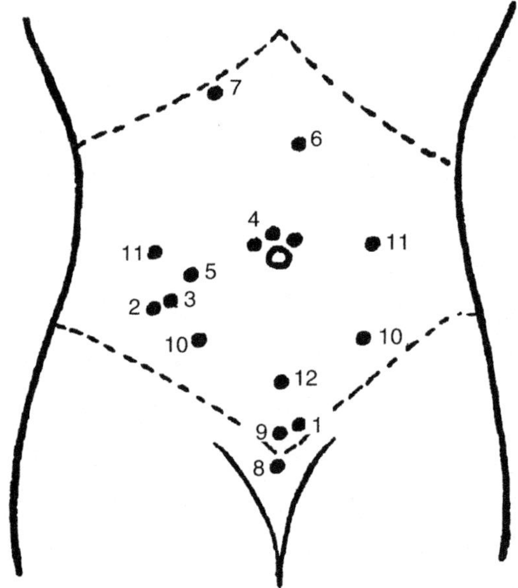

Figure A–1 Anterior reflexes. 1, internal rectal sphincter; 2, ileocecal valve; 3, appendix; 4, small intestine; 5, pyloric valve; 6, pancreas head; 7, gallbladder; 8, urethra; 9, bladder/prostate; 10, ovaries; 11, kidneys; 12, uterus.

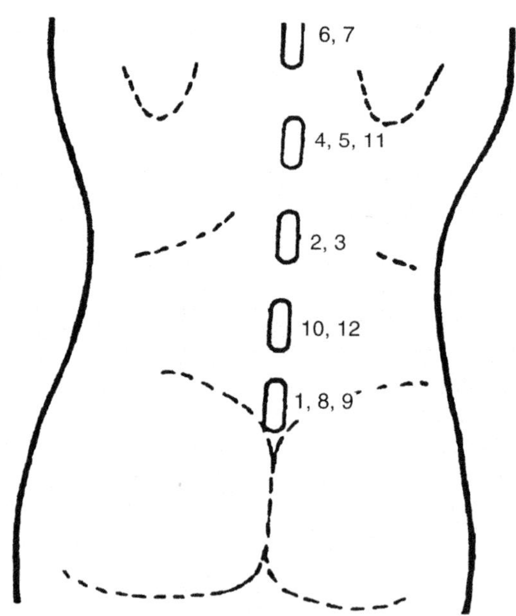

Figure A–2 Posterior contact areas. 1, internal rectal sphincter; 2, ileocecal valve; 3, appendix; 4, small intestine; 5, pyloric valve; 6, pancreas head; 7, gallbladder; 8, urethra; 9, bladder/prostate; 10, ovaries; 11, kidneys; 12, uterus.

sponse in muscle strength. Hence the organ-muscle relationship.

With further testing, Goodheart found that in the presence of organic problems the reflexes would be present and the muscle would be inhibited from normal function. If the muscle was injured, however, organic function was not affected. Goodheart theorized that the common denominator is that the reflex, when stimulated, improves the lymphatic drainage in both the organ and the muscle. Hence the name used in applied kinesiology: neurolymphatic reflexes.

METHODOLOGY

The foregoing is my interpretation of the work of Bennett, Chapman, and Goodheart and does not necessarily reflect the theories as originally presented. In the attempt to prove or disprove the theory, the neurolymphatic reflexes were not considered, only muscle weakness, fixations, and NVD.

To prove or disprove the organ-muscle relationship, it was necessary also to prove or disprove the fixation and NVD theories. Several things had to be considered:

- If a patient with organic symptoms presented with a muscle weakness, would the fixation be present? Would the NVD reflex be present?

- If a fixation is persistent, returning time after time, and other postural and functional faults have been corrected, would the muscle related to the organ that is related to the fixation be weak?

- If distortions in the posture can be related to one muscle or muscle group, would investigation find that the fixation is present? With further investigation, would the patient have clinical or subclinical symptoms of organic problems?

- If a muscle is inhibited from functioning as a result of an organ dysfunction, would the muscle respond if the NVD reflexes were used?

- If a muscle is inhibited from functioning as a result of an organ dysfunction, would the muscle respond to adjustment of the fixation?

I used several methods to find the answers. Students in several postgraduate classes were instructed to dine on spicy Mexican or Italian food for lunch. Upon their return to class, all the muscles related to digestion were tested and retested during the remaining 3 hours after the meal. This was not a scientific study because both the students and the examiners were aware of the test. Nevertheless, each time this method was used the majority of the muscles that presented weak corresponded with the organ required to function at that time during digestion. As the 3 hours passed and the food passed, the muscles associated with the stomach returned to normal, and those associated with the pancreas, small intestine, and so forth progressively weakened and then returned to normal. It would seem reasonable that, if the muscle is inhibited when the organ is overworked, it should be affected during any dysfunction.

All patients with known (or at least diagnosed) organic symptoms were checked for fixation, NVD reflexes, and muscle weakness. Fixations were found in the majority of the cases with proven organ problems (on ultrasound, radiography, computed tomography, etc). In several cases where fixations were not present, investigation proved the original diagnosis to be incorrect, with the new diagnosis later being confirmed on surgery. The NVD reflexes were present in most proven organic cases. One exception was the presence of stones in the gallbladder. The reflex was not always present without symptoms. A reasonable explanation is that, where stones are present and are not blocking the duct, the reflex would not be triggered. Gallstones are present in many individuals who have never experienced symptoms and are an incidental finding on another investigation or surgery. The muscles were affected in almost all the proven organ problems. In the majority of the proven organic cases, fixation, NVD reflex, and muscle inhibition were all present.

Patients who presented with persistent fixations in an area related to an organ were investigated as thoroughly as possible for other structural faults. If the fixations were still persistent, the patients were investigated for organic problems. The number of clinical and subclinical problems found was great enough to justify the use of persistent fixation as a major sign of organic disease. Some patients without obvious signs and symptoms limited this investigation. The patients could not ethically be referred for investigation without justification. Of course, some persistent fixations could have been, and probably were, compensatory for problems not found on the examination.

One procedure used on several occasions with classes of both students and doctors of chiropractic in a workshop setting is appropriate for this text because it involved the knee.

Without explanation, the students were instructed to examine each other in the erect posture, to include flexion-hyperextension of the knees, and to examine in the supine posture with the legs relaxed and suspended by the heels (for those hyperextended without weight bearing). Those with bilateral hyperextension were eliminated from the test. Using only those cases with unilateral hyperextended knees (20), the students were instructed to test the popliteus muscles bilaterally. Ninety-six percent of the hyperextended knees (mostly left knees) tested weak compared with the opposite knee. Careful palpation in the supine position found fixations at T4–5 in all cases. In two groups I adjusted each student in the supine position, and in two other groups the students were adjusted by the examiners, both with similar results. Seventy-seven percent (21) of those adjusted revealed upon reexamination that both the weakness and the hyperextension were eliminated. Of the remainder, 6 responded when NVD was used. One failed to respond; he reported that he had recently had an injury to the knee.

One can only conclude that, if the gallbladder is under stress,

- a fixation will be present at T4–5
- the popliteus muscle will test weak
- the affected knee will be hyperextended
- the NVD reflexes will be present
- by adjusting the T4–5 fixation, a response may be expected by the weak popliteus muscle (with no direct neurologic explanation) most of the time
- use of the NVD reflex (passive) after all else fails may produce improved function of the popliteus muscle (with no neurologic explanation) and possibly will help gallbladder function

The value of the above testing is proved often. When an examination reveals a hyperextended knee, a tight, sensitive area is usually present under the right rib cage, and a persistent T4–5 fixation is present. Inquiry into symptoms of gallbladder dysfunction many times surprises patients because they usually do not believe that a relationship exists between the gallbladder symptoms and their structural problems. With the use of organ-muscle relationships and subsequent investigation into the organ problems, the treatment program must be improved.

OPINION

Nothing is absolute. Each reflex, fixation, and muscle test requires judgment on the examiner's part to determine the reflex, the degree of fixation, and/or the loss of normal strength. Accuracy again depends on the amount of experience and ability of the examiner. To cloud the issue further, patient reaction varies from individual to individual.

Most signs and symptoms accepted by the medical community also require the judgment of the examiner and patient reaction. One study in Australia (where, with socialized medicine, one would expect fewer needless surgeries) showed that only 57% of the appendices removed from female patients were pathologic. Other studies in California showed even a lower percentage of accuracy.[6] The accepted signs and symptoms of nausea, elevated temperature, rebound over McBurney's point, and elevated white cell count were the criteria used to determine the necessity for surgery.

If the area of fixation (T12–L1) had been checked, if the NVD points had been palpated and found sensitive, and if the quadratus lumborum muscle had been tested and found lacking in its normal strength, could needless surgery have been prevented? Would the percentage of pathologic appendices be higher? No one can answer those questions after the fact. If the examiner has the advantage of the additional signs and symp-

toms provided by the fixation, NVD, and organ-muscle relationships, however, the diagnosis must certainly be more accurate.

There definitely is validity to the existence of an organic place, and this should be taught in palpation and examination and as a part of diagnosis together with accepted diagnostic signs and symptoms. NVD reflexes are valuable in the diagnosis and treatment of organic problems and should be taught as a part of diagnosis as well as technique. The organ-muscle relationship is sufficiently correct to include it as one of the signs and symptoms of organic disease and as part of structural analysis.

Using the three theories as a cross-check, some of the muscles proposed by applied kinesiologists proved clinically incorrect, but the majority proved correct. Only those proved correct are discussed here. Most of the NVD points coincided with the affected muscles and fixations. The fixations were found to be consistently correct in known, proven organic problems. None of the above is intended to endorse or discredit applied kinesiology. The neurolymphatic reflexes were not used as a part of the tests because my intention was to cross-check NVD. Therefore, the validity of treatment through use of the neurolymphatic reflexes was not a consideration.

A knowledge of normal muscle function is necessary to enable the examiner to detect malfunction and/or distortion. Determining the cause requires investigation and should include orthopedic testing, neurologic testing, palpation for fixations, muscle testing, and testing of all the reflexes known to be helpful in arriving at a correct diagnosis. The use of organ-muscle relationships, fixations, and NVD reflexes helps in determining that an organic problem exists, pinpointing the organ involved and adding to existing accepted medical diagnostic signs and symptoms. Their use can only enhance the diagnostic ability of our profession.

The examples used above are related to muscles affecting the knee. They may also affect the foot and ankle. One muscle and one muscle group that relates directly to the foot and ankle is the anterior tibialis, which is associated with the urethra. In the upright examination, the Achilles tendon may appear concave medially. The patient will report that he or she feels the body weight on the inside of the foot. If this is verified by manual testing, inquiry into possible incontinence or, in a male patient, possible prostate symptoms, should be made.

Another muscle group is the *dorsiflexor and everters* (the extensor digitorum longus, the peroneus tertius, and, to some degree, the peroneus brevis). In the upright position the foot will appear to have most of the weight on the outside. The patient will report that he or she feels the body weight on the outside of the foot. If this is verified by manual testing, inquiry into possible bladder problems should be made. It must be repeated that the above are signs and symptoms and must be used accordingly as part of the diagnosis.

REFERENCE

1. Palmer DD. *The Science, Art and Philosophy of Chiropractic.* Portland, OR: Portland Printing House Co.; 1910.

2. Biron WA, Welles BF, Houser RH. *Chiropractic Principles and Technic.* Chicago, Ill: National College of Chiropractic; 1939.

3. Bennett TJ. *A New Clinical Basis for the Correction of Abnormal Physiology.* Des Moines, IA: Foundation for Chiropractic Education and Research; 1967.

4. Owens C. *An Endocrine Interpretation of Chapman's Reflexes.* Colorado Springs: American Academy of Osteopathy; 1937.

5. Goodheart G. Applied Kinesiology Notes. Presented at Applied Kinesiology Seminars; 1972–1976.

6. Chang A. An analysis of the pathology of 3003 appendices. *Aust NZ J Surg.* 1981; 151(2):169–178.

Notes

Notes

Notes

Notes

Notes

Notes

Printed in Dunstable, United Kingdom